COMMUNITY HEALTH NURSING

CONCEPTS AND PRACTICE

Barbara Walton Spradley, R.N., M.N.

Public Health Nursing, School of Public Health,
University of Minnesota, Minneapolis

COMMUNITY

HEALTH NURSING

CONCEPTS AND PRACTICE

LITTLE, BROWN AND COMPANY · BOSTON

Library of Congress Catalog Card No. 80-84746

ISBN 0-316-80748-6

Printed in the United States of America

HAL

Cover design by Weymouth Design

To Jim, my husband and best friend

CONTENTS

PREFACE

Community health nursing is an evolving, challenging field of nursing practice, yet one that is not always clearly understood. *Community Health Nursing: Concepts and Practice* was written to capture the essence of community health nursing, to clarify its meaning for the practitioner, and to share enthusiasm for a field whose complex nature demands and fosters creativity, leadership, and innovation. It is a basic text designed to give undergraduate nursing students a comprehensive introduction to the field of community health nursing. It examines the unique contribution that this clinical practice area makes to our health care system.

Community health nursing has undergone many changes since its inception in the late 1880s, but some important components persist. Health maintenance and prevention of illness, emphasized by so-called health nurses as early as 1860, remain essential elements of community nursing. Seeking out clients and taking nursing service to them in their own environment is still of primary importance. Concern for population groups, which long ago stimulated Lillian Wald to provide nursing service to the sick poor, is receiving considerable attention in current community health nursing practice. Yet changes within the field have been numerous and varied. The nursing profession, including community health nursing, has broadened its perspective to stress a holistic approach to client needs. There is ever-increasing emphasis placed on health promotion through encouraging optimal levels of wellness in clients, in addition to encouraging health maintenance. Nurses now engage in community health planning, use and conduct epidemiologic research, encourage client self-care, and work collaboratively with a much broader range of professional and nonprofessional health team members than they have in years past. Expanded scientific knowledge has made community health nurses more sensitive to the influence of the physical, social, and psychological environment on family and community health and has sharpened their assessment and intervention skills. These nurses are becoming leaders and change agents in community health.

Many transitions in community health nursing have arisen from increased knowledge related to health and health care. These changes in practice have been and are today a direct response to client needs. It is a healthy sign when a service profession can maintain a flexible orientation that not only seeks out but acts on a constant flow of new information derived from and about those whom it serves.

This same responsiveness is reflected in changing nursing curricula. Nurse educators recognize a need to shift from a disease-oriented and hospital-based curriculum to one that emphasizes the promotion of health and the prevention of illness. Students are acquiring broader theoretical and conceptual bases for their practice. Their intellectual skills are being sharpened and their political and social awareness made more acute. Community health, while assuming a significantly larger role in health care, has also become a strategic focal area in nursing curricula, thus challenging and attracting more graduates to choose this field of nursing practice.

Community health nursing is a unique clinical practice area within nursing, not because of where it is practiced but because of what it is: It is an indivisible synthesis of nursing theories and public health theories and principles. Consequently, it is not defined or limited geographically but reaches out to meet the needs of the public in all environments. It is a field in which the nurse's primary mission is to promote and preserve the health of *populations.* Community health nurses promote wellness and prevent illness among population groups (or *aggregates*) of all sizes, ranging from families to entire communities, wherever they may be. A population orientation, essential to public health practice, requires a shift in thinking from the traditional, individualistic approach that nurses are trained to use. However, individuals are not ignored in the process of looking at communities. Rather, nurses are concerned about all those individuals who collectively make up a community, while at the same time they consider the community's needs of which those individuals are a part.

At present, community health nursing practice is strongly influenced by external forces. Funding limitations and reimbursement policies from third party payers often dictate how nurses spend their time. The home care boom has forced public health nursing agencies to compete with proliferating proprietary groups. Boards of health, legislative groups, and other policy setters are frequently ignorant or unconvinced of the value of preventive services and the contribution that community health nurses can make to widespread health care and health maintenance. Even within the profession, some nurses lack adequate vision or resources to help this field realize its potential.

Although the work of community health nurses is frequently impeded by such obstacles, there is evidence that, in many places, nurses are transforming their practice from basic nursing to true community health nursing. For example, when making a home visit, nurses not only provide expert care to the individual in need, stressing illness prevention and health promotion, but also attempt to serve the whole family as client by considering its needs as a complete unit. Family nursing and nursing to an entire group as client are growing fields of practice. Research focused on population groups has been common for many years, and now nursing service to population groups (e.g., all the elderly in a high-rise apartment building, or pregnant teenagers in a high school) is beginning to take hold. Despite the limits imposed on their practice by both internal and external forces, these nurses have succeeded in combining public health care and nursing to provide a specialized and much needed service to the community.

Community Health Nursing: Concepts and Practice defines community health nursing and demonstrates its application. It was written primarily for undergraduate nurses, some of whom will choose community health nursing as their field of specialization. Others who do not will enhance their own professional practice in any area by assimilating and applying basic community health nursing concepts and principles. This text will also be useful to practicing community health nurses, nurse educators, and all those who wish to expand their understanding of this field.

The book is organized into four major parts, each designed to give the reader a different perspective on community health nursing. Part One, Conceptual Foundations, introduces the reader to the field of community health generally and to community health nursing specifically. Important concepts such as health, community, population-oriented nursing, and culture are defined and discussed at length. Part Two, Tools for Practice, concentrates on the specific means by which community health nurses carry out their work, including an explanation of how the nursing process is applied to community health nursing practice. The nurse-client relationship, often long-term in community health, is discussed in a contractual framework. Health teaching, crisis intervention and prevention, and epidemiology and biostatistics are also basic tools with which the community health nurse must be equipped. Part Three, Care of Communities, describes four population levels of clients in community health nursing—families, groups, organizations and population groups, and communities. The nature and dynamics of each client level are studied in depth, and methods of assessing the health of and working with that population are presented. This part is richly illustrated with examples from community health nursing practice. Finally, Part Four, Expanding the Nurse's Influence, examines the nature of both leadership and planned change, and demonstrates how the nurse can rise to meet the responsibility and challenge of being a leader and change agent in community health.

B.W.S.

ACKNOWLEDGMENTS

I gratefully acknowledge the help of many individuals and organizations during the completion of the manuscript. Special thanks go to Chris Campbell, formerly of Little, Brown and Company, who encouraged me to start the book, and to Julie Stillman, my editor, for seeing me through the project with well-timed positive reinforcement. I am grateful to Ann West, Lois F. Hall, and Elizabeth Welch, all of Little, Brown and Company, for manuscript critique and preparation.

Many nurses in community health shared their time and expertise. In particular, I wish to thank Barbara O'Grady, Mary Lou Christenson, and Barbara Thune Schommer of Ramsey County Nursing Service; Esther Tatley of Chisago County Nursing Service; Yvonne Hargens and Kathy Lucas Johnson of the Bloomington Health Department; and Mary Jane Madden, formerly with the St. Louis Park Medical Center of Minneapolis.

Nursing faculty from several schools were also helpful. I especially thank Jean Martinson and Pat Brost Bartscher from the College of St. Catherine in St. Paul; Nancy Malcolm from Augsburg College, Minneapolis; and Sharon Danielsen, Barbara Reynolds, and Marla Salmon White from the University of Minnesota School of Public Health, Minneapolis, for responding to my ideas and sharing resources.

Finally, I am grateful to the many special people whose interest, support, ideas, and encouragement sustained and energized me throughout the writing of the book. Sincere thanks go to Karen and Robert Veninga, Joan and Thomas Correll, Eleanor M. Anderson, Marty Rossman, and Anedith Nash. I am especially grateful to my three daughters, Sheryl, Deborah, and Laura, who have shown patience and understanding with their working mother for many years. Most of all, I am indebted and forever grateful to my husband, James, who spent endless hours listening to and critiquing my ideas and writing, who provided vital support, typed portions of the manuscript, and who, drawing on his own considerable writing expertise, served as my at-home editor. His contribution is enormous and invaluable.

ONE

CONCEPTUAL FOUNDATIONS

ONE

COMMUNITY HEALTH

COMMUNITY INFLUENCE

Human beings are social creatures. All of us, with rare exceptions, live out our lives in the company of other people. An Eskimo lives in a small, tightly knit community of close relatives; a rural Mexican lives in a small village with hardly more than two hundred members. In complex societies most people find their lives influenced by many overlapping communities such as their professional society, political party, neighborhood, and city. Even those who try to escape community membership always begin their lives in some type of group and usually continue to depend on groups for material and emotional support. Communities are an essential and permanent feature of human experience.

The communities in which people live have a profound influence on their collective health and well-being. It is well known, for example, that the rate of alcoholism is very low among members of the Orthodox Jewish community. This religious and cultural community has firm rules and procedures for drinking which define its significance and control its use. Consequently, alcoholism among Orthodox Jews is practically unknown [11]. A recently identified illness, Legionnaires' disease, was named after its emergence to public attention at a national convention of the American Legion. This community, a voluntary organization with members in many parts of the country, was, for a brief period, peculiarly affected by a disease. Although many people tend to think of health and illness as individual matters, it has been established that they are also community matters. Communities can influence the spread of disease, provide barriers to protect members from health hazards, organize in ways to combat outbreaks of infectious disease, and promote practices that contribute to individual and community health.

ROLES AND FUNCTIONS IN COMMUNITY HEALTH

These facts are the basis for a challenging field of practice—community health. Many different professionals work in community health to form a complex team. The city planner designing an urban renewal project necessarily becomes involved in community health. The social worker counseling on child abuse or the use of chemical substances among adolescents is involved in community health. A physician treating patients affected by a sudden outbreak of hepatitis and seeking to find the source is engaged in community health practice. Prenatal clinics, meals for the elderly, genetic counseling centers, legislation to restrict smoking in public places, educational programs for the early detection of cancer, and hundreds of other activities are all part of the community health effort.

Professional nurses are an integral part of community health practice. Their roles and activities are so varied that it is impossible to describe the "typical" community health nurse. They work in every conceivable kind of community health agency from state public health departments to community-based advocacy groups. Their duties range from examining infants in a well-baby clinic or teaching elderly stroke victims in their homes to carrying out epidemiologic research or engaging in health policy analysis and decision making. Community health nursing is a specialty area. It combines all the basic elements of professional, clinical nursing with community health practice. This book examines the unique contribution that community health nursing makes to our health care system. Our discussion of the concepts and theories that make community health nursing an important specialty within nursing begins with the broader field of community health, which provides the context as well as essential content for community health nursing practice.

Community health, also known as public health, is sometimes misunderstood. Even many health professionals tend to think of community health in limiting terms such as sanitation, poverty area clinics, and massive efforts to prevent health problems. Although these are a part of its ever broadening practice, community health is much more. In order to understand the nature and significance of this field, it is necessary to look more closely at the concepts of community and health.

COMMUNITY

Broadly defined, a community is a collection of people who share some important feature of their lives. Some communities, such as a tiny village in Appalachia, are composed of people who share almost everything. They live in the same location, work at a limited number of jobs, attend the same churches, and make use of the single health clinic and visiting physician or nurse. Other communities, such as the American Legion, are large, scattered, and composed of people who may share only their interest and involvement in that particular group. Although most communities share many aspects of their experience, three primary criteria are useful for identifying communities that relate to community health practice: geography, common interest, and health problem.

GEOGRAPHY

A community is often defined by its geographic boundaries. A city, town, or village is a geographic community. Consider the community of Hayward, Wisconsin. Located in northwestern Wisconsin, it is set in the north woods environment, far removed from any urban center, and in a climatic zone characterized by extremely harsh winters. With a population of less than 2,500, it is considered a rural community. The population has certain identifiable characteristics such as age and sex ratios, and its size fluctuates with the seasons; summers bring hundreds of tourists and seasonal residents. Hayward is a social system as well as a geographic location. The families, schools, hospital, churches, stores, and government institutions are linked in a complex network. This community, like others, has an informal power structure; it has a communication system which includes gossip, the newspaper, the Co-op store bulletin board, and the radio station. In one sense, then, a community consists of a collection of people located in a specific place, and is made up of institutions organized into a social system.

Local communities such as Hayward vary in size. A few miles south of Hayward lie several other communities, including Northwoods Beach and Round Lake, but these three, along with other towns and isolated farms, form a larger community called Sawyer County. If you worked for a health agency serving only Hayward, that community would be of primary concern. However, if you worked for the Sawyer County Health Department, you would focus on this larger community. A community health nurse employed by the State Health Department in Madison, Wisconsin would have an interest in Sawyer

County and Hayward, but only as one small part of the larger community of Wisconsin.

Frequently, a single part of a city can be treated as a community. In Seattle, for example, the Skid Row district near the waterfront is a community of many transients. For certain purposes in community health, it is useful to identify a geographic area as a community.

COMMON INTEREST

A community can also be identified by a common interest. A collection of people, widely scattered geographically, can have an interest that binds the members together. The members of a church in a large metropolitan area, a group of migrant workers, or the members of a national professional organization can all be treated as communities. Sometimes within a fairly small geographic area, a group of people become a community by promoting their common interest. The younger families in the northern part of Sawyer County, Wisconsin, may emerge as a community through a common interest in the needs of their children for better schools. The residents in an industrial community may develop a common interest in air or water pollution issues while others who work but do not live there may not share that interest. The kinds of shared interests that lead to the formation of communities are almost infinitely varied (Fig. 1-1).

PROBLEM SOLVING

Frequently in community health practice a community is an area with fluid boundaries within which a problem can be identified and solved. The shape of this community varies with the size of the geographic area affected and the number of resources needed to address a problem. Such a community is called a "community of solution" [7]. A water pollution problem may involve several counties whose agencies and personnel must work together to control upstream water supply, industrial waste disposal, and city water treatment. This group of counties forms a community of solution around a health problem. In another instance, several schools may collaborate with law enforcement and health agencies to study patterns of students' drug use and possible preventive approaches. The boundaries of this community of solution form around the schools and agencies involved. Figure 1-2 depicts some communities of solution related to one city.

Community health workers, including the community health nurse, need to understand the complex nature of communities. What are the characteristics of the people in terms of age, sex, race, and socioeco-

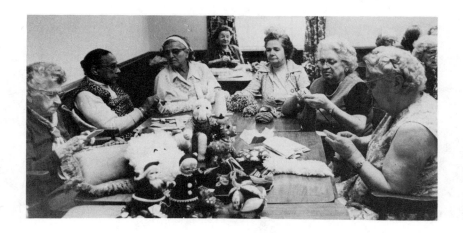

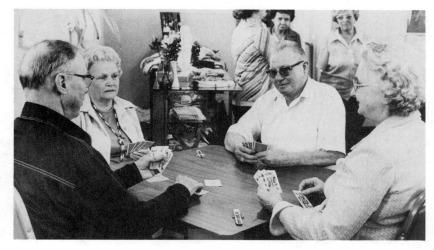

Figure 1-1. Senior citizens frequently form their own communities for the purpose of shared service projects and meaningful social relationships. (Courtesy of the *Mt. Vernon News.*)

nomic level? How does the community interact with other communities? What is its past history? Is the community undergoing rapid change? Many of these questions as well as the tools needed to assess a community for health purposes are discussed in Chapter Fourteen.

HEALTH

In 1946, the World Health Organization defined health as a state of complete physical, mental, and social well-being and not merely as the absence of disease or infirmity. Our understanding of the concept of health builds on this classic definition. We recognize that health is not just the absence of illness but the presence of a positive capacity to lead

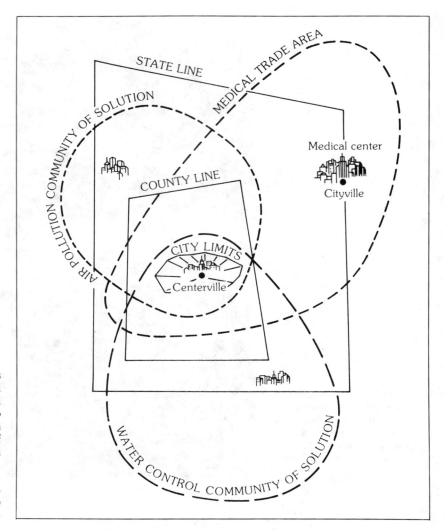

Figure 1-2. A city's communities of solution. State, county, and city boundaries (shown in solid lines) may have little or no bearing on health solution boundaries. (From a report of the National Commission on Community Health Services, *Health Is a Community Affair.* Cambridge, Mass.: Harvard University Press, 1967. Reprinted by permission.)

an energetic, satisfying, and productive life. We value a strong emphasis on well-being or "wellness" as we have come to know it. We are growing to understand health broadly through holistic perspectives.

Yet health is an elusive concept. For each person it has acquired dozens of meanings in the course of ordinary conversations. As children, we were encouraged to eat proper foods in order to grow strong and healthy. We later heard of people who "lost" their health. Under the treatment of physicians these people may have "regained" their health. Like barnacles slowly accumulating on the hull of an ocean barge, multiple meanings became attached to the concept of health. Although health is widely accepted as desirable, the exact nature of health is often unclear and ambiguous. In order to clarify the concept for our use in considering community health practice, the distinguishing features of health shall be briefly characterized; then the implications of this concept for the activities of professionals in the field can be examined more fully.

A RELATIVE CONCEPT

Health is a relative, not an absolute, concept. Our language tends to impose on us a black-and-white way of thinking about health. Most people contrast health with illness or disease. A person has one condition or the other—that is, a person can move from one category to the other, from sick to well again—in an absolute sense. This kind of thinking must be set aside if we are to grasp the nature and significance of community health practice.

Health, according to the concept used in this text, always involves many levels. We are all familiar with degrees of illness. We classify a person with terminal cancer or end-stage renal disease as very ill. Someone else recovering from a cholecystectomy is less ill while yet another person with infectious mononucleosis may be mildly ill. These are degrees or levels of illness. In the same manner we can identify degrees of wellness. From a mildly well person who functions minimally with a disease such as chronic arthritis to a robust 70-year-old person who is functioning at an optimal level of wellness, we see variations in degrees of health. Health always involves a continuum—a range of degrees—from optimal health at one end to death or total disability at the other (see Figs. 1-3, 1-4). The health of an individual, family, group, or community moves back and forth along this continuum throughout life.

By thinking of health relatively, as a matter of degree, we can avoid the strong tendency to polarize its meaning and thus limit our practice. Traditionally, the majority of health care was focused on treatment of acute and chronic conditions at the illness end of the continuum. Gradually the emphasis shifted to include attention to the health end of the continuum. Community health practice ranges over the entire continuum; it always works to improve the degree of health in individuals, families, groups, and communities. However, community health practice particularly emphasizes the promotion and preservation of health and the prevention of illness.

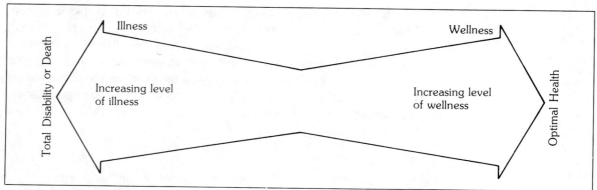

Figure 1-3. The health–illness continuum. The level (degree) of illness increases as one moves toward total disability or death; the level of wellness increases as one moves toward optimal health. This continuum shows the relative nature of health and illness. At any given time a person can be placed at some point along the continuum.

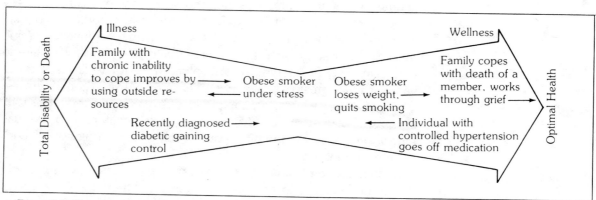

Figure 1-4. Dynamic nature of the health–illness continuum. A person's relative health is usually in a state of flux, either improving or deteriorating. This diagram of the health–illness continuum shows several examples of families and individuals in changing states of health and illness.

10

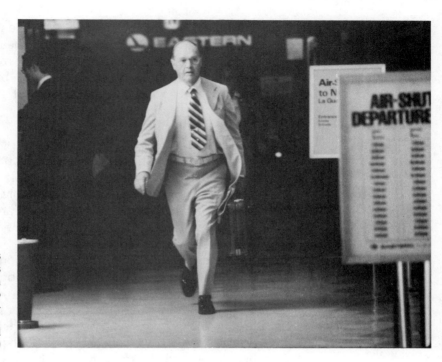

Figure 1-5. Rushing to catch his air shuttle, this businessman is experiencing work stress and an unhealthy lifestyle that is likely to move his health state to the illness end of the continuum. (Photograph by Dirck Halstead for *Time* © 1978, Time, Inc.)

A STATE OF BEING

Health refers to a state of being. Individuals and communities have many different qualities and characteristics. We might describe a person in such terms as energetic, outgoing, enthusiastic, beautiful, caring, loving, and intense. Together, these qualities become the essence of a person's existence; they describe a state of being. Similarly, a specific geographic community might be characterized as congested, deteriorating, unattractive, dirty, and disorganized. These characteristics suggest diminishing degrees of vitality. Again, they describe a state of being.

Health, as a set of qualities or a state of being, involves the total person or the total community. That is, all the dimensions of life affecting everyday functioning determine an individual's or a community's health. Physical, psychological, spiritual, and sociocultural experiences influence one's present condition. Thus, an individual's placement on the health–illness continuum can only be known if we consider that person from a holistic perspective (Fig. 1-5). Health is a relative state of well-being; illness is a relative state of ill-being.

As we consider an aggregate of people in terms of health, it sometimes becomes useful to speak of the "health of a community." With aggregates as well as individuals, health as a state of being does not merely involve the physical condition but includes psychological, spiritual, and sociocultural factors as well.

SUBJECTIVE AND OBJECTIVE DIMENSIONS

Health involves subjective and objective dimensions. Subjectively, a healthy person is one who "feels well," who experiences the sensation of a vital, positive state. Healthy people are full of life and vigor, capable of physical and mental productivity. They feel minimal discomfort and displeasure with the world around them. Again, people experience varying degrees of vitality and well-being. The state of feeling well fluctuates. Some mornings we wake up feeling more energetic and enthusiastic than other mornings. How a person feels varies day by day, even hour by hour; nonetheless, it can be a strong indicator of that person's health state.

Health also involves the objective dimension of ability to function. A healthy individual or community is one that can carry out necessary activities and achieve enriching goals. Unhealthy people not only feel ill but are limited, to some degree, in their ability to carry out daily activities. Indeed, levels of illness or wellness are largely measured in terms of ability to function [10]. A person confined to bed is labelled sicker than an ill person managing self-care. A family that meets its members' needs is healthier than one that has poor communication patterns and is unable to provide adequate physical and emotional resources. Degree of functioning is directly related to state of health.

The ability to function can be observed. A man dresses and feeds himself and goes to work. Despite financial exigencies, a family nourishes its members through a supportive emotional climate. A community fails to provide adequate resources and services for its members. These performances, to some degree, can be regarded as indicators of health status.

Underlying performance are the values an individual, family, or community places on actions. Some activities such as walking and taking care of personal needs are functions almost everyone values. Other actions (for example, sports such as running) have more limited appeal. In assessing the health of individuals and communities, the community health nurse can observe their ability to function but must also know their values, which may contrast sharply with those of the professional.

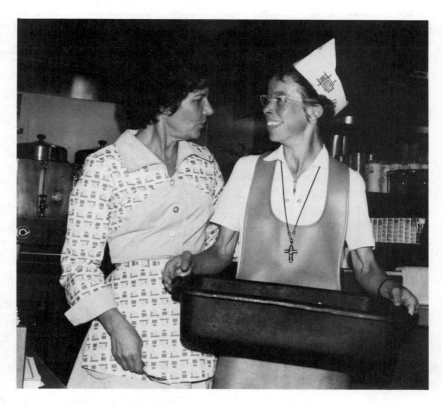

Figure 1-6. This retarded young adult, functioning well within her capacity demonstrates that a high level of health may be present despite disability. (From M. Blackwell, *Care of the Mentally Retarded.* Boston: Little, Brown, 1979.)

Subjective (feeling well or ill) and objective (function) dimensions together provide us with a clearer picture of people's health. When they feel well and demonstrate functional ability they are close to the wellness end of the health–illness continuum (Fig. 1-6). Even those with a disease such as arthritis or diabetes may feel well and perform well within their capacity. These people can be considered healthy. Figure 1-7 depicts the relationships between the subjective and objective views of health.

HEALTH AS A RESOURCE

Health can be viewed as an important resource, both of individuals and communities. The relationship between health and community has been summarized by Henkel [4]:

1. *The health and well-being of an individual physically, emotionally, and socially is one of his most important assets;*
2. *through judicious use of this asset he will be able to achieve more effectively his goals in life;*

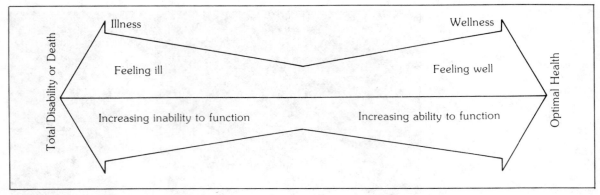

Figure 1-7. Subjective and objective views of the health–illness continuum.

3. *to develop this asset to the greatest possible level requires the concerted and cooperative efforts of many people;*
4. *society as a whole will ultimately benefit from healthy citizens.*

The implications of this view of health have far-reaching consequences for persons engaged in health care. No longer can we justify concentrating the majority of our efforts exclusively on healing the sick or even on the prevention of disease. For centuries health work has focused on the illness end of the health–illness continuum. We now live in an age when it is not only possible to promote health but our mandate and responsibility to do so [12].

As important as health promotion is the need for health assessment. When one considers health status from the perspective just discussed, its measurement becomes more feasible as well as necessary. Health promotion and health assessment are essential aspects of community health nursing and are discussed in detail in later chapters.

ELEMENTS OF COMMUNITY HEALTH PRACTICE

We have examined the definitions of community and of health. Together, these concepts provide the foundation for understanding community health. In acute care the health of an individual is the primary focus. Community health broadens that focus to concentrate on families, groups, and the community at large. The community becomes the recipient of service, and health becomes the product. Viewed from another perspective, community health is concerned with the interchange between population groups and their total environment and the impact of that interchange on health.

Just as a whole is greater than the sum of its parts, the health of a community is more than the sum of the health of its individual citizens.

A community that achieves high-level wellness is composed of healthy citizens, functioning in an environment that protects and promotes health. Community health, as a field of practice, seeks to provide the organizational structure, resources, and activities needed to accomplish the goal of an optimally healthy community.

What is the difference between community health and public health? In theory there is none. However, the term *public* is often associated with efforts of government agencies, governed by law and financed by taxes, while private health agencies are funded through private sources. Community health practice encompasses both. It is organized cooperative efforts aimed at promoting physical, emotional, and social health by all health agencies and individuals in the community.

One of the challenges community health practice faces is to remain responsive to community health needs. As a result, its structure is complex; numerous health services and programs are currently available or will be developed in the future. Examples include health education, family planning, accident prevention, environmental protection, immunization, nutrition, early periodic and developmental screening, school programs, mental health, industry, and occupational health.

Community health practice can best be understood by examining six basic elements, which together encompass its services and programs: (1) promotion of healthful living, (2) prevention of health problems, (3) treatment of disorders, (4) rehabilitation, (5) evaluation, and (6) research.

PROMOTION OF HEALTHFUL LIVING

Promotion of healthful living is now recognized as one of the most important elements of community health practice. Health promotion programs and activities include many forms of health education, demonstration of healthful practices, and efforts to provide a greater number of health-promoting options. Health education, although a useful tool, has limited significance alone unless accompanied by desire, opportunity, and resources that encourage more healthful practices [6]. In Maryland an intensive health education effort to teach families about safety and to reduce childhood injuries at home made no significant difference [2]. A similar effort in New York City to reduce childhood injuries from window falls combined home visits, health education, follow-up, and provision of free window guards (supplied by the Health Department) with highly successful results [9].

Demonstration of such healthful practices as eating more nutritious foods and exercising more regularly is often performed by individual health workers. In addition, groups and health agencies that support the rights of nonsmokers, encourage physical fitness programs for all ages, or demand that food products be properly labelled demonstrate the importance of these practices and create public awareness.

The goal of health promotion is to raise individuals', families', groups', and communities' levels of wellness. Community health accomplishes this goal through a three-pronged effort: (1) to increase understanding of health, (2) to raise community standards for health, and (3) to assist in developing more positive health practices. More specifically, the U.S. Public Health Service has outlined 15 action areas in *Healthy People: The Surgeon General's Report on Health Promotion and Disease Prevention* [12]:

Preventive health services
  Family planning
  Pregnancy and infant care
  Immunizations
  Sexually transmissible diseases
Health protection
  Toxic agent control
  Occupational safety and health
  Accidental injury control
  Fluoridation of community water supplies
  Infectious agent control
Health promotion
  Smoking cessation
  Reduction of alcohol and drug abuse
  Exercise and fitness
  Stress control

It is difficult to provide health-promoting options, that is, opportunities to make more healthful choices, without re-examining and, in many instances, restructuring organizational patterns and policies as well as increasing personal and societal resources. At the local level, many health agencies are offering services at hours more convenient to their clientele and, in some cases, are providing transportation or other means of easier access to service. Furthermore, community residents are forming stronger bonds of partnership with health workers in order to understand and solve their own health problems, as well as to assume greater responsibility for achieving positive health for themselves and their communities.

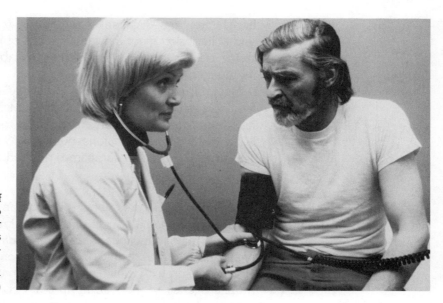

Figure 1-8. Early detection of warning signs that might lead to coronary artery disease or other illness is an important part of this health maintenance organization's preventive program. (Courtesy of the Harvard Community Health Plan, Boston.)

PREVENTION OF HEALTH PROBLEMS

Prevention of health problems constitutes a major part of community health practice. Prevention means anticipating and obviating problems or discovering them as early as possible in order to avert or minimize possible disability and impairment. It is practiced in an infinite number of ways in community health. For example, a nutritionist who instructs a group of obese women to follow a well-balanced diet during weight loss is preventing the complications of nutritional deficiency. A community health nurse who encourages an elderly couple to install safety devices, such as a grab bar by the bathtub or a hand rail on the front steps, is preventing injuries from falls. Local health departments help control and prevent communicable diseases such as rubeola or poliomyelitis by providing regular immunization programs. Hypertension screening centers, which are forming in many communities, help identify a high-risk group and encourage early treatment.

Health assessment of individuals, families, and communities is an important part of preventive practice (Fig. 1-8). One must determine health status in order to anticipate problems and select appropriate preventive measures. A social worker who discovers that a young mother has herself been a victim of child abuse institutes early treatment for the mother to prevent abuse and foster adequate parenting of her children. If assessment of a community reveals inadequate facilities and activities to meet the future needs of its increasing population of senior citizens, agencies and groups collaborate to plan and develop the needed resources.

Health problems are most effectively prevented by maintaining healthy lifestyles and healthy environments. To these ends, community health practice directs many of its efforts to provide safe and satisfying living and working conditions, nutritious food, and clean air and water. This area of practice is sometimes referred to as preventive medicine.

TREATMENT OF DISORDERS

Treatment of disorders, which focuses on illnesses and health problems, is the remedial aspect of community health practice. The first of its three major functions is to provide *direct service* to people with health problems. A family, unable to afford the purchase of a wheelchair for a son with multiple sclerosis, is provided one through a community agency. If the wife in an older couple is newly diagnosed as diabetic, home visits from a community health nurse, for assistance with diet planning, administration of insulin, and personal care, are arranged. A neighborhood health center forms an educational and support group for people needing to lose weight. Many kinds of community agencies provide direct health or health-related services.

Second, the remedial aspect of community health practice includes *indirect service* by assisting people with health problems to obtain treatment. In many instances a community agency may not be able to provide needed care and instead will refer the individuals or groups concerned to a more appropriate resource. A young woman with postpartum bleeding, assisted by the community health nurse, gets an immediate appointment with a physician at the local clinic. A social worker helps a family that is plagued by personal and economic problems to enter a family therapy and counseling program. A number of community agencies provide information and referral services.

Third, treatment of disorders also includes the development of *programs to correct unhealthy conditions*. One community with a high incidence of alcoholism and drug abuse initiated a chemical dependency counseling and treatment center. In another community, the health department developed new regulations for industrial waste disposal as a result of increased pollution of the water supply. Individual community members and health workers also take corrective action to remedy situations such as a case of apparent child abuse, poor nutrition in a school's lunch program, or inhumane conditions and treatment in a nursing home.

REHABILITATION

Rehabilitation, the fourth element of community health practice, focuses on reducing disability and, as much as possible, restoring function. People with handicaps that are congenital or acquired through illness or accident such as stroke, heart condition, amputation, or mental illness can be helped to regain some measure of lost function or to develop new compensating skills (see Fig. 1-9). For example, a factory worker who lost his leg in an industrial accident received good medical and nursing care, prosthetic fittings, and physical and occupational therapy; he thus retrained to assume successfully an office job.

In community health, the need to reduce disability and restore function applies equally to families, groups, and communities as well as to individuals. Many groups form for rehabilitative purposes, such as Alcoholics Anonymous, halfway houses for discharged psychiatric patients, or postmastectomy clubs. Rehabilitation services are often needed and sought by whole communities such as a ghetto area that desires to provide decent, safe playgrounds for its children.

As an element of community health practice, rehabilitation becomes increasingly significant when disease trends and changes in life expectancy are considered. Chronic conditions have replaced acute as the major causes of morbidity; these include such cripplers as cardiovascular disease and cancer, the increased incidence of accidents, and environmentally caused conditions. As a result, the need for long-term care and rehabilitation has increased, stimulated further by a greater proportion of elderly persons in the population.

EVALUATION

Evaluation is the means by which community health practice is analyzed and improved. Evaluation of health and health care should be an integral part of every kind of health service from individual practice to national and international programs. Whether done on the single case or program level, evaluation helps solve problems and provides direction for future health care efforts; its goals are to determine needs and the success of present activities, as well as to develop improved services. In one community, evaluation of mental health services revealed a need for more comprehensive psychiatric emergency care on a 24-hour basis. If a psychiatric crisis occurred dur-

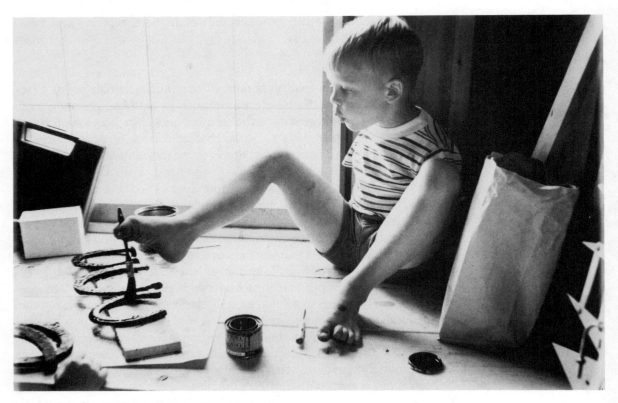

Figure 1-9. A young boy paints horseshoes for a family game with his feet. Through rehabilitation he has learned to compensate for the loss of his arms in a farm accident. (From C. Schuster and S. Ashburn, *The Process of Human Development: A Holistic Approach.* Boston: Little, Brown, 1980. Photograph by Carl Subitch.)

ing the night, police were the only persons available to help and jail the only place where the mentally ill could be taken. The deficiency was corrected by providing 24-hour psychiatric emergency service in the community mental health center. A community health nurse, in another instance, developed a contract with a family to whom she was making home visits. The parents wanted to learn how to cope with their adolescent boys. Specific, written objectives and a plan for measuring the outcomes enabled the couple and the nurse to evaluate the successful completion of this helping relationship.

RESEARCH

Research, a critical element of community health practice, provides a means for solving problems and exploring improved methods of health service. Community health conducts and utilizes scientific investigations at all levels from federal agencies such as the U.S. Public Health Service to state and local groups conducting research. Biostatistics and epidemiology are the primary measurement and analytic sciences associated with community health practice. Chapter Nine addresses these sciences in more detail.

Researchers in community health investigate the characteristics and patterns of illness and health. Conditions such as food poisoning, trauma, alcoholism, lung cancer, child abuse, drug dependency, or suicide are studied for possible causes and means of prevention. Health and healthful behavior are analyzed, for example, in nutrition projects and studies of normal human growth and behavior, for better understanding of ways to promote healthful living.

Community health researchers explore ways to improve health care. After a survey in Berkeley revealed many deficiencies in day care centers, specific recommendations for improvement of health services for children enrolled in day care centers were made [1]. A team of community health nurses in North Carolina studied nursing intervention with high-risk school children for the purpose of improving school nurse practice [5]. Other research projects might focus on the effectiveness of drug treatment programs, long-term stroke rehabilitation, or improved treatment approaches to obesity.

Community health researchers also examine the impact of social and environmental changes on health and health services delivery. For example, one study focused on the possible causes of wife-battering [8], while another concentrated on the epidemiology and prevention of drowning [3]. A growing number of studies center around needs and care of the elderly. Others investigate ways to improve health services planning and policy development through such efforts as studies of community needs and program utilization.

ORGANIZATION OF COMMUNITY HEALTH SERVICES

Although there are numerous agencies and individuals that provide health services in the United States, they can be classified under one of two types of organization, government or private.

GOVERNMENT HEALTH AGENCIES

Government health agencies, the tax-supported arm of the community health effort, perform an important function in community health practice. They are the official public health and welfare agencies whose areas of jurisdiction and types of service are dictated by law. They coordinate activities that often can be carried out only by group or community-wide action, for example, proper sewage disposal or the provision of sanitary water systems. Government health agencies develop facilities and programs for special groups, such as native Americans, migrant workers, and military personnel and veterans, whose health care is not the direct responsibility of any one state or locality. Many community health activities require an authoritative legal backing to ensure enforcement, another useful function of official agencies, of control in such areas as environmental pollution, highway safety practices, and harmful use of drugs. Official agencies provide important record-keeping services, which include the collection of vital statistics, research, consultation, and sometimes financial support to other community health groups.

Many different government agencies contribute to the health of a community. Most obvious are the city or county health departments, which provide a variety of direct and indirect health services, including community health nursing. Other tax-supported agencies that also give health or health-related services are the welfare department, department of public works, public schools and hospitals, police department, county agricultural service, and local housing authority.

PRIVATE HEALTH SERVICES

Private health services include proprietary (for profit) and voluntary (not for profit) health and welfare agencies as well as private practice; they comprise the non-tax-supported dimension of community health care.

Private health services are complementary and supplementary to government health agencies. They often meet the needs of special groups, such as people with cancer or heart disease; they offer an avenue for private enterprise or philanthropy; they are freer from restrictions than government agencies to develop innovations in health care; and they have been spurred to development, in part, by impatience or dissatisfaction with government programs. Their financial support comes from donations and fees. Examples of voluntary agencies include the American Cancer Society, Blue Cross–Blue Shield, and the Visiting Nurse Association. Some nursing homes or private home care services are examples of proprietary agencies.

Private practice is another part of non-tax-supported community health services. Physicians, dentists, nurses, veterinarians, pharmacists, optometrists, and many other specialists provide important services for individuals and communities. Private practice is primarily supported on a fee for service basis, that is, the client pays for the service after it has been rendered.

HEALTH CARE ECONOMICS

Financing of health care significantly affects community health practice. It influences the kind and quality of services offered as well as the way those services are utilized. Many factors can enter into a discussion of health care economics. Two shall be considered.

First, because of its financial incentives, the traditional American health care system tends to promote illness. Health care providers are primarily rewarded for treating problems, not for preventing them. The surgeon who advises a potential hemorrhoidectomy patient to increase the fiber in his diet may be losing a surgical fee. Hospitals have more income when their beds stay full of sick or injured people. The bulk of most reimbursable health services center around hospital, physician, nursing home, ambulatory, and skilled nursing care in the home. These services generally tend to be illness-oriented; the individual must play the role of patient in these settings. Health promotional activities such as comprehensive prenatal, maternal, and infant care; health education; childhood immunizations; and home services to enable the elderly to live independently are not covered by many insurers.

A system that financially supports illness care affects community health practice in several ways. The number and severity of health problems in a community increase when individuals postpone care because visits to the doctor or clinic mean greater expense, expense that they often cannot afford. In response to increased illness care, a greater proportion of community health practice is spent on treatment of disorders and rehabilitation, thus limiting the time and resources for, as well as minimizing the importance of, prevention and health promotion.

A second economic consideration is the health care system's trend toward a more health-oriented financial incentive structure. This is evident in the growth of health maintenance organizations (HMOs), which, as their name suggests, concentrate on the maintenance of good health. Members generally prepay and then receive comprehensive health services at the expense of the HMO. Since its operational cost is less when clients remain healthy, a HMO has the incentive to offer preventive and health-promoting services such as early treatment of symptoms, regular physical examinations, and health teaching. A health-oriented financial incentive structure affects community health practice by decreasing the proportion of remedial activities and increasing the emphasis on prevention and particularly the promotion of healthful living. Various approaches to national health insurance, for example, plans assuring comprehensive health care coverage for all

Americans, are incorporating the encouragement of preventive services and prepayment methods.

COMMUNITY HEALTH CHARACTERISTICS

Several characteristics of community health practice deserve special emphasis:

1. Community health practice, unlike the individualized focus of acute health care, has a group orientation. It is concerned with the health status of people in the aggregate, people who are parts of many groups. This interest includes all of the variables—physical, psychological, cultural, social, and biologic—that impinge on health and influence behavior.
2. In community health practice the promotion of health and prevention of illness are of first-order priority. There is minimal emphasis on curing.
3. Community health practice uses measurement and analysis. The need to collect and examine data before sound decision making is fundamental to community health practice. Analysis of health states, environmental factors, health-related services, economic patterns, and social policy are among the many foci of community health evaluation and research.
4. Community health practice utilizes the principles of management and organization necessary for effective management of health care and organization of services.

SUMMARY

Community health is much more than environmental programs and massive efforts to control communicable disease. To comprehend the nature and significance of community health we must understand the concepts of community and of health.

A community, broadly defined, is a collection of people who share some important feature of their lives. More specifically, it is helpful in community health practice to identify communities in terms of three criteria: geography, common interest, and health problem. Sometimes a community, such as a city, county, or neighborhood, is formed by geographic boundaries. At other times a community may be identified by its common interest; examples are a religious community, a group of migrant workers, or a gathering of residents concerned about air pollution. A community may also be defined as a community of solution, that is, a pooling of efforts by people and agencies toward solving some health-related problem.

Health is an abstract concept which can be understood more clearly when we recognize its distinguishing features. First, health is a relative, not an absolute, concept. People are not either sick or well in an absolute sense but have levels of illness or wellness. These levels may be plotted along a continuum ranging from optimal health to total disability or death. This is known as the health–illness continuum. Thus, a person's state of health is dynamic, varying from day to day and even hour to hour.

Second, health is a state of being. That is, the characteristics of a person, family, or community can be said to describe the essence of their existence. These characteristics portray people and therefore suggest the presence or absence of vitality. As a state of being, health also involves the total person. All the dimensions of life—physical, psychological, social, and spiritual—affect health.

Third, health has both subjective and objective dimensions. The subjective aspect involves feeling well; the objective aspect refers to the ability to function. How one feels can indicate one's state of health. At the wellness end of the health–illness continuum, people feel well; at the illness end, they feel ill. The ability to function, which is observable and often used to measure health status, may be present anywhere along the continuum. Most often, performance diminishes dramatically toward the illness end.

Community health practice is concerned with preserving and promoting the health of the community. It incorporates six basic elements: (1) promotion of healthful living, (2) prevention of health problems, (3) treatment of disorders, (4) rehabilitation, (5) evaluation, and (6) research.

Community health services can be classified as either governmental or private. Government agencies are tax-supported and their services are dictated by law. They serve public interests such as providing services to veterans and keeping statistics. Private health services, on the other hand, may be proprietary (for profit) or voluntary (not for profit). They include private practice and are financed through donations and fees.

Financial incentives in the health care system have tended to promote illness instead of wellness since treatment of the sick is rewarded. More recent approaches, for example, prepaid health care plans such as HMOs, demonstrate a trend toward a more wellness-oriented financial incentive structure.

Important characteristics of community health practice include its emphasis on aggregates, promotion of health and prevention of illness, use of measurement and analysis, and effective management and organization.

REFERENCES

1. Chang, A., Zukerman, S., and Wallace, H. Health services needs of children in day care centers. *Am. J. Public Health* 68:373, 1978.
2. Dershewitz, R., and Williamson, J. Prevention of childhood injuries: A controlled clinical trial. *Am. J. Public Health* 67:1148, 1977.
3. Dietz, P., and Baker, S. Drowning: Epidemiology and prevention. *Am. J. Public Health* 64:303, 1974.
4. Henkel, B. *Community Health* (2nd ed.). Boston: Allyn and Bacon, 1970. P. 2.
5. Long, G., et al. Evaluation of a school health program directed to children with history of high absence. *Am. J. Public Health* 65:383, 1975.
6. Milio, N. A framework for prevention: Changing health-damaging to health-generating life patterns. *Am. J. Public Health* 66:435, 1976.
7. National Commission on Community Health Services. *Health is a Community Affair.* Cambridge, Mass.: Harvard University Press, 1967. P. 2.
8. Parker, B., and Schumacher, D. The battered wife syndrome and violence in the nuclear family of origin: A controlled pilot study. *Am. J. Public Health* 67:760, 1977.
9. Spiegel, C., and Lindaman, F. Children can't fly: A program to prevent childhood morbidity and mortality from window falls. *Am. J. Public Health* 67:1143, 1977.
10. Terris, M. Approaches to an epidemiology of health. *Am. J. Public Health* 65:1037, 1975.
11. U.S. Department of Health, Education, and Welfare, National Institute of Mental Health. *Alcohol and Alcoholism.* Washington, D.C.: Government Printing Office, 1967. P. 26.
12. U.S. Department of Health, Education, and Welfare, Public Health Service. *Healthy People: The Surgeon General's Report on Health Promotion and Disease Prevention.* Washington, D.C.: Government Printing Office, 1979.

SELECTED READINGS

Anderson, O. Health-Services Systems in the United States and Other Countries: Critical Comparisons. In E. Jaco (Ed.), *Patients, Physicians and Illness: A Sourcebook in Behavioral Science and Health* (2nd ed.). New York: Free Press, 1972.

Brown, J. *The Health Care Dilemma.* New York: Human Sciences Press, 1978.

Braden, C. *Community Health: A Systems Approach.* New York: Appleton-Century-Crofts, 1976.

Dunn, H. *High-Level Wellness.* Arlington, Va.: Beatty, 1961.

Hart, S., et al. *Maintaining Health: An Adventure in Transition.* New York: National League for Nursing, 1972.

Lauzon, R. An epidemiological approach to health promotion. *Can. J. Public Health* 68:311, 1977.

Leininger, M., and Buck, G. (Eds.). *Health Care Issues.* Philadelphia: Davis, 1974.

Lerner, M. Conceptualization of health and social well-being. *Health Serv. Res.* 8:6, 1973.

Milio, N. *The Care of Health in Communities.* New York: Macmillan, 1975.

Milio, N. A framework for prevention: Changing health-damaging to health-generating life patterns. *Am. J. Public Health* 66:435, 1976.

National Commission on Community Health Services. *Health is a Community Affair.* Cambridge, Mass.: Harvard University Press, 1967.

National League for Nursing. *Community Health—Strategies for Change.* New York: National League for Nursing, 1973.

Parsons, T. Definitions of Health and Illness in the Light of American Values and Social Structure. In E. Jaco (Ed.), *Patients, Physicians, and Illness: A Sourcebook in Behavioral Science and Health* (2nd ed.). New York: Free Press, 1972.

Terris, M. Approaches to an epidemiology of health. *Am. J. Public Health* 65:1037, 1975.

Torrens, P. *The American Health Care System: Issues and Problems.* St. Louis: Mosby, 1978.

U.S. Department of Health, Education, and Welfare, Public Health Service. *Healthy People: The Surgeon General's Report on Health Promotion and Disease Prevention.* Washington, D.C.: Government Printing Office, 1979.

Two

The Nature of Community Health Nursing

Within the family of nursing specialties, community health nursing sometimes seems like an awkward adolescent. It has undergone an identity change from "public" to "community" health nursing which is not yet complete in the minds of some. With practitioners working in so many different settings, its professional character has not taken final shape, yet surely the current debates about this field suggest a growing, dynamic profession. This chapter examines the emerging nature of community health nursing. After defining the field, it traces historic development, examines several influential factors in that development, and then discusses the major characteristics of contemporary community health nursing.

DEFINING COMMUNITY HEALTH NURSING

Community health nursing can be defined as a field of practice that applies knowledge and skills from nursing and public health toward the promotion of optimal health for the total community.

Contrary to the popular image, community health nursing does not serve only clients in the community (those outside the acute care setting). As we shall see, nurses with other specialties have moved into the community, while some community health nurses work in hospitals. Community health nursing makes its unique contribution to health care by the nature of its practice, which combines basic concepts from nursing and public health. Increasingly it is being recognized as a subspecialty of both these fields [13]. Finally, community health nursing emphasizes the promotion of health and the prevention of illness for communities and groups as well as for families and individuals.

29

HISTORIC DEVELOPMENT

Community health nursing as practiced today did not appear like a new automobile off the assembly line. It has developed in response to identified health needs of consumers, and as the philosophy and concepts of community health nursing have become more clearly understood and applied. Its development, which has been influenced by changes in nursing and society, can be traced through several stages. This chapter examines both these stages and their societal causes.

STAGES OF DEVELOPMENT

Any review of public health nursing during the last century will reveal uneven changes. Innovations and new philosophies that developed in New York State, for example, spread slowly to other parts of the country. Even today, the functions of a community health nurse can differ sharply from one town to another or from an urban to a rural area. With this disparity in mind, we can still identify three general stages in the development of community health nursing: (1) the district nursing stage, (2) the public health nursing stage, and (3) the emergence of community health nursing.

DISTRICT NURSING (1860–1900)

Organized home nursing care started as a voluntary service for the poor. In 1859, William Rathbone, an English philanthropist, became convinced of the value of home nursing as a result of private care given to his wife [7]. He was the first to promote the establishment of a visiting nurse service for the sick poor in Liverpool. In the United States, the first visiting nurses were employed by the New York City Mission in 1877. In 1885, district nursing associations were founded in Buffalo and, in 1886, in Boston and Philadelphia. These district associations served the sick poor exclusively, since patients with enough money had private home nursing care. Before their establishment, care of the sick poor had fallen to various religious and charitable groups which delivered sporadic and limited health care.

Although district nurses primarily cared for the sick, they also taught cleanliness and wholesome living to their patients, even in that early period. Florence Nightingale, who assisted William Rathbone by training home visiting nurses, referred to them as health nurses. Her ideas and methods helped influence home nursing practice in England and the United States. The work of district nurses focused almost exclusively on the care of individuals. They recorded temperatures and

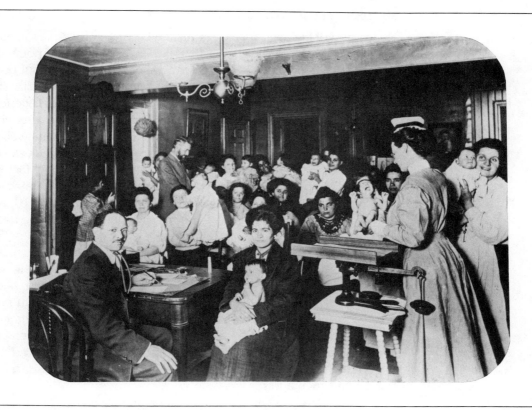

Figure 2-1. Examination of infants was part of early health department programs in which district nurses played a major role. (Courtesy of the Visiting Nurses' Association, Boston Collection.)

pulse rates and gave simple treatments under the immediate direction of a physician. They also instructed family members in personal hygiene, healthful living habits, and the care of the sick. Nursing educational programs at that time did not truly prepare nurses for these functions.

The early district nursing services were formed by voluntary organizations (Fig. 2-1). Funding came from contributions and, in some instances, from fees charged to patients on an ability to pay basis. The nursing services were administered by lay boards; even the actual nursing care was supervised by lay persons. In 1893, Lillian Wald initiated a district nursing service in New York City which, in contrast, provided nursing care under the supervision of nurses. Her service was associated administratively with the health department, an official agency, although most district nursing services at that time remained voluntary.

PUBLIC HEALTH NURSING (1900–1970)

By the turn of the century, district nursing began to broaden its focus to include the health and welfare of the public, not just of the poor. This new emphasis was part of a more general consciousness about public health. A growing sense of urgency about improving the health of all people led to an increase in the number of voluntary health agencies. These agencies supplemented the often ineffective work of government health departments. Specialized programs such as infant welfare, tuberculosis clinics, and venereal disease control were developed, causing a demand for nurses in establishments that included factories and schools. In 1902, the first school nurse in the United States was employed by the New York City Board of Education. By 1910, new federal laws made states and communities accountable for the health of their citizens.

The role of the district nurse expanded during this stage. Lillian Wald, a leading figure in this expansion, was the first to use the term *public health nursing* [3]. District nursing had pioneered in health teaching [2], disease prevention, and promotion of good health practices. Now, with a growing recognition of familial and environmental influences on health, public health nurses broadened their practice even more. Nurses working outside the hospital setting increased their knowledge and skills in specialized areas such as tuberculosis, school health, and mental disorders.

Then the family began to emerge as the unit of service. The multiple problems faced by many families started the trend toward nursing care generalized enough to meet a diversity of needs and provide continuity of care. By the 1920s public health nursing was acquiring more professional stature, in contrast to its earlier linkage with charity. It assumed greater leadership in improving and expanding health services and in increasing the standards of nursing education and practice. Public health nurses gradually gained more autonomy in such areas as bedside care and instruction of good health practices to families and community groups. Their collaborative relationships with other community health groups grew as the need to avoid gaps and duplication of services became apparent. Public health nurses also started to keep better records of their caregiving.

During this stage, the institutional base for public health nursing shifted to the government. Public health nursing services, which emphasized health guidance but also provided care for the ill, were offered through local health departments. As a result, rural public health nursing also expanded. Some of the district nursing services, now

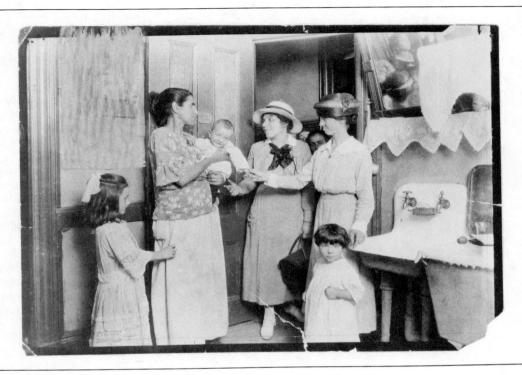

Figure 2-2. The public health nurse, carrying her bag of equipment and supplies, made regular home visits to provide physical and psychologic care as well as health teaching to families. (Courtesy of the Visiting Nurses' Association, Boston Collection.)

known as visiting nurse associations (VNAs), remained under the direction of voluntary agencies and offered their own nursing services of bedside care. In some places, city or county health departments joined administratively and financially with VNAs to provide a combination of services, such as bedside care and health guidance to families.

The public health nursing stage was characterized by service to the public, although the family was recognized as the primary unit of care (Fig. 2-2). Official health agencies, which placed greater emphasis on disease prevention and health promotion, provided the chief institutional base.

EMERGENCE OF COMMUNITY HEALTH NURSING (1970–PRESENT)

The emergence of community health nursing heralded a new era. The strengths of traditional public health nursing combined with a new consciousness of service to the total community. By the mid-sixties a number of events had occurred to cause concern about the nature of public health nursing:

1. Nursing schools, recognizing the importance of public health content, began to require courses in public health for all baccalaureate graduates. This prerequisite meant that graduates were expected to incorporate public health principles into nursing practice, regardless of their sphere of service. Consequently, some people questioned whether public health nursing retained any unique content.
2. A second source of confusion over the definition of community health nursing arose from the fact that hospital nurses followed community cases and public health nurses followed hospital cases. Hospital walls seemed permeable, for community health nurses were not the only nurses practicing in the community.
3. Many new kinds of community health workers appeared and the role of the community health nurse expanded. This development raised several important questions. Should community health nursing, which had become generalized in practice, return to a new specialization? Should it incorporate more specialized skills, such as physical assessment, into its generalized practice?
4. Accelerated changes in health care delivery, technology, and social issues made increasing demands on community health nurses' ability to adapt to new patterns of practice. By the mid-seventies various community health nursing leaders had identified knowledge and skills needed for more effective community health nursing practice [12]; this information had only begun to be incorporated in nursing school curricula.

Still, the direction in which community health nursing was moving had become clear—to care for, not in, the community [6]. Its primary responsibility was the health of the whole community; thus its focus turned to more comprehensive health care and diversity of programs. This shift made the term *community health nursing* more functional than the term *public health nursing;* this text, however, uses the two interchangeably. Community health nursing meant population-oriented nursing of problems along the entire range of the health–illness continuum, although health promotion was increasingly emphasized. Community health nurses were carving out new roles for themselves, including independent practice. Collaboration and interdisciplinary team work were recognized as crucial to effective community nursing. Practitioners served in many kinds of agencies and institutions, such as senior citizen centers, ambulatory services, mental health clinics, and family planning programs, as well as in many nonhealth settings; they followed clients before, during, and after hospitalization. Documentation of nursing care, program evaluation, peer review, and definitive community nursing research were of high priority. This field of nursing had begun to assume its responsibility as a full professional partner in community health (Fig. 2-3).

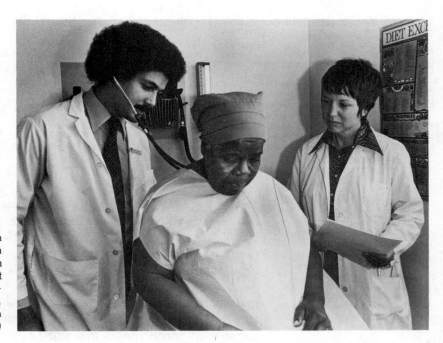

Figure 2-3. Community health nurses work collaboratively with physicians and other health team members to promote client health. (Courtesy of the Harvard Community Health Plan, Boston. Photograph by Sandra Shriver.)

Table 2-1 summarizes the most important changes that have occurred during community health nursing's three stages. It shows these changes in terms of focus, type of nursing, service emphasis, and institutional base.

SOCIETAL INFLUENCES

Many factors influenced the growth of community health nursing. To understand better the nature of this field, it is helpful to recognize the forces that began and continue to shape its development. Five are particularly significant: advanced technology, progress in causal thinking, changes in education, the changing role of women, and the consumer movement.

ADVANCED TECHNOLOGY

Advanced technology has contributed in many ways to shaping the practice of community health nursing. For example, technologic innovation has greatly improved health care and nutrition, thus increasing life expectancy. Consequently, community health nurses direct much of their efforts toward meeting the needs of older persons and working with chronic conditions. Advanced technology has also been a strong force behind industrialization, large-scale employment, and urbaniza-

Table 2-1. Development of Community Health Nursing

Stages	Focus	Type of Nursing	Service Emphasis	Institutional Base (Agencies)
District nursing (1860–1900)	Sick poor	Individual-oriented	Curative; beginning of preventive	Voluntary; some government
Public health nursing (1900–1970)	Needy public	Family-oriented	Curative; preventive	Government; some voluntary
Emergence of community health nursing (1970–present)	Total community	Population-oriented	Health promotion; illness prevention	Many kinds; some independent practice

tion. We are now primarily an urban society; health planners project that 80 percent of the United States population will live in urban areas by the year 2000 [10]. Population density leads to many health-related problems, particularly the spread of disease and increased stress. Community health nurses are learning how to combat these urban health problems. In addition, changes in transportation and high job mobility have affected the health scene. As people travel and relocate, they are separated from families and traditional support systems; community health nurses frequently help people cope with the accompanying stress. New products, equipment, and methods in industry have also increased environmental pollution and industrial hazards. Community health nurses have become involved in related research, occupational health, and preventive education. Finally, technologic innovation has helped promote medicine's complex diagnostic and treatment procedures, thus making illness-oriented care more dramatic and desirable, as well as more costly. Community health nurses face a challenge to demonstrate the physical and economic value of wellness-oriented care.

PROGRESS IN CAUSAL THINKING

Progress in causal thinking in the health sciences has significantly affected the nature of community health nursing. The germ theory of disease causation, established in the late 1800s, was the first real breakthrough in control of communicable disease. Nurses incorporated the teaching of cleanliness and personal hygiene into basic nursing care (Fig. 2-4). A second advance in causal thinking was initiated by the tripartite view which called attention to the interactions between a causative agent, a susceptible host, and the environment. This information offered community health nursing new ways to control and prevent health disorders. For example, nurses could decrease

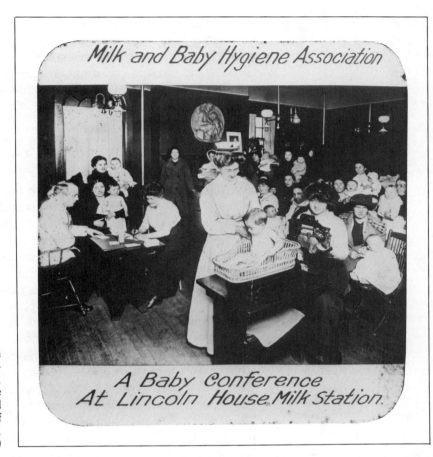

Figure 2-4. Early public health nurses, consistent with the scientific knowledge of their day, taught mothers the importance of keeping their babies clean and properly nourished. (Courtesy of the Visiting Nurses' Association, Boston Collection.)

the vulnerability of an individual (host) by teaching the person a healthier lifestyle. They could instigate measles vaccination programs as a means of preventing the organism (agent) from infecting children. They could promote proper disinfection of a school's swimming pool (environment) to prevent disease. Further progress in causal thinking led to the recognition that not just one but many factors contribute to a disease or health disorder. A food poisoning outbreak that is associated with a restaurant is caused not only by the salmonella organism but also by improper food handling and storage, lack of adherence to minimum food preparation standards, and lack of adequate health department supervision and enforcement.

Community health nurses can control health problems by examining all possible causes and then attacking strategic causal points. Current causal thinking has led to a broader awareness of unhealthy conditions; in addition to disease, problems such as trauma and environmental pollution are major targets of concern. As a result, work-related stress, environmental hazards, chemical food additives, and alcohol and nicotine consumption during pregnancy are all examples of considerations in community health nursing practice.

CHANGES IN EDUCATION

Changes in education, especially those in nursing education, have had an important influence on community health nursing practice. Education, once an opportunity for a privileged few, has become widely available; it is now considered a basic right and a necessity for a vital society. When people's understanding of their environment grows, an increased understanding of health is usually involved. For the community health nurse, health teaching has steadily assumed greater importance in practice. For the learner, education has led to much more responsibility. As a result, people feel that they have a right to know and question the reasons behind the care they receive. Community health nurses have had to shift from planning *for* clients to collaborating *with* clients.

Education has had other effects. The scientific approach, considered basic to progress, has created a dramatic increase in knowledge. The wealth of information relevant to community health nursing practice means that nursing students have more content to assimilate while practicing community health nurses have to make greater efforts to keep abreast. In contrast to earlier times when nurses worked as apprentices in hospitals or health agencies and perfunctorily followed orders, there are now educational programs, including many in continuing education, which prepare nurses to think for themselves in the application of theory to practice. Community health nursing has always required a fair measure of independent thinking and self-reliance; now community health nurses need skills in such areas as family and community assessment, decision making, and collaborative functioning. As the result of expanding education, community health nurses have had to re-examine their practice and clarify their roles.

CHANGING ROLE OF WOMEN

The changing role of women has profoundly affected nursing and community health nursing. In the past century, the women's rights movement has made considerable progress. Women have achieved the right to vote and have gained greater economic independence by entering the labor force. There are many more women with higher education and consequently more influence. The percentage of women in professions such as medicine, law, or engineering has increased, although it is proportionately smaller than that of men. Many women are managing the dual careers of job and family. These gains have increased the number of women entering nursing, whose professional responsibilities and recognition have also improved.

Changes resulting from the women's rights movement continue to occur. Nurses still struggle for equality—equality of job selection, equal pay for equal work, and equal opportunity for advancement outside the nursing hierarchy. If community health nurses are to influence the field of community health, they need status and authority equal to that of their colleagues. This step will require nurses to demonstrate their competence and learn to be assertive in assuming roles as full professional partners. In community health, as in society generally, women hold very few administrative or policy-making positions. Although the majority of nurses are female, a much higher proportion of male than female nurses serve in leadership capacities. The women's movement has contributed to community health nursing's gains in assuming leadership roles, but a need for much greater influence and involvement remains.

CONSUMER MOVEMENT

The consumer movement has also affected the nature of community health nursing. Consumers have become more militant, as evidenced in various boycotts and tax revolts. They are demanding their rights in many areas, including health care, regardless of sex, race, color, or socioeconomic level. Consumers now assert their right to be informed about, and to participate in, decisions that affect them. This movement has stimulated some basic changes in the philosophy of community health nursing. Health care consumers are viewed as active members of the health team, rather than as passive recipients of care. They may contract with the community health nurse for personal or family care, represent the community on the Health Board, or act as ombudsmen, that is, investigate complaints and report findings, to protect the quality of care in the local nursing home. This assumption of consumers' responsibility for their own health means that the community health nurse assists more often than supervises the client's care.

The consumer movement has also contributed to increased concern about the quality of health services. Quality assurance programs, peer review, and tighter evaluation are now part of most health care accreditation requirements. Community health nursing has been led to improve its evaluation of services and programs. Many community health nursing agencies have begun to implement forms of peer review.

The consumer movement has increased the demand for more humane, personalized health care. Dissatisfied with fragmented services offered by impersonal health workers, consumers now seek holistic care. A group of senior citizens living in a high-rise apartment building need more than a series of social workers, nutritionists, recreational therapists, nurses, and other callers ascertaining a variety of specific needs and starting a proliferation of programs. Community health nurses, as members of the health team, increasingly aim at providing coordinated, comprehensive, and personalized services.

CHARACTERISTICS OF COMMUNITY HEALTH NURSING

Thus far this chapter has defined community health nursing and examined events and influences that have shaped its present practice. Now the nature of community health nursing can be observed more closely. Six characteristics of community health nursing are especially salient: (1) it is a field of nursing; (2) it combines public health with nursing; (3) it is population-oriented; (4) it emphasizes health; (5) it involves interdisciplinary collaboration; and (6) it promotes client participation.

FIELD OF NURSING

Community health nursing is a field of nursing; its basic knowledge and skills are those of professional nursing practice. It seeks to give humanistic, accessible, and holistic care. For instance, community health nurses are nursing when they express concern for a group of mothers and tired children sitting on hard chairs for three hours in a clinic hallway, or when they consequently change the appointment scheduling policy and establish a comfortable waiting area. They engage in nursing when they institute a discharge planning system with local hospitals to provide continuity of care. When they visit older clients in their homes to give personal care, instruction, and comfort, they are again nursing.

Community health nursing is a nursing speciality; nursing theory forms its foundation but community health nursing adds concepts, knowledge, and skills from other fields to become a distinctive practice.

ELEMENTS OF PUBLIC HEALTH

In addition to nursing theory, community health nursing incorporates public health content. Knowledge of the following elements of public health is basic to community health nursing:

1. The history of public health
2. The philosophy behind its current practice
3. The means for measurement and analysis, which include epidemiologic concepts and biostatistics, of community health problems
4. The concept of community—how to assess needs and provide service at the total community level
5. The principles basic to leadership, management, and change

There are many ways in which community health nursing incorporates public health knowledge into its practice. For example, some school nurses in Cincinnati, who were working with city health authorities, were concerned with the failure of many children to receive adequate immunization. They used health statistics, specifically a review of school immunization records, to determine immunization needs of school children. Next they set up a successful immunization program which met the needs of the community [1]. They effectively combined biostatistics with a community focus to carry out their goals.

Another nurse, who was working in a city jail emergency room and inpatient ward [4], noticed that prisoners (most of whom were alcoholics) appeared to have very low self-esteem, which consequently impeded their health progress. She designed an experimental program in which staff (nurses, physicians, and police officers) treated the patients with greater respect. The results were improved care and increased patient self-respect. By studying these patients' needs through an epidemiologic approach, she was combining public health with nursing.

As community health nurses carefully analyze their caseloads, assess needs, establish priorities, and plan, implement, and evaluate care, they are utilizing public health management and organization principles. For example, one community health nurse discovered a concern in the community whose needs she was assessing about the high incidence of dental decay among its school children. Because of the relationships she had already established within the community, she was able to help form a committee that studied the problem and initiated a pilot dental health program in one school, to be evaluated a year later. She continues to assist this group in its efforts [5].

Each of the nurses mentioned here has demonstrated an important characteristic of community health nursing, the combination of fundamental public health concepts and nursing.

POPULATION EMPHASIS

The central mission of public health practice is to improve the health of population groups [8]. Community health nursing shares this essential feature: it is population-oriented, concerned with the personal and environmental health of population groups. A population may consist of a community health nurse's caseload or all the patients in a clinic. It may be a scattered group with common characteristics, such as people at high risk of developing coronary heart disease or all the unwed mothers in the county. It may include all the people living in a district, census tract, city, or nation. In fact, the terms *population* and *community* (as defined in Chapter One) can be used interchangeably.

Working with individuals and families is also a part of community health nursing; however, such work must incorporate a strong emphasis on population-oriented nursing, a feature which distinguishes it from other nursing specialties. The difference is in degree. Basic nursing focuses on individuals and community health nursing focuses on aggregates [16], but the many variations in client needs and nursing roles inevitably cause some overlap. Figure 2-5 shows these distinctions between basic and community health nursing.

A population-oriented focus requires the observation of relationships. When working with individuals, families, or groups, the community health nurse does not consider them separately but rather in relationship to the rest of the community. When a case of hepatitis is diagnosed, for example, the community health nurse does more than simply treat it. The nurse tries to stop spread of the infection, locate the possible source, and prevent its reoccurrence in the community. As a result of their population-oriented focus, community health nurses seek to discover possible groups with a common health need, such as expectant mothers, or groups at high risk of developing a common health problem, such as potential diabetics or child abuse victims. Community health nurses continually look for ways to increase environmental quality. They work to prevent health problems by, for example, promoting safety measures in school playgrounds or offering more nourishing, easily prepared meals for nursing home residents. A population-oriented focus involves a whole new outlook and set of attitudes. The community is the client; service is provided to multiple and overlapping groups.

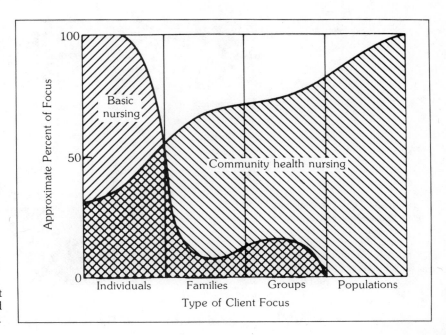

Figure 2-5. Difference in client focus between basic nursing and community health nursing.

HEALTH EMPHASIS

Another distinguishing characteristic of community health nursing is its emphasis on health, or wellness. Chapter One discussed the health–illness continuum. Acute care nursing and medicine deal primarily with the illness end of that continuum since they treat health problems. In contrast, community health nursing has a primary charge to prevent health problems from occurring and to promote a higher level of health. For example, although a community health nurse may assist a woman at home with postpartum fatigue and depression, the nurse also works to *prevent* such problems among other mothers by establishing a prenatal class and encouraging proper rest, nutrition, adequate help, and reduction of stress (*see* Fig. 2-6). Individualized care is important in community health practice, but prevention of aggregate problems reflects more accurately its philosophy and benefits a larger number of people.

Community health nurses concentrate on the health end of the health–illness continuum in a variety of ways. They teach proper nutrition or family planning, demonstrate aseptic technique for home care of a wound, encourage regular physical and dental checkups, start exercise classes or physical fitness programs, and promote healthy inter-

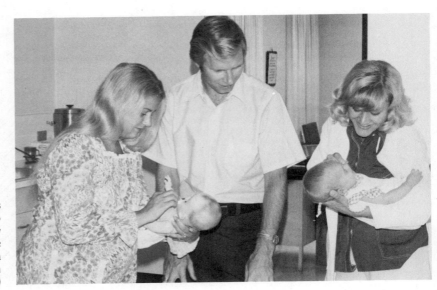

Figure 2-6. This prenatal class offers couples an opportunity to gain skill in caring for a new baby, demonstrated by the nurse, while practicing with a doll. (Courtesy of the American Red Cross.)

personal relationships. Their goal is to help the community reach its optimal level of wellness.

This emphasis on health changes the community health nursing role from a reactive to a proactive stance. It places a greater responsibility on community health nurses to search for cases that require their intervention. In clinical nursing and medicine, the patients seek out professional assistance because they have health problems. As Williams puts it, "patients select themselves into the care system, and the providers' role is to deal with what the patients bring to them" [16]. Community health nurses, in contrast, seek out potential health problems. They identify high risk groups and institute preventive programs. They watch for early signs of child neglect or abuse and intervene when any occur, often long before a request for help is made. They look for possible environmental hazards in the community, such as smoking in public places, and work with appropriate authorities to correct them. A health emphasis requires taking initiative and making sound judgments, which are characteristics of an effective community health nurse.

INTERDISCIPLINARY COLLABORATION

Community health nurses work as full members of a health care team. Such coordination and cooperation are required in a practice that deals with population groups. Individualized efforts and specialized programs, when planned in isolation, can lead to fragmentation and gaps in health services. For example, without collaboration, a well-child clinic may be started in a community that already has a strong early and periodic developmental screening and testing (EPDST) program; at the same time, community prenatal services may be nonexistent. Interdisciplinary collaboration is also important in individualized practice, since nurses need to plan with and keep informed the physician, social worker, physical therapist, or other involved health professional; however, it is an even greater necessity in working with population groups.

Effective collaboration requires team members who are strong individuals. A variety of opinions and ideas, together with a commitment to team goals, lead to the best solutions. Community health nurses who think and act independently make a great contribution to the team effort. In appropriate situations, community health nurses function autonomously, making independent judgments. They also function interdependently, working with members of other disciplines, such as serving on community advisory boards or health planning committees.

Interdisciplinary collaboration requires clarification of each team member's role, a primary reason for community health nurses to understand the nature of their practice. When planning a city-wide immunization program with a community group, for example, community health nurses can explain the ways they might contribute to the program's objectives. They can offer to contact key lay individuals with whom they have established relationships in order to help influence community acceptance of the program. They can share their knowledge of the public's preference about times and locations to offer the program. They can help organize and give the immunizations, thus assuring humanistic service, as well as influence planning for follow-up and continuity of care.

CONSUMER PARTICIPATION

A characteristic of community health nursing which is sometimes overlooked is the encouragement of consumer participation in health care. Our examination of the consumer movement discussed consumers' rights to health care and to involvement in health care's decision-making. However, consumers are frequently intimidated by health professionals and uninformed about health and health care. They do not know what information to ask for and are hesitant to act assertively. A Mexican-American woman brought her two-year-old son, who had symptoms resembling scurvy, to a clinic. Recognizing a vitamin C deficiency, the physician told her to feed the boy large quantities of orange juice but gave no explanation. Several weeks later, she returned; the child was much worse. After questioning her, the nurse discovered that the mother had been feeding the child large amounts of an orange soft drink, not knowing the difference between that and orange juice. Obviously the quality of care is affected when the consumer does not understand and cannot participate in the health care process.

The goal of public health, "to protect, promote, and restore people's health" [14, p. 3], requires a partnership effort. Just as learning cannot take place in schools without student participation, the goals of public health cannot be realized without consumer participation. Community health nursing's efforts toward health improvement can go only so far. Clients' health status and health behavior will not change unless they accept and apply community health nurses' proposals.

Community health nurses encourage consumer participation in several ways. They can promote the client's autonomy. Without realizing it, health professionals can easily cause their clients to depend upon them. Although providing nurturance and guidance sometimes meets the professional's needs, it may prove a great disservice to clients who need to be self-reliant. An elderly couple had been receiving three visits a week from a community health nurse for assistance with the wife's surgical dressing changes and bath. During the visits the nurse taught the husband how to perform these procedures. She also showed him how to prepare simple, nutritious meals and together they arranged with a meals-on-wheels service to bring the couple's dinners for a few weeks. She encouraged them to contact other community resources for assistance with shopping, housework, and transportation to the doctor's office. She reduced her visits to one a week, then to one a month, and, when the couple agreed that they were able to manage on their own, the relationship ended. Independence and feelings of self-worth are closely related. By treating people as independent adults, with trust and respect, community health nurses help promote self-reliance and the ability to function independently.

Community health nurses encourage consumer participation by promoting clients' sense of responsibility for their own health. When consumers feel that their health and that of the community are their, and not the health professionals', responsibility, they will take a much more active interest in promoting it [15]. The process of taking responsibility for developing one's own health potential is called *self-care* [9, 11], a concept which has gained considerable prominence in recent years. Nurses foster self-care by treating clients as adults capable of managing their own affairs, not, as Norris puts it, "as weak, needy, unintelligent, . . . bad, irresponsible children" [11, p. 486]. Nurses can encourage clients to negotiate health care goals and practices, make their own appointments, contact their own resources, and learn ways to monitor their own health.

Consumer participation is promoted when clients are treated as partners on the health care team. The goal is collaborating with clients rather than working for clients. As consumers are treated with respect and trust and, as a result, gain confidence and skill in self-care—promoting their own health and that of their community—their contribution to health care services will become increasingly valuable. The consumer perspective in planning and delivering health services makes those services relevant to consumer needs. Community health nurses encourage the involvement of consumers by soliciting their ideas and opinions, by inviting them to participate on health boards and committees, and by using contracts for care that give them equal authority in choosing services.

SUMMARY

Community health nursing works to promote optimal health for the total community; it achieves this goal by applying knowledge and skills from nursing and from public health.

Historically, the specialty of community health nursing developed through three stages. The district nursing stage began in 1860 with voluntary home nursing care for the poor. Sometimes called health nurses, these specialists treated the sick and taught wholesome living to patients. The public health nursing stage began in 1900 and lasted until about 1970. It was characterized by a consciousness of the general public and their health care. The institutional base shifted to the government. The family became the primary unit of care. The community health nursing stage began around 1970 and has continued to the present. Nursing schools began to require courses in public health for all baccalaureate graduates. This stage made it clear that community nursing involved more than merely working in the community. Roles expanded in many different directions.

Five major societal influences have shaped the development of community health nursing. Advanced technology has solved some health care problems; thus nurses' attention has shifted to problems such as aging, chronic illness, and prevention. Progress in causal thinking has broadened our perspective to multiple causes, including stress, environmental hazards, and the community structure. Changes in education have led community health nurses to emphasize collaborating with clients rather than planning for clients. The changing role of women has helped to open new avenues of leadership for nurses in community health. Finally, the consumer movement has increased the public's concern for quality health service. As consumers have assumed responsibility for their own health, the community health nurse has become, in many instances, a catalyst to assist clients toward autonomy in health.

There are six important characteristics of community health nursing:

1. It is a field of nursing, a specialty within the larger discipline.
2. It combines the specialized knowledge of public health with nursing practice.
3. It is population-oriented and does not deal only with individual clients.
4. It emphasizes health rather than disease or illness.
5. It involves interdisciplinary collaboration, that is, teamwork with other professionals.
6. It promotes client participation by fostering a sense of responsibility among people for their own health.

REFERENCES

1. Anthony, N., et al. Immunization: Public health programming through law enforcement. *Am. J. Public Health* 67:763, 1977.
2. Brainard, A. M. *The Evolution of Public Health Nursing.* Philadelphia: Saunders, 1922. P. 208.
3. Bullough, V., and Bullough, B. *The Care of the Sick: The Emergence of Modern Nursing.* New York: Neale, Watson, 1979. P. 145.
4. Chavigny, K. Self-esteem for the alcoholic: An epidemiologic approach. *Nurs. Outlook* 24:636, 1976.
5. Flynn, B., et al. One master's curriculum in community health nursing. *Nurs. Outlook* 26:633, 1978.
6. Freeman, R. The Dilemma of Public Health Nursing Today. In D. Roberts and R. Freeman (Eds.), *Redesigning Nursing Education for Public Health: Report of the Conference.* Bethesda, Md.: United States Department of Health, Education, and Welfare Pub. No. (HRA) 75–75, 1973. P. 14.
7. Kalisch, P., and Kalisch, B. *The Advance of American Nursing.* Boston: Little, Brown, 1978. P. 228.
8. Kark, S. L. *Epidemiology and Community Medicine.* New York: Appleton-Century-Crofts, 1974. P. 319.
9. Levin, L. Self-care: An emerging component of the health care system. *Hosp. Health Serv. Admin.* 23:17, 1978.
10. Matek, S. J. Some Key Features in the Emerging Context for Future

Health Policy Decisions in America. In D. Roberts and R. Freeman, (Eds.), *Redesigning Nursing Education for Public Health: Report of the Conference.* Bethesda, Md.: U.S. Department of Health, Education, and Welfare Pub. No. (HRA) 75–75, 1973. P. 25.

11. Norris, C. M.   Self-care. *Am. J. Nurs.* 79:486, 1979.

12. Roberts, D., and Freeman, R. (Eds.).   *Redesigning Nursing Education for Public Health: Report of the Conference.* Bethesda, Md.: U.S. Department of Health, Education, and Welfare Pub. No. (HRA) 75–75, 1973. Also see October 1978 issue of *Nursing Outlook* for several perspectives on preparation for community health nursing.

13. Ruth, M. V., and Partridge, K.   Differences in perception of education and practice. *Nurs. Outlook* 26:622, 1978.

14. Sheps, C. G.   *Higher Education for Public Health: A Report of the Milbank Memorial Fund Commission.* New York: Neale, Watson, 1976.

15. Watkin, D.   Personal responsibility: Key to effective and cost effective health. *Fam. Community Health* 1:1, 1978.

16. Williams, C. A.   Community health nursing—what is it? *Nurs. Outlook* 25:250, 1977.

SELECTED READINGS

Archer, S. E., and Fleshman, R. P.   Community health nursing: A typology of practice. *Nurs. Outlook* 23:358, 1975.

Brainard, A. M.   *The Evolution of Public Health Nursing.* Philadelphia: Saunders, 1922.

A Conceptual Model of Community Health Nursing. Kansas City, Mo.: American Nurses Association, 1980.

Freeman, R.   *Community Health Nursing Practice.* Philadelphia: Saunders, 1970.

Freeman, R.   The Dilemma of Public Health Nursing Today. In D. Roberts and R. Freeman (Eds.), *Redesigning Nursing Education for Public Health: Report of the Conference.* Bethesda, Md.: U.S. Department of Health, Education, and Welfare Pub. No. (HRA) 75–75, 1973.

Fromer, M. J.   *Community Health Care and the Nursing Process.* St. Louis: Mosby, 1979.

Goodson, J.   Demonstrating Excellence in a Community Nursing Service. In A. Warner (Ed.), *Innovations in Community Health Nursing.* St. Louis: Mosby, 1978.

Hays, B. J., and Mockelstrom, N. R.   Consumer survey: An approach to teaching consumer participation in community health. *J. Nurs. Educ.* 16:30, 1977.

Kalisch, P., and Kalisch, B.   *The Advance of American Nursing.* Boston: Little, Brown, 1978.

Kinlein, M. L.   On the front: nursing and family and community health (editorial). *Fam. Community Health* 1:57, 1978.

Leahy, K., Cobb, M., and Jones, M. *Community Health Nursing* (3rd ed.). New York: McGraw-Hill, 1977.

Levin, L. Self-care: An emerging component of the health care system. *Hosp. Health Serv. Admin.* 23:17, 1978.

Norris, C. M. Self-Care. *Am. J. Nurs.* 79:486, 1979.

Novello, D. J., et al. *Consumerism and Health Care.* New York: National League for Nursing, 1978.

Roberts, D., and Freeman, R. (Eds.). *Redesigning Nursing Education for Public Health: Report of the Conference.* Bethesda, Md.: U.S. Department of Health, Education, and Welfare Pub. No. (HRA) 75–75, 1973.

Ruth, M. V., and Partridge, K. Differences in perception of education and practice. *Nurs. Outlook* 26:622, 1978.

Scott, J. M. The changing health care environment: Its implications for nursing. *Am. J. Public Health* 64:364, 1974.

Standards: Community Health Nursing Practice. Kansas City, Mo.: American Nurses Association, 1973.

Tinkham, C., and Voorhies, E. *Community Health Nursing: Evolution and Process.* New York: Appleton-Century-Crofts, 1972.

Wales, M. *The Public Health Nurse in Action.* New York: Macmillan, 1941.

Watkin, D. Personal responsibility: Key to effective and cost-effective health. *Fam. Community Health* 1:1, 1978.

Williams, C. A. Community health nursing—what is it? *Nurs. Outlook* 25:250, 1977.

THREE

ROLES AND SETTINGS FOR PRACTICE

There was a day when uniformed public health nurses and home visits summed up the roles and settings of community health nursing, but that day is gone. In its place we find professional community health nurses practicing in a wide variety of settings, such as family planning clinics, industrial plants, and elementary schools, who are no longer restricted to giving treatment. Instead their roles range from educators and organizers to agents of change. The last chapter discussed the nature of community health nursing, how it developed and the characteristics that form a conceptual foundation for its practice. Now we shall consider the specific application of these concepts in the form of various roles assumed by community health nurses, as well as the kinds of settings in which these roles are practiced.

ROLES

Community health nursing incorporates a variety of roles; one could say that we wear many hats while conducting our day-to-day practice. At times, one role is primary; for example, a community health nurse may assume a set of responsibilities in a specialized role such as full-time researcher. More often, however, a number of roles are assumed simultaneously. Several factors influence the roles played by community health nurses. The organization with which the nurse is affiliated often has policies that govern activity. Consumers use community health nursing services differently, depending on their perceptions of nursing. Sociocultural norms, which vary from one group to another, will affect certain community health nurse functions. For example, some groups' values about acceptable female behavior will influence role choices. Political and legal restrictions also set limitations and determine directions for community health nursing practice. Perhaps the most important factor in determining roles will be the community health nurse's own values and ability to adapt to changing health needs. To clarify and expand our understanding of the way community health nursing is practiced, we shall examine seven major roles: (1) care provider, (2) educator, (3) advocate, (4) manager, (5) collaborator, (6) leader, and (7) researcher.

CARE PROVIDER

The most familiar role is provider of care. However, giving nursing care takes on new meaning in the context of community health. The target of service expands beyond the individual to include families, groups, and communities. Nursing care is still designed for the special needs of the client; however, when that client is a group of people, care takes different forms. It requires different skills to assess collective needs and tailor service accordingly. For instance, a community health nurse receives a referral to visit a family with multiple problems. The call is initiated by the eleven-year-old son's frequent absence from and misbehavior at school. Together, the nurse and family design a plan of care that includes counseling for the whole family. It is a response to questions such as what are the family's resources and problems and what are their perceptions of the situation.

HOLISTIC CARE

We recognize that nursing care is holistic, but in community health this approach means viewing the client as a larger system. The client, most often a family or group, is a composite of people whose relationships and interactions with each other must be considered in totality; holistic care must emerge from this perspective. For example, a community health nurse may be working with a group of pregnant teenagers living in a juvenile detention center. The nurse would consider the girls' relationships with each other, their parents, the fathers of their unborn children, and the detention center staff. The nurse would evaluate their age level, developmental needs, and knowledge of pregnancy, delivery, and issues related to the choice of keeping or giving up the baby. The girls' reentry into the community and their future plans for school or employment would also be considered. Holistic care would go far beyond the physical condition of pregnancy and childbirth.

FOCUS ON HEALTH

The role of care provider in community health is also characterized by its focus on health. As we discussed in Chapter One, the community health nurse provides care along the entire range of the health–illness continuum but especially emphasizes promotion of health and prevention of illness. Nursing care includes seeking out clients in order to offer preventive services, rather than waiting for them to come for help after problems arise. Community health nurses identify people who are interested in achieving a higher level of health and work with them to accomplish that goal. They may help a family or group learn how to shop for and eat more nutritious foods, or work with a weight loss group. They may hold seminars on handling stress for a men's club. They may assist a family with a terminally ill member at home to develop healthier attitudes toward dying and death.

NECESSARY SKILLS

The community health nurse uses many different skills in the care provider role. In nursing's early years, the skills most often used were those associated with physical care. Such skills are still very important as a result of earlier hospital discharges and a growing number of elderly persons in the population. As time went on, skills in observation, listening, communication, and counseling became integral to the care provider role. There was an increased emphasis on psychological and sociocultural factors. Most recently, environmental considerations, for example, awareness of problems caused by pollution or of emotional stress related to urban congestion, have created a need for new skills such as assessment and intervention at the community level.

EDUCATOR

It is widely recognized that health teaching is part of good nursing care and one of the major functions of the community health nurse. Health education is especially significant for two major reasons. First, the clients in the community are usually not in an acute state of illness and are better able to absorb and act on health information. For example, a class of expectant parents, unhampered by significant health problems, can grasp the relationship of diet to fetal development. They will understand the value of specific exercises to the childbirth process and then perform those exercises. Second, the health educator role is significant because people in the community have acquired a higher level of health consciousness. Through plans ranging from the President's physical fitness program to local antismoking campaigns, people are recognizing the value of health and are increasingly motivated to achieve higher levels of wellness. When a middle-aged businessman, for example, is discharged from the hospital following a heart attack, he is likely to be more interested in learning how to prevent occurrence of another attack. He can learn how to reduce stress, gradually develop an appropriate exercise program, and alter his eating habits. Families with young children are often interested in learning about normal child growth and development; many young parents want to raise happier, healthier children. An increasing number of business companies are promoting the health of their employees through active health education programs. They recognize that healthy workers mean less absenteeism and higher production levels. Some companies even provide exercise areas and equipment for employee use.

All nurses teach patients about personal care, diet, and medications. Community health nurses, however, go beyond these topics to educate people in a great many areas. People in the community need and want to know about a wide variety of topics. How do you toilet train a two-year-old? What foods should you avoid when you have coronary atherosclerosis? How do you manage an alcoholic spouse? What do you do with adolescent rebellion? What is the best way to lose weight and keep it off? How can you organize the community to work for clean air? What are health consumers' rights? The range of topics taught by community health nurses extends from personal health care and management of leisure to environmental health and community organization.

As educators, community health nurses seek to facilitate client learning. They share information with clients informally, often in the clients' homes (Fig. 3-1). They act as consultants to individuals or groups. They may hold formal classes to increase people's understanding of health and health care. Community health nurses utilize established community groups in their teaching. For example, they may teach parents about signs of drug abuse at a PTA meeting, discuss safety practices with a group of industrial workers, or give a presentation on the importance of early detection of child abuse to a health planning committee considering the funding of a new program. At times, the community health nurse facilitates client learning through referral to more knowledgeable sources or through use of experts on special topics. The community health nurse also facilitates clients' self-education; in keeping with the concept of self-care, clients are encour-

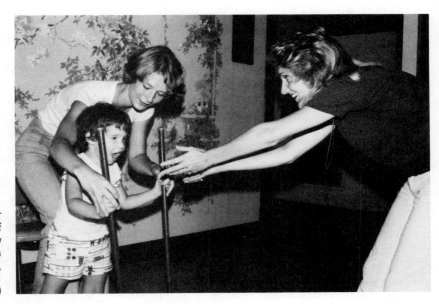

Figure 3-1. Teaching this mother how to help her child is one of the many ways that community health nurses serve as health educators. (From M. Blackwell, *Care of the Mentally Retarded.* Boston: Little, Brown, 1979.)

aged and helped to use appropriate health resources and to seek out health information for themselves. The emphasis throughout the health teaching process continues to be placed on illness prevention and health promotion.

ADVOCATE

Patients' rights are an important issue in health care today. Every patient has the right to receive just, equal, and humane treatment. In our present society, the health care system is often characterized by fragmented and depersonalized services. Clients, especially poor ones, are frequently unable to achieve their rights. They become frustrated, confused, and degraded, unable to cope with the system on their own.

GOALS

Kosik has described two underlying goals in client advocacy [4]. One is to help clients gain greater independence. The community health nurse shows clients what services are available, which they are entitled to, and how to obtain them until they can discover this information for themselves. A second goal is to help make the system more responsive and relevant to the needs of clients. By calling attention to inadequate or unjust care, the community health nurse can influence change (Fig. 3-2).

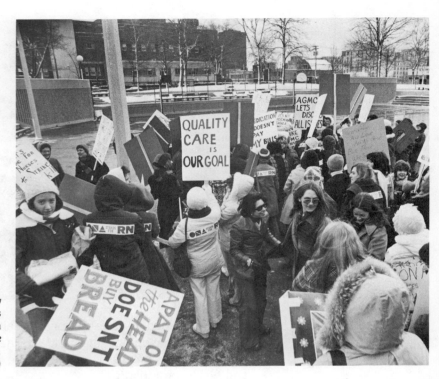

Figure 3-2. Insisting on quality services is one way that nurses serve as client advocates. (From P. Kalisch and B. Kalisch, *The Advance of American Nursing.* Boston: Little, Brown, 1978.)

Consider the experience of a family that shall be called the Martins. Gloria Martin and her three small children had gone to the Westside Clinic on Wednesday. On Tuesday morning, the baby, Tony, had suddenly started to cry. Nothing would comfort him. Gloria called the clinic and was told to come in the next day; the clinic did not take appointments and was too busy to see any more patients that day. The rest of that day and night Tony cried almost incessantly. On Wednesday there was a 45-minute bus ride and a 3½-hour wait in the crowded reception room, punctuated by intake workers' interrogations. The children were restless, and the baby was crying. Finally they saw the physician. Tony had an inguinal hernia that could be gangrenous. The doctor admonished that the baby should have been brought in sooner; now immediate surgery was necessary. Someone at the clinic told Gloria that Medicaid would pay for it. Someone else told her that she was ineligible because she was not a registered clinic patient. By now all the children were crying. Gloria had been up most of the night. She was frantic, confused, and felt that no one cared. This family needed an advocate.

ACTIONS AND CHARACTERISTICS

As an advocate, the community health nurse pleads the cause of another by speaking and acting on that person's or group's behalf. There are times when health care clients need someone to explain what services to expect and which they ought to receive. They need someone to guide them through the complexities of the system, and someone to assure the satisfaction of their needs.

The advocate role requires at least four important characteristics. First, advocates must be assertive. In the Martins' dilemma a community health nurse took the initiative to identify their needs and find appropriate solutions. She contacted the right people and helped them establish eligibility for coverage of surgery and hospitalization costs. She helped Gloria make arrangements for the hospitalization and care of the other children. A second characteristic of the advocate role is willingness to take risks, to go out on a limb, if need be, for the client. The community health nurse was outraged at the kind of treatment that the Martins had received—the delays in service, the impersonal care, and the surgery which could have been prevented. She wrote a letter describing the details of the Martins' experience to the clinic director, the chairman of the clinic board, and the nursing director. It resulted in better care for the Martins and a series of meetings aimed at changing clinic procedures and providing better initial screening. A third characteristic of advocates is their ability to communicate well, to bargain thoroughly and convincingly. The community health nurse helping the Martins was able to state the problem clearly and argue for its solution. Finally, the advocate role requires the ability to identify sources of power and tap them for the client's benefit. By contacting the most influential people in the clinic and appealing to their desire for quality service, the nurse concerned with the Martins was able to facilitate change.

MANAGER

Community health nurses, like all nurses, are managers of client care. In community health this role may involve such activities as managing family care, handling a case load, administrating a clinic, or conducting a community health planning project.

PLANNING

The manager role in community health nursing utilizes three functions in particular: planning, organizing, and coordinating. Planning, the first and most basic function, enables the manager to decide on an objective (client care goals) and to achieve it (nursing process). The nurse begins by studying the situation and drawing up a detailed plan. Community health nurses, as managers, need time for planning, which involves determining client concerns and needs, establishing objectives, and deciding on an appropriate course of action. When starting a therapy group with recovering drug addicts, for example, the nurse sits down with the entire group to discuss their present situation and ambitions. What would they like to accomplish in group therapy? What topics would they like to cover? How would they like to approach them—through discussion or role-playing? When and where would they like to meet? In the process of making these decisions, nurses are planning, that is, mapping out a course of action based on predetermined goals.

ORGANIZING

The second function of the community health nurse manager role is organizing. Organizing means structuring activities and placing people into a functioning whole aimed at attaining stated objectives [5]. A manager must arrange matters so that the job can be done; people, activities, and relationships have to be assembled in order to put the plan into effect [6]. In the process of organizing, the nurse provides a framework for the various aspects of service so that each will run smoothly and accomplish its purpose. The framework is a part of service preparation. When a community health nurse manages a well-baby clinic, for instance, the organizing function involves making certain that all equipment and supplies are present, required staff are hired and on duty, and staff responsibilities are clearly designated.

COORDINATING

Coordinating, the third function of the community health nurse manager role, means bringing people and activities together so that they function in harmony while pursuing desired objectives. Like the matching of a movie film's sound track with its pictures, coordination involves assembly and synchronization. It occurs during planning and implementation of service. On a nurse-patient or nurse-family level, some coordination is almost always necessary (Fig. 3-3). The nurse may arrange an early demonstration of walking on crutches by the physical therapist, time a home health aid's visit to coincide with an older woman's preferred bath schedule, or bring an eight-year-old boy

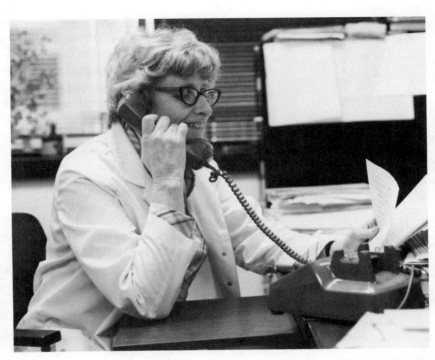

Figure 3-3. As a manager, the nurse coordinates client care so that needed resources are available at the right time. (From M. Blackwell, *Care of the Mentally Retarded.* Boston: Little, Brown, 1979.)

and his parents together with his teacher and the learning disabilities specialist to discuss ways to approach his learning problems.

Coordinating becomes a more complex activity at the community level. Consider a community health nurse working with a group of citizens and health professionals who are interested in starting a mobile health center for a two-county area. Their objective is to make health service more accessible to residents. The nurse will need to contact many individuals, arrange meetings, explore funding sources, tap community leaders, and help maintain the group's focus on its objective. Once the project is in operation, the nurse, as manager, will have a continuing responsibility to coordinate it.

The manager role, at times, involves other functions, such as leading, staffing, supervising, motivating, and controlling service activities. While performing all these functions community health nurses most often are participative managers; that is, they participate with clients or staff, or both, in planning and carrying out services.

COLLABORATOR

Community health nurses seldom practice in isolation. Our work involves many other people, including other nurses, physicians, social workers, physical therapists, nutritionists, attorneys, and secretaries. As a member of the health team, the community health nurse assumes the role of collaborator. To collaborate means to work jointly with others in a common endeavor, to cooperate as partners. Successful community health practice depends on this collegiality. Everyone on the team, including the community health nurse, has an important and unique contribution to make to the health care effort. As on a championship football team, the better each member plays his position and cooperates with other members, the more likely the health team is to win.

Interdisciplinary collaboration has been discussed in Chapter Two as a vital characteristic of community health nursing. The collaborator role is simply an application of that concept. For example, one family needed to find a good nursing home for their 83-year-old grandfather. The community health nurse and family, including the grandfather, made a list of desired features that included a shower; he did not like baths. The daughter, son-in-law, and community health nurse, working with a social worker, located and visited several homes. The grandfather's physician was contacted for medical consultation and the grandfather made the final selection. In another situation, the community health nurse collaborated with the city council, police department, neighborhood residents, and manager of a senior citizens' highrise apartment building to help a group of elderly people organize and lobby for safer streets. In a third example, a school nurse noticed a boy with a high absentee record and low grades. Counseling was started after joint planning with his parents, teacher, school psychologist, and family physician.

The community health nurse collaborator role requires skills in communicating, in interpreting the nurse's unique contribution to the team, and in acting assertively as an equal partner. The collaborator role may also involve functioning as a consultant (Fig. 3-4).

LEADER

The leadership role is not always obvious in community health nursing, but community health nurses are increasingly becoming active leaders. When they guide decision making, stimulate interest in health promotion, initiate therapy, direct a preventive program, or influence health policy, they are assuming a leadership role. It tends to be a role of influence and persuasion more than of directorship.

The leader role, as distinct from the manager role, serves a unique purpose. Its main function is to effect change; thus the community

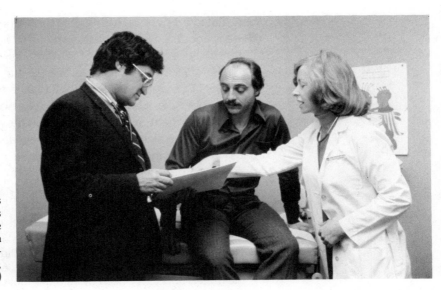

Figure 3-4. The nurse often has unique knowledge about clients which, as a collaborator, she shares with other health team members. (Courtesy of the Harvard Community Health Plan, Boston.)

health nurse becomes an agent of change. The nurse in the leader role influences people to think and behave differently about their health and the factors contributing to it. For example, a community health nurse who made home visits to a young mother suggested that the mother invite her neighbors over for coffee and discussion about health topics of interest. The group met once a month and expanded as the community health nurse increased their desire for more information.

The leader role assumes a different form in another situation. A community health nurse was eager to start a mental health program, which she and her nursing colleagues felt was needed, through her agency. But certain individuals on the health board were opposed to adding any new programs because of cost. Her approach was to gather considerable supportive data to demonstrate the program's need and cost effectiveness. She lunched individually with key board members in order to convince them of the need. She prepared written summaries, graphs, and charts and, at a strategic time, presented her case at a board meeting. The mental health program was approved and implemented.

RESEARCHER

The researcher role is an integral part of community health nursing practice. But, it may be asked, how can research be combined with practice? It is true that research often involves a complex set of activities conducted by persons with highly developed and specialized skills. But there is another way to view research and it is from this perspective that community health nurses are researchers.

Research literally means to search—to investigate, discover, and interpret facts. This questioning attitude is a basic prerequisite to good nursing practice. There have probably been many times when you revisited a patient and noticed some change in his condition such as restlessness or skin color. Consequently, you wondered what was causing this change and what could be done about it. In everyday practice, community health nurses encounter numerous situations that challenge them to ask questions. Consider the following examples:

"Mr. Hansen is still very weak on his right side since his CVA [cerebrovascular accident]. I wonder if he really understands how to do his exercises?"

"Little Marc seems unusually quiet and I see another bruise on his left arm. Could this possibly be the beginning of child abuse?"

"This prenatal class is dragging; am I going too fast, is there some conflict in the group, or do they need more opportunity for expressing themselves?"

"While driving through this part of the city, I haven't seen a single playground for miles. I wonder where the kids play?"

Each of these questions places the community health nurse in the role of researcher. They express the fundamental attitude of every researcher, *a spirit of inquiry.*

A second attribute, careful *observation,* is also evident in the examples just given. The community health nurse develops a sharpened ability to notice things as they are, deviations from the norm, and even subtle changes that suggest the need for some nursing action.

Coupled with observation is *open-mindedness,* another attribute of the researcher role. After observing Mr. Hansen's weakness, the community health nurse postulates that Mr. Hansen may not understand how to do his exercises but keeps an open mind to other possibilities. He can demonstrate his exercises and, if that is not the problem, perhaps he needs some different activities to strengthen the weak muscles. In the case of little Marc, the community health nurse's observations suggest one possible cause, child abuse. But open-mindedness requires consideration of other alternatives and, as a good researcher, the nurse explores these as well.

The community health nurse also uses *analytic* skills in this role. In the prenatal class example, the nurse has already started to analyze the situation by trying to determine its cause and effect relationships. Successful analysis depends on how well the data has been collected. Insufficient information can lead to false interpretations so the community health nurse is careful to seek out the needed data. Analysis, like a jigsaw puzzle, involves studying the pieces and fitting them together until the meaning of the whole picture can be described.

Finally, the researcher role involves *tenacity*. The community health nurse persists in an investigation until facts are uncovered and a satisfactory answer is found. Noticing an absence of playgrounds and wondering where the children play is only a beginning. The nurse, concerned about the children's safety and need for recreational outlets in the district, gathers data about location and accessibility of play areas as well as felt needs of community residents. A fully documented research report may result. If the data support a need for additional play space, the report can be brought before the proper authorities.

Community health nurses practice the researcher role at many levels. Up to this point we have focused primarily on simple kinds of investigations to emphasize that research is an essential and integral part of community health nursing practice. However, the attributes that have been described are basic to research practice at any level. In addition to everyday inquiries, community health nurses often participate in agency or organizational studies to determine such matters as the effectiveness of a screening program or the need for a new family planning clinic. Some community health nurses also initiate more complex research of their own or in collaboration with other health professionals. The researcher role, at all levels, helps to determine needs, evaluate effectiveness of care, and develop theoretical bases for community health nursing practice (Fig. 3-5).

SETTINGS FOR PRACTICE

We have just examined community health nursing from the perspective of its major roles. Now we can place the roles in context by viewing the settings in which they are practiced. The numbers and kinds of places for community health nursing practice are too varied to make it practical to examine them all. For purposes of discussion, however, they can be grouped into six categories: (1) homes, (2) ambulatory settings, (3) schools, (4) occupational health settings, (5) residential institutions, and (6) the community at large.

HOMES

One of the most frequently used settings for community health nursing practice is the home. In the home setting all of the community health nursing roles, to varying degrees, are performed. Clients discharged from acute care institutions, such as hospitals or mental health facilities,

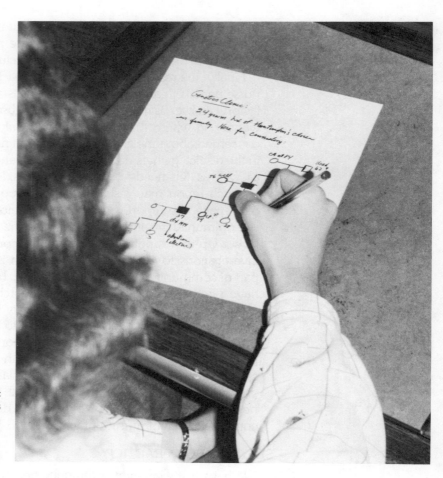

Figure 3-5. Tracing genetic linkages is one aspect of this nurse researcher's investigation. (From M. Blackwell, *Care of the Mentally Retarded.* Boston: Little, Brown, 1979.)

are regularly referred to community health nursing for continued care and follow-up. Here the nurse can see the client in a family and environmental context, and service can be individualized to the client's particular needs. For example, Mr. White, 67 years of age, was discharged from the hospital with a colostomy. Doreen, the community health nurse from the county public health nursing agency, immediately started home visits. She met with the Whites to discuss their needs as a family and to plan for Mr. White's care and adjustment to living with a colostomy. Practicing the care provider and educator roles, she reinforced and expanded on the teaching started in the hospital for colostomy care, that is, bowel training, diet, exercise, and proper use of equipment. As part of a total family care plan, Doreen provided some forms of physical care for Mr. White as well as counseling, teaching, and emotional support for both the Whites. In addition to consulting with the physician and social services, she arranged and supervised home health aid visits that gave personal care and homemaker services; she thus utilized the manager, leader, and collaborator roles.

The home is a setting for health promotion as well. Many community health nursing visits focus on assisting families to understand and practice healthier living. They may, for example, include preparation for parenting, infant care, child discipline, eating right, getting proper exercise, coping with stress, or managing grief and loss.

The character of the home setting is as varied as the clients whom the community health nurse serves. In one day a community health nurse may visit an elderly well-to-do widow in her luxury home, a middle income family in their modest bungalow, and a transient in his one room fifth story walk-up apartment. In each home situation, community health nurses can view their clients in perspective and, therefore, better understand their limitations, capitalize on their resources, and tailor health services to their needs. In the home, unlike most other health care settings, clients are on their own turf. They feel comfortable and secure in the familiar surroundings and are thus often better able to understand and apply health information. Client self-respect can be promoted since the client is host while the nurse is a guest in the home setting.

AMBULATORY SETTINGS

Ambulatory settings include a variety of places in which community health nurses practice. Each is a place where clients *come* for day service; in other words, they seek out or are referred to these health services for care that does not include overnight stays. Clinics are an example of an ambulatory setting. Sometimes multiple clinics, offering medical, surgical, orthopedic, dermatologic, and many other services, are located in the outpatient department of hospitals or medical centers. They may also be based in a comprehensive neighborhood health center. A single clinic, such as a family planning or well-child clinic, may be found in a location more convenient for clients, for example, a church basement or empty store front. Some kinds of day care centers, such as those for physically handicapped or emotionally disturbed adults, utilize community health nursing services. Additional ambulatory settings include health departments and community health nursing agencies where clients may come for assessment and referral or counseling.

Offices are another type of ambulatory setting. Some community health nurses provide service in conjunction with medical practice; for example, a community health nurse associated with a HMO sees clients in the office and undertakes screening, referrals, counseling, health education, and group work. Others establish their own independent practice by seeing clients in their offices as well as making home visits [2, 3].

Another type of ambulatory setting includes places where services are offered to selected groups. For example, community health nurses practice in migrant camps, Native American reservations, and remote mountain and coal-mining communities. Again, in each ambulatory setting all the community health nursing roles are utilized to varying degrees.

SCHOOLS

Schools of all levels comprise a major group of settings for community health nursing practice. Nurses from community health nursing agencies frequently serve private schools of elementary and intermediate levels. Public schools are served by the same agencies or by community health nurses hired through the public school system. Community health nurses may work with groups of children in preschool settings, such as Montessori schools, as well as in vocational technical schools, junior colleges, and college and university settings. Specialized schools, such as those for the handicapped, are another setting for community health nursing practice.

Community health nurse roles in school settings are expanding. School nurses, whose primary role was initially care provider, are widening their practice to include much more health education, collaboration, and client advocacy. For example, one school had been accustomed to utilizing the nurse as a first-aid giver and record keeper; her duties were handling minor problems, such as headaches and cuts, and keeping track of such events as immunizations. This nurse determined to expand her practice and, after planning and preparation, implemented a series of classes on personal hygiene, diet, and sexuality; started a drop-in health counseling center in the school; and established a network of professional contacts for consultation and referral. Community health nurses in school settings are also beginning to assume manager and leader roles and recognize that the researcher role should be an integral part of their practice.

OCCUPATIONAL HEALTH

Business and industry provide another group of settings for community health nursing practice. Employee health has long been recognized as making a vital contribution to individual lives, productivity of business, and the well-being of the entire nation. Organizations now are expected to provide a safe and healthy work environment in addition to health insurance and health care. An increasing number of companies, recognizing the value of healthy employees, go beyond traditional health benefits to include health promotional efforts. Some businesses, for example, encourage healthy snacks like fruit instead of coffee at breaks and jogging during the noon hour. A few larger corporations have built exercise facilities for their employees, provide health education programs, and offer financial incentives for staying well.

Community health nurses in occupational health settings practice a variety of roles. Early industrial nursing, which started in 1895 when the first nurse was hired by an industry mostly involved visiting sick workers in their homes [1]. The care provider role was primary for many years as nurses continued to care for sick or injured employees at work. However, recognition of the need to protect employees' safety and later to prevent their illness, led to inclusion of health education. Now industrial nurses also act as employee advocates, assuring appropriate job assignments for workers and adequate treatment for job-related illness or injury. They collaborate with other health care providers and company management to offer better services to their clients and act as leaders and managers in developing new health services in the work setting, such as hypertension screening or weight control programs. Occupational health settings range from factories and industries, such as an automobile assembly plant, to business corporations and even large department stores. The field of occupational health offers a challenging opportunity, particularly in smaller businesses where nursing coverage is not provided.

RESIDENTIAL INSTITUTIONS

Facilities where clients reside form a fifth group of settings in which community health nursing is practiced. Clients may be housed temporarily in these institutions, as in a half-way house for recovering alcoholics, or on a relatively permanent basis, as in an in-patient hospice program for the terminally ill. Some of these institutions, for example, hospitals, exist solely to provide health care. Community health nurses based in a community agency maintain continuity of care for their clients by collaborating with hospital personnel, visiting clients in the hospital, and helping plan care during and following hospitalization. As part of their case loads, some community health nurses serve one or more hospitals on a regular basis by providing a liaison with the community, consultation for discharge planning, and periodic inservice programs to keep hospital staff updated on community services for their clients. Other community health nurses with similar functions are based in the hospital and serve the hospital community. A skilled-nursing-care home is another example of a residential facility providing health care that may utilize community health nursing services. In this kind of setting, where residents are usually elderly with many chronic health problems, the community health nurse functions particularly as advocate and collaborator to improve care. He or she will coordinate available resources to meet the needs of residents and their families, and help safeguard the maintenance of proper nursing home operating standards.

Community health nurses also practice in settings where residents are gathered for other purposes. Health care is offered as an adjunct to the primary goals of the institution. One example is the many camping programs for children and adults offered by churches and other community agencies, such as the Boy Scouts, Girl Scouts, or Y.M.C.A. As camp nurses, community health nurses practice all available roles, often under interesting and challenging conditions.

Residential institutions provide a unique kind of setting for community health nurses to practice health promotion. Their clients are a "captive" audience whose needs can be readily assessed and whose interests can be stimulated. These settings offer community health nurses the opportunity to generate an environment of caring and optimal quality services.

COMMUNITY AT LARGE

Unlike the five already discussed, the sixth setting for community health nursing practice is not confined to a specific location or building. When nurses work with groups, populations, or the total community, they may practice in many different places. For example, a community health nurse, as care provider and health educator, may work with a parenting group in a church or town hall. Another nurse, as client advocate, leader, and researcher, may study the health needs of a neighborhood's elderly population by collecting data throughout the area and meeting with resource people in many places. Again, the community at large becomes the setting for practice of a nurse who serves on health care planning committees, lobbies for health legislation at the state capitol, or runs for a school board position.

While the term *setting* implies place, it is important to remember that community health nursing practice is not limited to a specific arena. Community health nursing is a specialty of nursing that can be practiced anywhere.

SUMMARY

Community health nursing incorporates many roles and is practiced in many settings. Seven major roles, when combined, describe community health nursing practice: care provider, health educator, client advocate, health service manager, health team collaborator, leader or initiator of change, and researcher. The types and number of roles that are practiced vary depending on the nurse, clients, and demands of the situation.

The settings of community health nursing practice are also many and varied, but they can generally be grouped into six categories: homes, ambulatory settings, schools, occupational health settings, residential institutions, and the community at large.

REFERENCES

1. Freeman, R. *Community Health Nursing Practice.* Philadelphia: Saunders, 1970. P. 325.
2. Goodson, J. Demonstrating Excellence in a Community Nursing Service. In A. Warner (Ed.), *Innovations in Community Health Nursing.* St. Louis: Mosby, 1978.
3. Greenidge, J., Zimmern, A., and Kohnke, M. Community nurse practitioners—A partnership. *Nurs. Outlook* 21:228, 1973.
4. Kosik, S. H. Patient advocacy or fighting the system. *Am. J. Nurs.* 72:694, 1972.
5. Longest, B. *Management Practices for the Health Professional.* Reston, Va.: Reston Pub., 1976. Pp. 44, 105.
6. Plachy, R. Delegation and Decision-Making. In S. Stone et al. (Eds.), *Management for Nurses: A Multidisciplinary Approach.* St. Louis: Mosby, 1976. P. 60.

SELECTED READINGS

Archer, S., and Fleshman, R. Community health nursing: A typology of practice. *Nurs. Outlook* 23:358, 1975.

Fromer, M. J. Functions of the Community Health Nurse. In M. J. Fromer (Ed.), *Community Health Care and the Nursing Process.* St. Louis: Mosby, 1979.

Goodson, J.   Demonstrating Excellence in a Community Nursing Service. In A. Warner (Ed.), *Innovations in Community Health Nursing*. St. Louis: Mosby, 1978.

Greenidge, J., Zimmern, A., and Kohnke, M.   Community nurse practitioners—A partnership. *Nurs. Outlook* 21:228, 1973.

Hitchcock, J.   Working in a nonhealth-oriented setting. *Nurs. Clin. North Am.* 5:251, 1970.

Keller, M. J.   Health Needs and Nursing Care of the Labor Force. In M. J. Fromer (Ed.), *Community Health Care and the Nursing Process*. St. Louis: Mosby, 1979.

Kosik, S. H.   Patient advocacy or fighting the system. *Am. J. Nurs.* 72:694, 1972.

Lysaught, J. P.   Distributive Nursing Practice: Development and Fusion of Roles. In J. P. Lysaught, *Action in Nursing*. New York: McGraw-Hill, 1974.

Oda, D.   The Role of the Community Nurse in School Systems. In S. Archer and R. Fleshman (Eds.), *Community Health Nursing: Patterns and Practice*. North Scituate, Mass.: Duxbury Press, 1975.

Pacifico, P. B.   The dynamic and expanded role of nurses in community health nursing. *Phillippine J. Nurs.* 46:86, 1977.

Quinn, M. and Reinhardt, A.   Community Health Nursing: New Directions for Practice. In A. Reinhardt and M. Quinn (Eds.), *Family-Centered Community Nursing: A Sociocultural Framework*. St. Louis: Mosby, 1973.

Skrovan, C., Anderson, E. J., and Gottschalk, J.   Community nurse practitioner: An emerging role. *Am. J. Public Health* 64:847, 1974.

Standards: Community Health Nursing Practice.   Kansas City, Mo.: American Nurses Association, 1973.

Warner, A. (Ed.).   *Innovations in Community Health Nursing*. St. Louis: Mosby, 1978.

Williams, C. A.   Community health nursing—What is it? *Nurs. Outlook* 25:250, 1977.

FOUR

CULTURE AND COMMUNITY

For most health professionals, individual differences are a treasured value. We are delighted to see children grow and develop in unique ways. We applaud someone's creative achievement. We each have preferences about the kind of food we eat, the way we dress, and how we decorate our living quarters. The right to be ourselves and different from others is highly valued. But although individuality is part of our culture, we recognize limits to the range of acceptable differences. People whose behavior falls outside of that range become "deviants" or "misfits." Our culture approves moderate social drinking but not alcoholism. Why are some behaviors acceptable and others not? Why do so many health professionals have difficulty converting their clients to new ways of thinking and acting? Explanations can be found by examining the concept of culture and its application to community health nursing practice.

THE MEANING OF CULTURE

Culture refers to the ideas, values, and behavior that are shared by members of some social group. It is a design for living, a way of life. More than simply custom or ritual, culture is a way of organizing and thinking about life. It gives people a sense of security about their behavior; without having to consciously think about it, they know how to act. Culture also provides the underlying values and beliefs upon which this behavior is based. For example, culture determines the value we place on achievement, independence, work, and leisure. It forms the basis for our definitions of male and female roles and determines our responses to authority figures. As anthropologist Edward Hall says, "culture controls our lives" [5, p. 38].

INFLUENCE ON BEHAVIOR

Every community, every social or ethnic group, has its own culture. Furthermore, all the individual members behave in the context of that specific culture. Each of us belongs to a group or set of overlapping groups that influences our thoughts and actions. Even very small elements of everyday living are influenced by our culture. For instance, culture determines the distance we stand from another person while talking. A comfortable talking distance for Americans is at least 2½ feet, while Latin Americans prefer a shorter distance, often only 18 inches for dialogue. Consider how culture influences our perception of time. When we make an appointment to see someone, we expect to be on time or not more than a few minutes late. To keep a person waiting (or to be kept waiting) for 45 minutes or an hour is insulting and intolerable. Yet there are other cultures and subcultures, including Native American and Asian groups, whose response to time is much more flexible; their members think nothing of waiting, or keeping someone else waiting, for an hour or two. Clearly, culture, as Benjamin Paul puts it, "is a blueprint for social living" [8, p. 233].

RELATIONSHIP TO HEALTH CARE

Culture, because it so profoundly influences thinking and behavior, is an essential dimension of health care. Just as physical and psychological factors determine clients' needs and attitudes toward health and illness, so too does culture. Kark emphasizes that "culture is perhaps the most relevant social determinant of community health" [7, p. 149]. Culture influences diet and eating practices and determines how children are raised. How people react to pain, cope with stress, deal with death, respond to health practitioners, and value the past, present, and future are all affected by culture. Yet the concept of culture is not always clearly understood or incorporated into health care. Many nursing care plans omit consideration of clients' cultural and social needs. Others may include them only after some painful experience at the client's expense, as is shown in the following illustration.

Maria Juarez, a 53-year-old Chicano widow, was referred to a community health nursing agency by a clinic. Her married daughter reported that Mrs. Juarez was having severe and prolonged vaginal bleeding and needed medical attention. The daughter had made several appointments for her mother at the clinic, but Mrs. Juarez had refused at the last minute to keep any of them.

After two broken home visit appointments, the community health nurse made a drop-in call and found Mrs. Juarez at home. The nurse was greeted courteously and invited to have a seat. After introductions, the nurse explained that she and the others were only trying to help. Mrs. Juarez had caused a lot of unnecessary concern to everyone by not cooperating, she scolded in a friendly tone. Mrs. Juarez quickly apologized and explained that she had felt fine on the days of her broken appointments and saw no need to "bother anyone." Questioned about her vaginal bleeding, Mrs. Juarez was evasive. "It's nothing," she said, "it comes and goes like always, only maybe a little more." She listened politely, nodding in agreement, as the nurse explained the need for her to see a physician. Her promise to come to the clinic the next day, however, was not kept. The staff labelled Mrs. Juarez unreliable and uncooperative.

Mrs. Juarez had been brought up to be a traditional Chicano woman. Her role was to be submissive and interested primarily in the welfare of her husband and children. She had learned long ago to ignore her own needs and, in fact, found it difficult to identify any personal wants. Her major concern was to avoid causing trouble for others. To have a medical problem, then, was a difficult adjustment. The pain and bleeding had caused her great apprehension. Many Chicanos have a particular dread of sickness and especially hospitalization [6]. Furthermore, her culture had taught Mrs. Juarez the value of modesty. "Female problems" were not discussed openly. This cultural orientation meant that the sickness threatened her modesty and created intense embarrassment. Conforming to Chicano cultural values, she had first turned to her family for support. Often it is only under dire circumstances that Chicanos seek help from others; to do so means sacrificing pride and dignity [14]. Mrs. Juarez agreed to go to the clinic because refusal would have been disrespectful. But her fear of physicians as well as her extreme reluctance to discuss such a sensitive problem kept her from going.

Mrs. Juarez was being asked to take action which violated a number of deeply felt cultural values. Her behavior was far from unreliable and uncooperative; with no opportunity to discuss and resolve the conflicts, she had no other choice.

CULTURAL DIFFERENCES

A major barrier to meeting Mrs. Juarez's needs was a failure to recognize cultural differences. In fact, many of the health care system's failures result from this shortsightedness [3]. It is most obvious that every group has its own culture when we contrast our way of life with a vastly different one, for example, that of some New Guinea tribe. We easily recognize culture when we see people sleep on the floor together in large extended family groups, eat monkey meat with their fingers from a common bowl, or seldom discipline young children.

Cultural differences, however, are equally strong in the United States. Although broad cultural values are shared by many of us, a rich diversity of subcultures also exists. The members of each subculture retain some of the characteristics of the society from which they came or in which their ancestors lived [12]. Some of their beliefs and practices, such as the food they eat, the language they speak at home, the way they celebrate holidays, or their ideas about sickness and healing, remain an important part of their everyday life (Fig. 4-1). Native American groups have retained some aspects of their traditional cultures. Mexican-Americans, Irish-Americans, Italian-Americans, Afro-Americans, Puerto Ricans, Chinese-Americans, and many other ethnic groups have their own subcultures. Furthermore, certain customs, values, and ideas are unique to the poor, the rich, the middle class, women, men, youth, and the elderly. Many deviant groups, such as narcotic addicts, criminals, homosexuals, and skid row alcoholics have developed their own subcultures. Regional subcultures, for instance, the Kentucky Mountain people, also have distinctive ways of defining the world and coping with problems. Even occupational and professional groups develop their own special languages and outlooks. Nurses, for example, have a special culture with unique vocabulary, values, clothes, and customs. Recognizing such cultural differences is a first step toward cultural understanding.

ETHNOCENTRISM

Another barrier to effective care for Mrs. Juarez was the judgment of her behavior by a middle-class standard. Good patients, many people believe, appreciate help from health professionals and comply with their requests. This kind of thinking is based on the assumption that "my way is right." It is easy to view one's own way of life as the best while those whose ideas differ are rejected as inferior, ignorant, or irrational. Such a belief is called *ethnocentrism* [9, 11]. Ethnocentrism

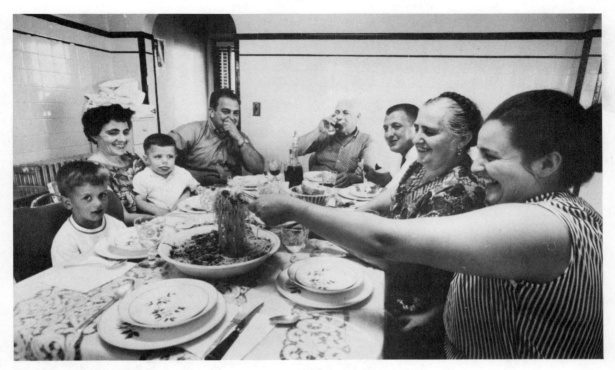

Figure 4-1. The deFranco family of Roseto, Pa., continue to enjoy traditional Italian meals. (Photograph by Russell Hamilton for *Time* © 1964, Time, Inc.)

creates biases and misconceptions about human behavior that can cause irreparable damage to interpersonal relationships. Mrs. Juarez was labelled unreliable and uncooperative because she failed to conform to prescribed patterns of correct behavior. Yet these same patterns contradicted Mrs. Juarez's value system. From her perspective, American health culture must have seemed equally strange and irrational. It is one thing to believe that your way is good for you, and it is another to insist that everyone else conform to it. Here lies the distinction between healthy cultural identification and ethnocentrism. Here also is another clue to the mystery of bridging cultural gaps; rather than apply moral judgments, one should understand and appreciate cultural differences.

CHARACTERISTICS OF CULTURE

In their study of culture, anthropologists and sociologists have made significant contributions to the field of community health. Five characteristics of culture are especially pertinent to consider in the effort to improve community health.

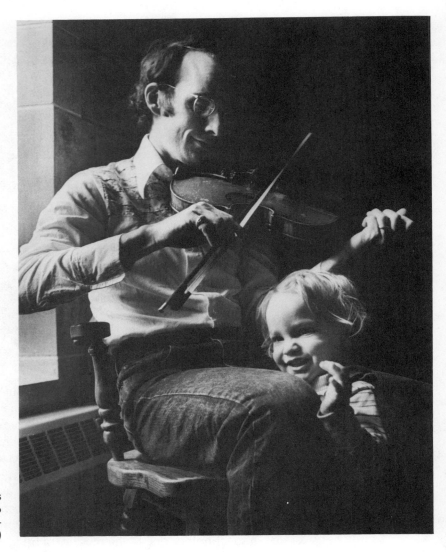

Figure 4-2. This child at his father's knee learns early to enjoy and value music. (Courtesy of the *Mt. Vernon News.*)

CULTURE IS LEARNED

Patterns of cultural behavior are acquired, not inherited. As Murdock explains, "cultural behavior is socially rather than biologically determined" [13, p. 258]. Each of us learns a cultural heritage through the process of socialization, sometimes called enculturation (Fig. 4-2). As a little girl grows up in a given society, she acquires certain attitudes, beliefs, and values. She learns how to behave in ways appropriate to

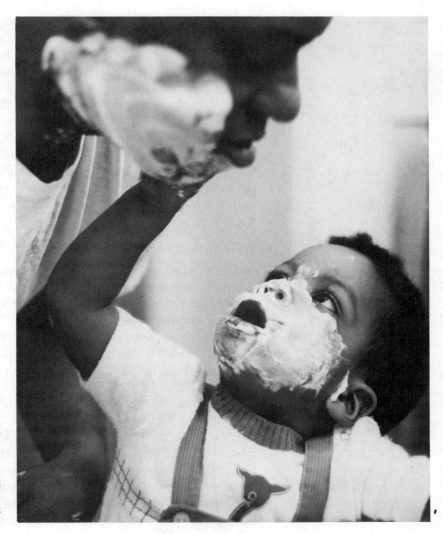

Figure 4-3. Children learn much of their culture and future roles through observation and imitation of adult behavior. The little boy imitating his father shaving is learning to identify with the male sex role. (Photograph by Burk Uzzle, Magnum.)

that society's definition of the female role. She is learning that culture (Fig. 4-3). Ruth Benedict summarizes this learning process [2, p. 2]:

The life-history of the individual is first and foremost an accommodation to the patterns and standards traditionally handed down in his community. From the moment of his birth the customs into which he is born shape his experience and behavior. By the time he can talk, he is the little creature of his culture, and by the time he is grown and able to take part in its activities, its habits are his habits, its beliefs his beliefs, its impossibilities his impossibilities.

Although culture is learned, the process and results of that learning are different for each person. Each individual has a unique personality and experiences life in a singular way; both these factors influence acquisition of culture. Families, social classes, and other groups within a society differ from one another, and this social variation has important implications for planned change. Since culture is learned, it is possible for parts of it to be relearned; people might change some cultural elements or adopt some new behaviors or values. In addition, Foster points out, "there will be differences in the ease and ability with which [people] continue to learn and in their flexibility in casting off old forms of behavior that conflict with new forms" [4, p. 18]. Some individuals and groups will be more willing to try new things than others and thus potentially influence change.

CULTURE IS INTEGRATED

Rather than an assortment of various customs and traits, a culture is a functional, integrated whole. As in any system, all the parts of a culture are interrelated and interdependent. Ruth Benedict, who first examined the systemic nature of culture, says, "A culture, like an individual, is a more or less consistent pattern of thought and action" [2, p. 46]. The various components of a culture, such as its social mores or religious beliefs, perform separate functions which depend upon and articulate in relative harmony with each other to form an operating whole. Benedict emphasizes that this cultural whole is greater than the sum of its individual parts [2, p. 47]. In other words, to understand culture, one cannot simply describe single traits. Each part must be viewed in terms of its relationships to the other parts and to the whole.

Our own culture is an integrated web of ideas and practices. For example, we promote three balanced meals a day, a practice tied to our belief that nutrition leads to good health and that prevention is better than cure. These cultural traits, in turn, are related to our values about health. Health, we say, is essential for, among other conditions, maximum energy output and productivity at work. Productivity is important since it enables us to compete effectively. These values are linked to religious beliefs about hard work and taboos against laziness. Nutrition, health, economics, religion, and family are the fibers of a web whose design and usefulness depends on their integration.

Another person's culturally determined behavior can be understood, therefore, by considering it in the context of that person's larger culture. For example, when a couple who are Jehovah's Witnesses refuse blood transfusions for their child, their action is neither irrational nor ignorant. Rather, it represents behavior consistent with the couple's cultural values and beliefs, and, in regard to their child's health, results from deeply held religious convictions. The single behavior of refusing blood transfusions, when viewed in context, is part of a larger religious belief system and a basic component of their culture.

The recognition that culture is integrated, that introducing a change in one part of a cultural system will affect other parts, influences community health nursing practice. Mrs. Juarez's cultural beliefs about modesty and self-effacement were related to her culture's definition of the woman's role which, in turn, influenced her interpersonal relationships. To change one practice was to affect many others. Likewise, the request from a nurse to submit to a physical exam with a male physician was equal to saying, "stop behaving like a woman!" Asking certain Native American groups to accommodate to our rigid appointment scheduling means requiring them to reframe their concept of time. It also violates their values of patience and pride. Before we attempt a change in a person's or group's behavior, we need to ask how that change will affect them through its influence on other parts of their culture. Extra time and patience or different strategies may be needed if change is still indicated. We may even find that our system can be modified to preserve the client's cultural values.

CULTURE IS SHARED

Culture is the product of aggregate behavior, not individual habit. Certainly, individuals practice a culture, but customs are phenomena shared by all members of the group (Fig. 4-4). Because it is collectively shared, culture has been called "superindividual." Murdock explains [13, p. 258]:

Culture does not depend on individuals. An ordinary habit dies with its possessor, but a group habit lives on in the survivors, and is transmitted from generation to generation. Moreover, the individual is not a free agent with respect to culture. He is born and reared in a certain cultural environment, which impinges upon him at every moment of his life. From earliest childhood his behavior is conditioned by the habits of those about him. He has no choice but to conform to the folkways current in his group.

Knowing that culture is shared helps us to understand human behavior. For example, a community health nurse tried unsuccessfully to convince an American mother to stop heavily oiling her infant's skin [17]. She discovered that the mother was acting in a tradition of her subculture which held that oil promoted good health. The fact that all

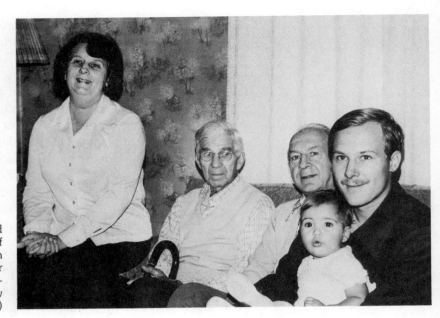

Figure 4-4. Culture is shared collectively by all members of the group. In this five generation family many aspects of their culture are transmitted to maintain cultural continuity. (Courtesy of the *Mt. Vernon News.*)

the other mothers in that religious group also used oil on their babies proved a powerful deterrent to the change requested by the nurse. Individual health behavior is always influenced by other people of the same culture. Thus, it becomes very difficult for one person to ignore some cultural practice when it will continue to be reinforced by other group members. In fact, group acceptance and a sense of membership almost always depend on conforming to shared cultural practices.

EFFECT ON COMMUNITY HEALTH NURSING

Community health nursing practice with groups and communities takes on added significance when it recognizes that culture is shared. Attempting to provide health care to one individual at a time limits community health nurses' effectiveness. Once a nurse leaves, the client must face all the informal cultural pressures that come from friends and family. On the other hand focus on an entire group can positively change that group's health behavior and thus affect individual practices. The pattern of oiling young infants, for instance, ceased when the nurse worked with the entire church group. She began with a well-recognized cultural strategy, that is, work through formal or informal leaders. She contacted the minister and discussed the cultural practice. He admitted that anointing with oil, a Biblical teaching, was one of their beliefs. When she explained her concerns, he agreed that a drop of oil on the head was all that was needed. He clarified this teaching in his next sermon and, as a result, additional health problems also cleared up when other members of the group stopped rubbing oil into wounds and infections [17].

In another example, a community health nursing instructor with several groups of nursing students successfully developed a series of health classes for a group of Indian women who lived on the northwest coast of Washington State [1]. As the group accepted teaching on subjects such as child care, treatment of burns, and prevention of colds, individual behavior was affected. A group focus also gives the nurse a broader picture of the culture being served and a better understanding of its health needs. Respect and trust of the entire group can be won, thus increasing the chance to improve health practices.

SHARED VALUES

One of the most important elements shared by a culture is its values. Each culture classifies phenomena "into good and bad, desirable and undesirable, right and wrong" [4]. When people respond in favor of or against some practice, they are reflecting their culture's values about that practice. One man may eagerly anticipate eating a steak for dinner. Another, who believes that eating meat is sacrilegious, will experience revulsion at the idea. Some American subcultures think that loud, vocal expressions are a necessary way to deal with pain. Others value silence and stoicism. Either way, values serve a purpose. Shared values give a culture stability and security; they provide a standard for behavior. Members therefore know what to think and how to act. Values are more deeply rooted than behaviors and consequently change more slowly.

CULTURE IS TACIT

Culture provides a guide for human interaction which is mostly unexpressed, or tacit. Members of a cultural group, without the need for discussion, know how to act and what to expect from one another. Culture provides an implicit set of cues for behavior, not a written set of rules. It "may be thought of as a memory bank where knowledge is stored, available immediately and usually without conscious effort, to guide us in the situations in which we routinely find ourselves" [4, p. 18]. Culture teaches us the proper tone of voice to use for each occasion. It tells us how close to stand when talking with someone (Fig. 4-5). We learn to make the responses appropriate to our sex, role, and status. We know what is right and wrong. All of these attitudes and

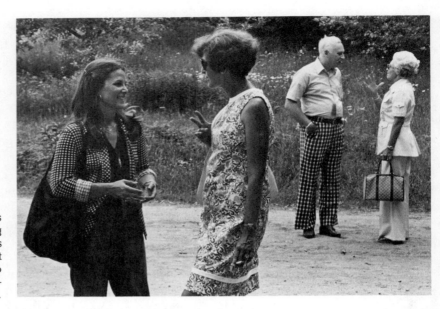

Figure 4-5. Culture influences everyday behavior by giving people a prescribed set of norms for their conduct. It has taught these women how far apart to stand during a casual conversation.

behaviors are so ingrained, so tacit, that we seldom, if ever, need to discuss them. We know. The same is true for each culture.

The difficulty comes when we cross cultural boundaries. No longer does our culture provide a guide map for behavior. The cues given by a person in another culture may mean something entirely different. Silence in a group meeting with Native American women was uncomfortable for some nurses but enjoyed by the Indian women, who valued patience and listening [4]. Offering food to a guest, in many cultures, is not merely a social gesture but an important symbol of hospitality and acceptance. To refuse, for any reason, is insulting and rejecting. Thus our behavior, albeit completely well-intentioned and appropriate for our own culture, can cause misunderstanding and damage to relationships in another.

Because culture is tacit, it is difficult to realize the number and types of behaviors of ours that may be offensive to people from other groups. It is also difficult to know the meaning and significance of their practices. Consequently, community health nurses have a two-fold task in developing cultural awareness; not only is it necessary to understand the clients' culture but also nurses' culture. Effective practitioners maintain awareness of the "taken-for-granted" aspects of their own culture. Cross-cultural conflict can be resolved through conscious efforts at developing awareness, patience, and acceptance of cultural differences.

CULTURE IS DYNAMIC

Every culture experiences constant change; none is entirely static. Within every cultural group are individuals who generate innovations. More importantly, there are members who see advantages in other people's ways and are willing to adopt new practices. Each culture, then, becomes an amalgamation of ideas, values, and practices from a variety of sources. This process depends, of course, on the extent of exposure to other groups. Nonetheless, every culture is in a dynamic state of adding or deleting components. Functional aspects are retained; less functional ones are eliminated. When we tend toward ethnocentrism, saying "our way is best," we should remind ourselves that our culture is largely a collection of borrowed traits. We owe much of our beliefs, actions, and possessions to other cultures.

The dynamic nature of culture is useful to community health nursing for several reasons. Cultures and subcultures do indeed change over time. Patience and persistence are probably key attributes to cultivate when working toward improvement of health behaviors. Another point to remember is that cultures change as their members see greater advantages in the "new ways." Convincing them of these advantages will have to be done in a language they understand and in the context of their own cultural value system. This is an important reason for nurses to develop an understanding of their clients' culture [10]. Furthermore, change within a culture is usually brought about by certain key individuals who are receptive to new ideas and able to influence their peers. Tapping this resource becomes imperative for successful change. Finally, the health culture can change too. Consider its changes in the past. We can learn a great deal from our clients and their cultures. And as we discover more effective ways of working with clients, we can and should modify our own practices.

CULTURE AND NURSING PRACTICE

Our examination of the meaning and nature of culture has shown the need to recognize cultural differences and understand our clients in the context of their cultural backgrounds. Practically speaking, however, how can the concept of culture be applied to everyday community health nursing practice? The following case studies give some insights.

CULTURE OF THE POOR

This first case study represents a community of people whose way of life is often not considered as a separate subculture (Fig. 4-6).

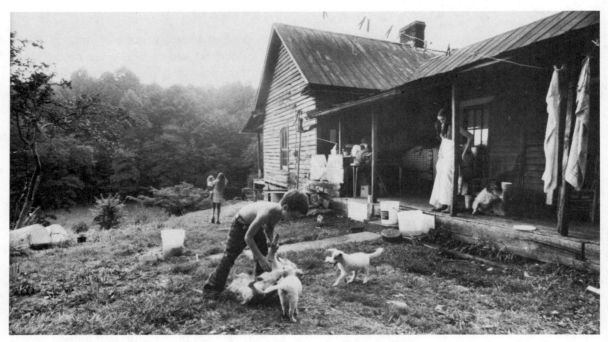

Figure 4-6. The poor have values, attitudes, and practices which give them a separate culture of their own. This Tennessee family enjoys the stability and security that its culture provides. (Photograph by Michael O'Brien. © 1976 Time, Inc.)

The Jacksons came to the attention of the city health center through a welfare referral. Albert, 42 years of age, had left each of his last three jobs after only a few days of employment. The case worker made a home visit and found Vera Jackson, a shy, thin, 38-year-old woman, with three of her children. The other three were in school. The small, two-bedroom apartment, part of a multiracial, low-income housing project, was "shabby, dirty, and cluttered," according to the referral. Albert seldom came home. Vera held the family together, supplementing the welfare checks through occasional day housework and a night cleaning job in an office building. She didn't know where Albert was, maybe somewhere drunk again. They had been in the city for eight months. Before that, Albert had done itinerant farm labor. Neither had finished high school. "We ain't stayed long anywheres, I guess," Vera told the case worker. Two of the children had bad colds, one of which was complicated by a deep, chesty cough. This boy felt feverish and the caseworker, concerned, arranged for Vera to take him to the health center.

The center's waiting room was crowded and noisy; staff hustled impatiently through the hallways. Vera's neighbor at the housing project had warned her, "That place don't like us poor folks." She and the children waited anxiously, then started to their feet when the loudspeaker blared out "Jackson." The nurse was friendly but brisk. "Mrs. Jackson," she inquired, "how are you?" There was no time for Vera to reply as the nurse launched into an explanation of the care and prevention of colds while checking the boy and taking his temperature. The physician, too, had many instructions. "These children should be on vitamins all the time," he commented. "Are they eating well-balanced meals?" Vera was confused. "Do you have any questions?" the nurse asked, handing her the antibiotics and some pamphlets on child growth and development. Vera shook her head. She felt too stupid to say anything, too embarrassed to admit she did not understand. A well-balanced meal, she thought, must mean not overfeeding the kids. That was no problem, considering the little they had to eat. She saw no point in vitamins. Why did they need to take something when they were well? She could not afford them anyway. She guessed that giving her son the medication at supper, their one "meal" a day, was what the doctor meant when he directed that the boy take it with each meal. Several days later the Jackson boy was hospitalized with pneumonia. Although he recovered, the Jacksons never returned to the health center.

CULTURAL DIFFERENCES

The culture of the poor is an enigma to most health professionals. It is seldom considered a separate subculture; consequently, the poor are assumed to have the same values and attitudes as middle-class professionals. On the contrary, the poor in our country are distinctive. Compared to health professionals, the poor think and respond in terms of sharply contrasting values, customs, and lifestyles. Most important, their ideas about health and illness differ from those of health professionals, and yet our system of health care tends to ignore this fact.

The poor differ from middle-class professionals in a variety of ways. For example, many poor people "live strictly and wholeheartedly in the present" [16]. Much of the health practitioner's emphasis, on the other hand, is preventive, thus future-oriented. Taking vitamins, eating right, and preventing colds all involve a future-orientation, an unimportant value in Mrs. Jackson's realm of understanding. A present-orientation influences the poor to seek immediate gratification rather than long-term gains.

Another difference is that the lives of the poor "are uncertain, dominated by recurring crises" [16]. The pressures and troubles of daily life are all they can cope with. Bad health is a part of that life, and they have learned to live with it. It was easier for Mrs. Jackson to live with family illness than to use up her few resources in trying to prevent or cure it. A sense of hopelessness and unworthiness prevents the poor from valuing their bodies, from taking care of themselves, from asserting their rights, and from asking questions. As Robertson states [15, p. 43]:

The poor are often characterized by low self-esteem. The culture of poverty is characterized by its members' lack of orientation to education, long-term experience of powerlessness, lack of self-esteem, sense of hopelessness regarding improvement of their socioeconomic status, and willingness to accept immediate gain rather than postpone satisfaction.

The depersonalized atmosphere of the health center only reinforced these feelings for Mrs. Jackson.

Mrs. Jackson's cultural differences needed recognition and acceptance. Her self-esteem needed to be increased, and her fear and suspicion of authority figures decreased. She required a relationship of trust with a caring person who understood her culture. Then, with patient assistance, she would have been able to change her values about health and assume greater responsibility for her own and her family's health.

CULTURE OF INTERNATIONAL CLIENTS

This case study involves clients transplanted from one culture to an entirely different culture; it presents an interesting challenge to the community health nurse (Fig. 4-7).

Armed with enthusiasm and pamphlets on prenatal diet and pregnancy, the community health nurse began home visits to the Kim family. Her initial plan was to discuss pregnancy and fetal development, teach diet, and prepare the mother for delivery. Mr. Kim, a graduate student, was present to interpret since Mrs. Kim spoke very little English. Their 2 boys, 3 years and 1½ years of age, played happily on the kitchen floor. The family offered tea to the nurse and listened politely as she explained her reasons for coming and added, "How can I be most helpful to you? What would you like from my visits?"

The Kims were grateful for this approach. Hesitant at first, they hinted at Mrs. Kim's fears of American doctors and hospitals; her first two children had been born in Korea. None of the family had any experience with Western medicine. They shared some concerns about adjustment to living in the United States. It was difficult to shop in American food stores with their overwhelming variety of foods, many

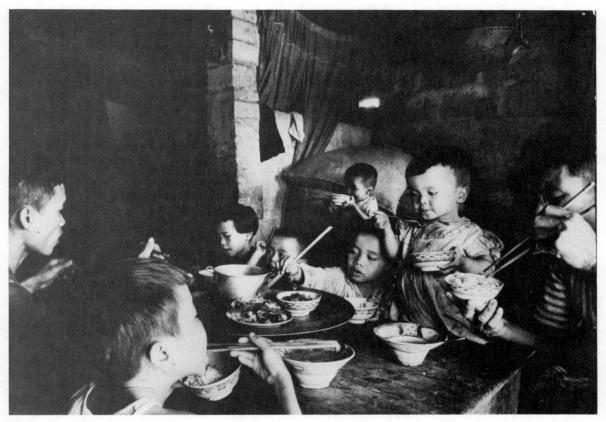

Figure 4-7. Clients transplanted from completely different cultures will continue to adhere to their own beliefs and practices. This Vietnamese family enjoys eating a traditional meal with chopsticks, one of many customs they will maintain until selected aspects of the new culture are gradually absorbed. (Photograph by John Dominis for *Life* © 1961, Time, Inc.)

of which the Kims found unfamiliar. Mrs. Kim, who had come from a family whose servants prepared the food, was an inexperienced cook. Servants had also cared for the children, and her role had been that of a "fine lady" in hand-tailored silk gowns.

Listening carefully, the nurse began to realize the striking differences between her own and her clients' cultures. Her care plans changed. In subsequent visits she determined to learn about Korean culture and base her nursing intervention on that knowledge. She learned about their traditional ways of raising children, male and female roles, and practices related to pregnancy and lactation. She respected their value of "saving face," and attempted never to offend their pride or dignity. As time went on, her interest and respect for their way of life won their trust. She inquired about their cultural practices before attempting any intervention. As a result, the Kims were receptive to her suggestions. Appropriate changes were made in Mrs. Kim's diet, for example, that were still compatible with her food preferences and cultural eating patterns. Because she was not accustomed to drinking milk, she increased her calcium intake by learning to prepare custards (which disguised the milk flavor) and to eat more green, leafy vegetables.

After five months, a strong, positive relationship had been established between this family and the nurse. Mrs. Kim delivered a healthy baby girl and looked forward to continued supportive visits from the community health nurse.

Although she had not initially considered the possibility of cultural barriers, the nurse soon recognized that subtle but important differences existed and thus changed her objectives. She proceeded to gain understanding and respect of this family's culture as a means toward improving their health. Whenever possible, she adapted her teaching and suggestions to comply with the Kims' culture. Implicitly, her message was, "Your culture is valuable and necessary for you. The parts of that culture that can continue to be useful, I will help preserve. The parts that are not functional for you in this new society, I will help you change, over time."

CULTURE OF A NATIVE AMERICAN GROUP

A third case study portrays another distinct culture. Its members live in the United States, assume many American values and practices, yet preserve large aspects of their own culture (Fig. 4-8).

As she drove up the dirt road and parked her car next to the community hall, Sandra felt apprehensive. She had been warned by the previous community health nurse that these Indian people were hard to work with. "They're all lazy and unappreciative. You can't get anywhere with them." It was only through the urging of an Indian community aide, Mrs. Brown, that a group of the women had reluctantly agreed to meet with the new nurse. They would see what she had to say.

Sandra's steps echoed hollowly as she walked across the wooden floor of the large room to the far corner where a group of women sat silently in a circle. Only their eyes turned; their faces remained impassive. Mrs. Brown rose slowly, greeted the nurse, and introduced her to the group. Swallowing her fear, Sandra smiled. She told them of her background and explained that she had not worked with Indian people before. There was a long silence. No one spoke. Sandra continued, "I'd like to help you if I can, maybe with problems about care of your children when they are sick or questions about how to keep them healthy, but I don't know what you need or want." Silence fell

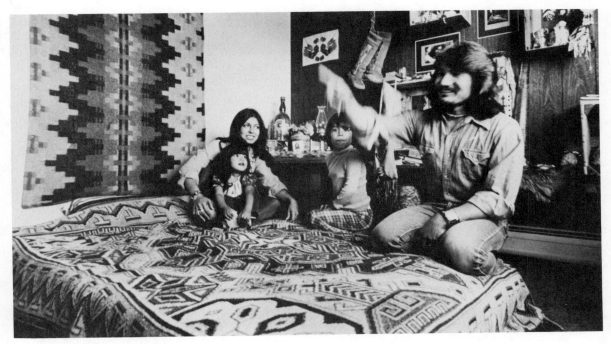

Figure 4-8. Many Americans, such as these Native Americans, come from culturally diverse backgrounds and retain large segments of their original culture. (Photograph by Henry Peck. © 1974 Time, Inc.)

again. She would like to learn from them, she repeated. Would they help her? Again, an uncomfortable silence ensued.

Then one woman began to speak. Quietly, but with deep feeling, she described several bad experiences with the previous nurse and the county social worker. Then others spoke up: "They *tell* us what we should do. They don't listen. They say our way is not good." Seeing Sandra's interest and concern, the women continued. One of their main concerns was their children's health. Another was the high incidence of accidents and injuries on the reservation. They wanted to learn how to give first-aid. Other concerns were expressed. The group agreed that Sandra could help them by teaching a first-aid class.

In the weeks that followed, Sandra taught several classes on first-aid and emergency care; she then began a series of sessions on child health. Each time she would ask the women to choose a topic for discussion and elicit from them their accustomed ways of dealing with each topic, for example, how they handled toilet training or taught their children to eat solid foods. Her goal was to learn as much as she could about their culture and incorporate that information into her teaching, which preserved as many of their practices as possible. Sandra also visited informally with the women in their homes and at community gatherings. She learned about their way of life, their history, and their values. For example, patience was highly valued. It was important to be able to wait patiently, even if a scheduled meeting was delayed as much as two hours. It was also important to wait for others to speak, which explained the Indian women's comfort with silences during a conversation. Other values influenced their way of life. Courage, pride, generosity, and honesty were all important determinants of behavior. These were also values by which they judged Sandra and other professionals. Sandra's honesty in keeping her promises enabled the women to trust her. Her generosity in giving her time, helping them occasionally with some household task, and arranging for child care during the classes, won their respect.

The women came to accept her, and Sandra was invited to eat with them and share in tribal get-togethers. The women criticized and advised her on acceptable ways to speak and act. Her openness and patience to learn and her respect for them as a people had paved the way to improving their health. At first, Sandra felt that her progress was very slow, but this slowness was actually an advantage. She had built a solid foundation of cross-cultural trust and, in the months that followed, she saw many changes in their health practices.

PRINCIPLES FOR PRACTICE

In the context of these cases and our earlier discussion of culture, several principles for nursing practice can be identified.

RECOGNIZE AND ACCEPT CULTURAL DIFFERENCES

Our beliefs and ways of doing things frequently contrast with those of our clients. A first step toward bridging cultural barriers is recognition of those differences. Mrs. Jackson's values and health practices sharply contrasted with those of the center's staff. Failure to recognize these differences led to breakdown in communication and ineffective care. Once differences in culture are recognized, it is important to accept them. A nurse's ways are valid for the nurse; clients' ways work for them. The nurse visiting the Kims avoided the dangerous trap of assuming that her way was best and consequently developed a fruitful relationship with her clients.

UNDERSTAND CULTURAL BASIS FOR CLIENT BEHAVIOR

Each of our client's actions, like our own, is based on underlying culturally learned beliefs and ideas. Mrs. Kim did not like milk because her culture had taught her that it was distasteful. The Indian women's response to waiting or keeping someone else waiting was influenced by their value of patience. Instead of making assumptions or judging client behavior, first discover the attitude behind that behavior [1]. Some culturally based reason is probably causing that client to engage in (or avoid) certain actions.

LISTEN AND LEARN BEFORE ADVISING

We do not change people's behavior by just giving suggestions or instructions. For Mrs. Jackson as well as the Native American women, this approach had, in fact, the opposite effect. Health teaching must be geared to the client's level of understanding and frame of reference. We accomplish this by finding out about the client first. Asking questions, listening, and observing help us to understand the client and his culture. Consequently, nursing intervention can be tailored to the client's needs.

EMPATHIZE WITH CULTURALLY DIFFERENT CLIENTS

In addition to learning their culture or subculture, we need to understand clients' points of view. We need to stand in their shoes, to identify with them. The ability to show interest, concern, and compassion enabled Sandra to win the affection and respect of the Native American women. It told the Kims that their nurse cared about them. These nurses participated in the feelings and ideas of their clients. Empathizing with clients gives them needed reassurance and often provides the motivation to adopt new health behaviors [15].

SHOW RESPECT FOR CLIENTS AND THEIR CULTURE

Respect is shown in many ways. When Sandra involved the Native American women in decisions and gave them choices, she was showing respect. When the nurse gave positive recognition to the importance of the Kims' culture, she was showing respect. Within the United States, people of different cultures and subcultures particularly need respect. Their ways are in contrast to the dominant culture. It is difficult for them to retain pride in their lifestyles, or in themselves, when constantly reminded that their ways are inferior. The message may be only implied or even unintentional. Such was the case for Mrs. Jackson. The health center's routine and manner of the staff were certainly not meant to intentionally show disrespect. They did, nevertheless, and Mrs. Jackson felt insignificant, inferior, and inadequate. Everyone needs respect to enhance pride, dignity, and self-esteem; it is an important contributor to good mental health.

BE PATIENT

It takes time to build trust and effect culture change. It can be difficult to establish the nurse-client relationship when it involves two different cultures. Trust must be won, and that may take weeks, months, or even years. Patience is essential. Time must be allowed for both the nurse and the client to learn how to communicate with one another, to test each other's trustworthiness, and to learn about each other. Change in behavior (learned aspects of the culture) occurs gradually. Some aspects of both the nurse's and the client's cultures can, and probably will, change. The Kims' nurse, for example, modified some of her usual practices and adapted them to the Kims' culture and needs. They, in turn, began to assume some American practices and values. However, the process took several months. Time and patience help to break down cultural barriers.

ANALYZE YOUR BEHAVIOR

Self-awareness is crucial for the nurse working with people from other cultures [10]. Remember your values are different than theirs. Are you aware of your own values, habits, and typical responses? How do you appear to your clients? The nurse who assisted Mrs. Jackson probably thought that she was being friendly, efficient, and helpful. In terms of her own culture, this nurse's behavior was intended to reassure clients and meet their needs. Unaware of the negative consequences of her behavior, she caused damage rather than met needs.

To gain skill in analyzing your behavior, two points are helpful to keep in mind. First, knowledge of the clients' culture helps you to know how they will interpret various behaviors. It tells you what responses are most appropriate to make. Second, establishing a relationship of trust with clients of different cultures opens doors of communication. As in Sandra's experience, trust creates a willingness to share reactions and constructively criticize behavior.

SUMMARY

In community health, each client, whether a family, group, or community, has its own culture. A culture is a design for living, and every culture is different. The unique culture of each group is essential for the functioning of that group. It serves as a guide for behavior, a map telling the people of that group how to live. Culture provides a set of values, which are the threads holding together the fabric of a society. It offers stability and security.

Several characteristics of culture are significant for community health nursing practice. It is *learned,* not acquired. Thus some elements can be relearned, and some practices changed. It is *integrated.* All of the many traits comprising a culture work together as a functioning whole. Specific cultural practices must be considered in the context of the client's larger culture. Changing one set of traits will affect other aspects of the culture. It is *shared.* Culture is a group phenomenon; it controls all the members' values and behavior. Attempts to change individual behavior may be ineffective; a group approach might be more productive. It is *tacit.* Culture tells people how to behave without the need for conscious thought. A collision between two different cultures can create considerable conflict and misunderstanding. Conscious effort is required to understand and accept cultural differences. It is *dynamic.* Every culture preserves its integrity by deleting nonfunctional practices and acquiring new components that will better serve the group. Consequently, it is possible to introduce improved health practices that are presented in a manner consistent with the clients' cultural values.

Some principles, drawn from an understanding of the concept of culture, can guide community health nursing practice:

1. Recognize and accept the differences between your clients' culture and your own.
2. Understand the cultural basis for your clients' behavior.
3. Listen and learn before giving advice.
4. Empathize with clients of different cultural backgrounds.
5. Show respect for clients and their culture.
6. Be patient: it takes time to build trust and effect cultural change.
7. Analyze your behavior in the context of the clients' culture.

REFERENCES

1. Aichlmayr, R. H. Cultural understanding: A key to acceptance. *Nurs. Outlook* 17:23, 1969.
2. Benedict, R. *Patterns of Culture.* Boston: Houghton Mifflin, 1934. Pp. 2, 46, 47.
3. Branch, M. Models for introducing cultural diversity in nursing curricula. *J. Nurs. Educ.* 15:7, 1976.
4. Foster, G. M. *Traditional Cultures and the Impact of Technological Change.* New York: Harper & Row, 1962. P. 18.
5. Hall, E. T. *The Silent Language.* Garden City, N.Y.: Doubleday, 1959. P. 38.
6. Herrera, T., and Wagner, N. Behavioral Approaches to Delivering Health Services in a Chicano Community. In A. Reinhardt and M. Quinn (Eds.), *Current Practice in Family-Centered Community Nursing.* St. Louis: Mosby, 1977.

7. Kark, S. L. *Epidemiology and Community Medicine.* New York: Appleton-Century-Crofts, 1974. P. 149.
8. Landy, D. *Culture, Disease and Healing: Studies in Medical Anthropology.* New York: Macmillan, 1977. P. 233.
9. Leininger, M. *Anthropology and Nursing: Two Worlds to Blend.* New York: Wiley, 1970. P. 19.
10. Leininger, M. Transcultural Nursing: A Promising Subfield of Study for Nurses. In A. Reinhardt and M. Quinn (Eds.), *Current Practice in Family-Centered Community Nursing.* St. Louis: Mosby, 1977.
11. MacGregor, F. C. *Social Science in Nursing.* New York: Wiley, 1960. P. 66.
12. Mead, M. Cultural Contexts of Nursing Problems. In F. C. MacGregor, *Social Science in Nursing.* New York: Wiley, 1960. P. 74.
13. Murdock, G. The Science of Culture. In M. Freilich (Ed.), *The Meaning of Culture: A Reader in Cultural Anthropology.* Lexington, Mass.: Xerox College Pub., 1972. P. 258.
14. Murillo, N. The Mexican-American Family. In N. Wagner and M. Haug (Eds.), *Chicanos: Social and Psychological Perspectives.* St. Louis: Mosby, 1971.
15. Robertson, H. R. Removing barriers to health care. *Nurs. Outlook* 17:43, 1969.
16. Strauss, A. L. Medical Ghettos. *Trans-Action* 4:10, 1967.
17. Taylor, C. The Nurse and Cultural Barriers. In D. Hymovich and M. Barnard (Eds.), *Family Health Care.* New York: McGraw-Hill, 1973.

SELECTED READINGS

Aichlmayr, R. H. Cultural understanding: A key to acceptance. *Nurs. Outlook* 17:23, 1969.

Asian Americans: The neglected minority. *Personnel Guidance J.* 51:385, 1973.

Bello, T. A. The third dimension: Cultural sensitivity in nursing practice. *Imprint* 23:36, 1976.

Benedict, R. *Patterns of Culture.* Boston: Houghton Mifflin, 1934.

Blackwell, J. E. *The Black Community: Diversity and Unity.* New York: Dodd, Mead, 1975.

Branch, M. Models for introducing cultural diversity in nursing curricula. *J. Nurs. Educ.* 15:7, 1976.

Brinton, D. Value differences between nurses and low income families. *Nurs. Res.* 1:15, 1972.

Bullough, B., and Bullough, V. *Poverty, Ethnic Identification and Health Care.* New York: Appleton-Century-Crofts, 1972.

Davitz, L. J., Sameshima, Y., and Davitz, J. Suffering as viewed in six different cultures. *Am. J. Nurs.* 76:1296, 1976.

DeGracia, R.   Cultural influences on Filipino patients. *Am. J. Nurs.* 79:1412, 1979.

Dubos, R.   The dangers of tolerance. *J. Sch. Health* 44:182, 1974.

Fire, M., and Baker, C.   A smile and eye contact may insult someone. *J. Nurs. Educ.* 15:14, 1976.

Foster, G. M., and Anderson, B. G.   *Medical Anthropology.* New York: Wiley, 1978.

Freeman, H. E., Levine, S., and Reeder, L. G.   *Handbook of Medical Sociology* (2nd ed.). Englewood Cliffs, N.J.: Prentice-Hall, 1972.

Hall, E. T.   *The Silent Language.* Garden City, N.Y.: Doubleday, 1959.

Kane, R. L., Kasteler, J., and Gray, R. (Eds.).   *The Health Gap: Medical Services and the Poor.* New York: Springer, 1976.

Kerr, L.   The poverty of affluence. *Am. J. Public Health* 65:17, 1975.

Kneip-Hardy, M., and Burkhardt, M.   Nursing the Navajo. *Am. J. Nurs.* 77:95, 1977.

Koshi, P. T.   Symposium on cultural and biological diversity and health care. *Nurs. Clin. North Am.* 12:1, 1977.

Leininger, M.   *Anthropology and Nursing: Two Worlds to Blend.* New York: Wiley, 1970.

Leininger, M.   The Culture Concept and its Relevance to Nursing. In M. Auld and L. Birum (Eds.), *The Challenge of Nursing: A Book of Readings.* St. Louis: Mosby, 1973.

Leininger, M. (Ed.).   *Barriers and Facilitators to Quality Health Care.* Philadelphia: Davis, 1975.

Leininger, M.   *Transcultural Nursing.* Somerset, N.J.: Wiley, 1978.

Lewis, O.   The Culture of Poverty. In B. A. Kogan (Ed.), *Readings in Health Science.* New York: Harcourt, Brace, Jovanovich, 1971.

MacGregor, F. C.   *Social Science in Nursing.* New York: Wiley, 1960.

Mackie, J. B.   The father's influence on the intellectual level of black ghetto children. *Am. J. Public Health* 64:615, 1974.

Mead, M.   Cultural Contexts of Nursing Problems. In F. C. MacGregor, *Social Science in Nursing.* New York: Wiley, 1960.

Mei-Li, L.   Folk beliefs of the Chinese and implications for psychiatric nursing. *J. Psychiatr. Nurs.* 14:38, 1976.

Milio, N.   *9226 Kercheval Street: The storefront that did not burn.* Ann Arbor, Mich.: U. Mich. Press, 1970.

Milio, N.   Values, Social Class and Community Health Services. In A. Reinhardt and M. Quinn (Eds.), *Family-Centered Community Nursing: A Sociocultural Framework.* St. Louis: Mosby, 1973.

Mitchell, A. C.   Barriers to therapeutic communication with black clients. *Nurs. Outlook* 26:109, 1978.

Murillo, N.   The Mexican-American Family. In N. Wagner and M. Haug (Eds.), *Chicanos: Social and Psychological Perspectives.* St. Louis: Mosby, 1971.

Paul, B. D. *Health, Culture and Community*. New York: Russell Sage Foundation, 1955.

Primeaux, M. Caring for the American Indian patient. *Am. J. Nurs.* 77:91, 1977.

Robertson, H. R. Removing barriers to health care. *Nurs. Outlook* 17:43, 1969.

Spradley, J. P. Public Health Services and the Culture of Skid Row Bums. In *Proceedings: Seminar on Public Health Services and The Public Inebriate*. Rockville, Md.: National Institute on Alcohol Abuse and Alcoholism, 1975.

Strasser, J. A. Urban transient women. *Am. J. Nurs.* 78:2076, 1978.

Stanley, S., and Wagner, N. (Eds.). *Asian-Americans: Psychological Perspectives*. Ben Lomond, Calif.: Science and Behavior Books, 1973.

Taylor, C. The Nurse and Cultural Barriers. In D. Hymovich and M. Barnard (Eds.), *Family Health Care*. New York: McGraw-Hill, 1973.

Wagner, N., and Haug, M. (Eds.). *Chicanos, Social and Psychological Perspectives*. St. Louis: Mosby, 1971.

TWO

TOOLS FOR PRACTICE

FIVE

THE NURSING PROCESS IN COMMUNITY HEALTH

Nurses who work to promote community health, like all nurses, accomplish their goal through a systematic, purposeful set of interpersonal actions—the nursing process [8]. Process means forward progression in an orderly fashion toward some desired result. In community health it involves a series of actions that enable the nurse to work with the client toward achieving the client's optimal health.

COMPONENTS

The nursing process incorporates several components or steps. Nursing theorists attach different labels to these components but all agree on the basic sequence of actions. The four most obvious components are assessment, planning, implementation, and evaluation. All of these depend on a fifth component, interaction. Current literature and practice give increasing emphasis to this element of the nursing process [2, 3, 6]. Nurse-client interaction is often an implied or assumed element in the process; for community health nursing, particularly, it is an essential first step.

INTERACTION

Community health nursing practice involves helping clients to help themselves. Listening to an elderly couple, teaching a class of expectant mothers, lobbying in the legislature for the poor, or working with parents to set up a dental screening program for children all involve relationships. The nurse may establish an initial relationship, maintain an existing one, or redefine a previous one. Whatever its stage of development, a relationship involves reciprocal influence and exchange—in a word, interaction. This mutual give and take between nurse and clients, whether a family, a group of mothers on an Indian reservation, or school children, is the first step in the nursing process.

NEED FOR COMMUNICATION

Interaction requires communication. When a community health nurse initially contacts a family, for example, any information she may have in advance can give only partial clues to that family's needs and wants. Unless they begin by talking and listening, the later steps in the nursing process will go awry. By open, honest sharing, the nurse will begin to develop trust and establish lines of effective communication. For instance, she will explain who she is and why she is there. She will encourage the family members to talk about themselves. Nurse and family together will discuss their relationship and clarify the desired nature of that alliance. Does the family want help in identifying and working on its health needs? Would its members like this nurse to continue regular contacts? What will their respective roles be? Effective communication, as a part of interaction, is essential to develop understanding and facilitate a free exchange of information between nurse and clients.

Interaction is reciprocal. Nurses must avoid the temptation either to do all the talking or to merely listen while a father or mother monopolizes the conversation. There is a dynamic exchange between two systems: the community health nurse represents one system, and the client the other. Whether the client is a handicapped family, a parent group, or an entire community, this exchange involves a two-way sharing of information, ideas, feelings, concerns, and ultimately, self. There is mutuality and cooperation.

Consider the following example. A dozen junior high school boys, most of whom were on the football team, met for several weeks with the school nurse to discuss physical fitness, nutrition, and other health topics. After their agreed-upon goals had been accomplished, the nurse wondered whether further meetings were needed. She raised the question and offered several topics, such as taking drugs and preventing injuries, for possible future sessions. The boys were not interested in these suggestions but, after more discussion, said they did want help with talking to girls. Renewed interaction was necessary as a first step in reapplying the nursing process.

Interaction paves the way for a helping relationship. As nurse and client interact, each is learning about the other. There is a period of testing before trust can be fully established. For the school nurse, establishing interaction had been more difficult at the time of her initial contact with the boys. They had been reluctant to talk, felt embarrassed to discuss personal subjects with a woman, and yet had strong interests in body building and personal appearance, strong enough to attract them to these optional sessions. Interaction began with a friendly exchange on nonthreatening topics and gradually deepened as the boys seemed ready to discuss personal subjects. Now it was relatively simple to talk about a new "problem" (to start the nursing process over again) because a helping relationship had already been developed. The nurse had a track record. The boys trusted, respected, and liked her so they were happy to interact around a new need.

GROUP LEVEL

Since community health practice focuses largely on the health of population groups, interaction goes beyond the one-to-one approach of clinical nursing [12]. The challenge that faces the community health nurse is a one-to-group approach. A family, a group of concerned neighbors, or a group of handicapped persons, are all collections of people with different concerns and opinions. Each person in a group is influenced by the thinking and behavior of the other group members. Nursing interaction with group-as-client demands an understanding of group behavior and group level decision making, and requires interpersonal communication at the group level. Thus, the task of interacting becomes more complex with a group than with an individual, but it also can be challenging and rewarding. Once community health nurses address themselves to understanding aggregate behavior, they can capitalize on the potential of group influence in order to make a far-reaching impact on the health of the total community. During this phase of the nursing process, however, the challenge lies with learning to interact effectively at the aggregate level. Later chapters will deal more specifically with communicating and working with groups.

Not only the first step, interaction is an integral, ongoing part of the nursing process (see Fig. 5-1). It is central to the process because nurse-client interaction forms the core of the relationship and information exchange. The effectiveness of each successive step, assessment, planning, implementation, and evaluation, depend on nurse-client interaction.

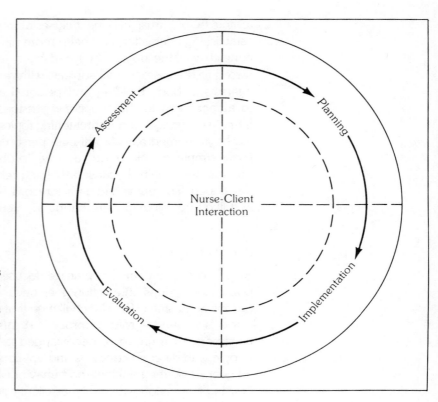

Figure 5-1. Nursing process components. Nurse-client interaction, a permeable structure, forms the core of the process. As nurse and client maintain a reciprocal exchange of information and trust through interaction, they can effectively assess client needs, and plan, implement, and evaluate care.

ASSESSMENT

After establishing ongoing interaction, the community health nurse is ready to determine client needs. Therefore, assessment is the next phase of the nursing process. According to Webster, assessment means judgment of the importance, size, or value of something; it is an act of appraisal. We judge client health status to discover existing or potential needs as a basis for planning future action.

Assessment involves three major activities: (1) collection of pertinent data, (2) interpretation of data, and (3) diagnosis. These actions overlap and are repeated constantly throughout the assessment. Thus, while diagnosing a family's need for counseling, you may simultaneously collect data on a persistent cough in a child and interpret previously collected data about nutritional deficiencies.

COLLECTION OF DATA

The nurse can collect a wide range of data in the process of assessing community clients. What information and how much to collect depend, in the first place, on the initial reason for nurse-client contact. A specific health problem, such as Down's syndrome in the family, obesity among a group of teenagers, or widespread pediculosis in a grade school, focuses the data collection on information related to the present problem and its resolution. If the initial reason for nurse-client contact is health promotion, as for a normal postpartum family, data collection can be broadened to include information such as family history, constellation, present health status, coping abilities, support systems, and parenting skills.

A second consideration in data collection involves actual versus potential needs. Assessment of multiproblem clients may force the community health nurse to focus only on existing (actual) needs because of limited time and resources. When possible, however, the community health nurse collects data aimed at uncovering potential needs in order to prevent problems from occurring (Fig. 5-2). Early and periodic screening of children or health screening for hypertension, glaucoma, and diabetes are examples of preventive assessment.

Community health nurses utilize many sources in data collection. We begin with clients since they are closest to their own situation and can frequently offer the most accurate insights and comprehensive information. Another source is people who know the client group well. In working with a family, the extended family members, friends, neighbors, and work associates may all be potential sources of information, pending client permission. Additional sources include health team members, client records, community agencies, books, and community health nurses themselves.

Data collection in community health requires the exercise of sound professional judgment, effective communication techniques, and special investigative skills. Observation is a basic technique; nurses constantly gather information this way. Seeing the home environment tells the nurse something about a family's socioeconomic level and ability to cope with present resources. Hearing interpersonal conflict among the members of a weight control group can give the nurse clues about possible client concerns and stress levels. Noticing the absence of a caring atmosphere in a nursing home may suggest a need for intervention. Observation, as a data-gathering technique, depends largely on nonverbal communication. The tone of a conversation may be friendly, hostile, or passive. A family may fail to keep appointments. A group's body language or a neighborhood's appearance convey a message. All offer information about clients.

A second technique for data collection is the interview. The interview

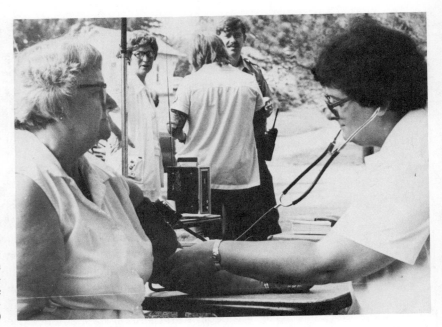

Figure 5-2. The nurse assesses individual, family, and community health through data collection. Here a free health screening program for hypertension gives the nurse important information on which to base future plans. (*Courtesy of the Mt. Vernon News.*)

involves a series of questions designed to elicit needed information. The community health nurse may conduct a formal interview during an early encounter to gather a health history and to encourage client expression. Informal directed questioning can sometimes provide even more data about client health status and needs. Communicating with clients serves as an important follow-up to observation. If you observe children with bruises that suggest possible abuse, a carefully planned informal interview may be useful. You may discover a mother who is isolated and under emotional stress. Then you can undertake co-operative nurse-client planning for dealing with the problem.

Listening is another important data collection technique. It is a skill which must be acquired through discipline and concentration. Too often we listen inattentively while we formulate our next question or allow our minds to wander. Good listening involves eye contact. It assures clients of our full interest and encourages greater expression of ideas and feelings. The community health nurse who is a good listener can gain a wealth of information about clients.

Other techniques for data collection include surveys, use of screening instruments, and use of records. Surveys, like interviews, provide specific information in response to selected questions. They can be especially useful for gathering data such as patterns of behavior among teenage alcoholics or battered women. Community health nurses also use surveys to assess neighborhood and community needs. Many kinds of standard screening instruments, including blood pressure apparatus, audiometers, scales, neurologic appraisal guides, and developmental tests, are useful for collecting data about clients.

INTERPRETATION OF DATA

This stage of assessment is analytic. Interpretation of data means analyzing the information gathered, drawing inferences or possible conclusions about the data's meaning, and validating those inferences to determine their accuracy. First the nurse separates the data into categories such as physical, mental, social, and environmental. In many instances, data base sheets used in community agencies provide a structure for gathering and analyzing data. Second, the nurse examines each category to determine its significant meaning. At this point the nurse may need to search for additional information to clarify the meaning of the present data. Next, inferences are made. The nurse has analyzed the data and come to a tentative conclusion about its meaning. But before making a diagnosis, the nurse must validate those assumptions. Are they accurate? Are they sound? The client should participate actively in data interpretation by clarifying feelings, explaining the circumstances surrounding the situation, and acting as a sounding board for testing assumptions. The nurse also uses other resources, such as other health team members to check out and confirm inferences. An example of data interpretation follows.

A community health nurse had been collecting data about a group of mothers who regularly attended a well-child clinic. Their responses to child health information and parenting classes had been considerably less than enthusiastic. Yet, when questioned, they expressed no dissatisfaction with the teaching program. After examining all the data, the nurse concluded that their social and supportive needs were far greater than their need for child care information. Merely gathering weekly at the clinic served an important function for them. She sat down with the mothers and discussed her findings. All agreed that they needed to get out of the house and be with people who had similar kinds of problems and interests.

In the situation just cited, data analysis led to drawing an inference, which was then validated. These are the important activities in interpretation of data. There is an ever-present danger in data interpretation, however, of making inaccurate assumptions and diagnoses. Many nursing care plans and activities have been based on a false idea of the

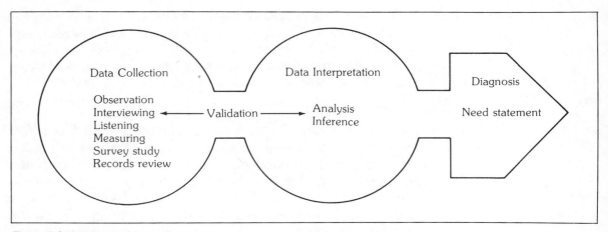

Figure 5-3. Assessment phase of the nursing process. Interpretation of data leads to diagnosis of client needs.

client's need, resulting in wasted and sometimes detrimental efforts. Thus, we cannot overemphasize the importance of validation. Data collection and data interpretation are sequential activities with validation serving as a bridge between them (see Fig. 5-3). When performed thoroughly, these steps lead to an accurate diagnosis.

NURSING DIAGNOSIS

The nursing diagnosis is the conclusion the nurse draws from interpretation of collected data. It is a statement of client need, sometimes called a problem statement. However, in community health, we do not limit our focus to problems; we consider the client as a total system and look for evidence of all kinds of needs that may influence client level of wellness. Needs cover the whole length of the health–illness continuum from a specific health problem, such as chemical dependency, all the way to opportunities for maximizing client health by filling needs such as improvement of parenting skills or development of better nutrition. Thus the statement of client need, the diagnosis, can focus on a wide range of topics.

Diagnoses differ in their scope. A broad diagnosis, such as the well-child clinic mothers need for emotional support, must be further broken down to become managable for planning care. The community health nurse in the above instance did further data collection and interpretation to develop a list of specific needs or diagnoses. Together, she and the mothers identified their feelings of inferiority as housewives, limited sexual satisfaction, and feelings of powerlessness about family decision making and spending of family money. A broad diagnosis is useful as a starting point. It can serve as a summary, as in the diagnosis of culture shock, nonsupportive parenting, or an unsafe school playground. Using the broad diagnosis as a base, the nurse can ask further questions, gather more data, and, with the client, develop a set of *specific diagnoses* to act on. Diagnoses that are already specific are ready for the planning step.

The nursing diagnosis changes over time because it reflects changes in client health status. Therefore, diagnoses need to be periodically reevaluated and redefined. The changing diagnosis can be a useful means of encouraging clients toward improved health because it gives them a clear standard against which to measure their progress.

PLANNING

The purpose of the planning phase is to determine how to meet client needs. Assessment discloses needs but does not prescribe the specific actions necessary to meet them. Knowing that the group of well-child mothers needed emotional support did not tell the nurse what to do about it. A diagnosis of culture shock for a family newly arrived from Cuba does not reveal what action to take. The nurse must plan.

Planning is a logical, decision-making process. It means designing an orderly, detailed program of action around specific goals. There is a systematic approach to planning which guides the community health nurse during this phase of the nursing process: (1) prioritize needs, (2) establish goals and objectives, and (3) write the care plan. As in the rest of the nursing process, the community health nurse collaborates with the client in each of these planning activities (Fig. 5-4).

SETTING PRIORITIES

Setting priorities means assigning rank order to client needs (diagnoses). One way to order needs is to group them into three categories—immediate, intermediate, and long-range—and then assign a priority to those in each group. Immediate needs are more urgent but not necessarily more important. For example, a meeting place was the most immediate need identified by a community health nurse and a group of senior citizens who wanted a class on exercise for the aging. Obviously their goal, to learn about appropriate exercises, was more important than finding a place to meet; however, the immediate need was requisite to accomplishing the long-range goal. Some needs are ranked as immediate because they are potentially hazardous or life-threatening, such as lack of eye protection in a school welding class. Other needs are ranked first because they are of greatest concern to the client. One family could not see how they would manage to lift and

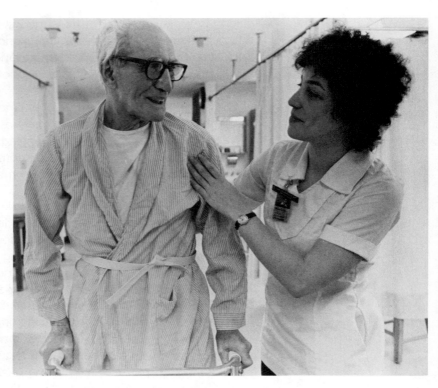

Figure 5-4. Clients should participate in planning for their home care even before hospital discharge. (Courtesy of Beth Israel Hospital, Boston. Photograph by Michael Lutch.)

move their grandfather, a new CVA. They selected his transportation as their highest priority. Other needs were identified but could not be addressed until this first concern had been alleviated.

ESTABLISHING GOALS AND OBJECTIVES

Goals and objectives are as crucial to planning as a target is to a missile-firing team. The nurse without planned objectives who visits a needy family cannot expect to accomplish anything. Needs must be translated into goals to give direction and meaning to the nursing care plan. Goals can first be stated broadly, to give an overview of the proposed end product and then divided into subgoals or objectives which describe specific desired outcomes and target dates. Objectives, as used here, are like stepping stones to help us reach the larger goal. For the family concerned about transporting their grandfather, their need, goal, and objectives were defined in the following manner.

Need
  Family does not know how to help grandfather move around the house after his discharge with a CVA from the nursing home.

Goal
Within a week after grandfather comes home, the family will be able to help him move about the house.
Objectives
1. On grandfather's first day home, the community health nurse will determine with the family its capabilities (including grandfather's) for helping him move about the house.
2. A physical therapist, making a joint home visit on the first day with the community health nurse, will recommend needed equipment and procedures to be used for helping grandfather move.
3. Recommended equipment will be installed by the end of the second day.
4. Each day, family members will practice lifting and moving procedures under the nurse's supervision.
5. By the end of the first week, family members will all be able to help grandfather move safely in and out of bed and to the bathroom, kitchen, and living room.

Development of objectives depends on a careful analysis of all the ways one could accomplish the larger goal. One needs to select the courses of action best suited to meeting the goals and then build objectives. For grandfather and family, other alternatives, such as keeping him in the nursing home longer, hiring an orderly to assist him at home, or confining him to bed with a strong exercise program, were considered and rejected. The grandfather's and family's choice was to rehabilitate him as soon as possible in his normal environment.

Some rules of thumb are helpful when writing objectives. Each objective should state a single idea. When more than one idea is expressed, as in an objective to obtain equipment and learn procedures, completion of the objective is much more difficult to measure. State each objective as an outcome. In other words, write the objective so that it describes one end result. For instance, objective 5 describes what the family will be able to do to help their grandfather move. This is a behavioral objective because it describes observable behaviors which can be measured. One can more readily evaluate objectives that include specifics like what will be done, who will do it, and when it will be accomplished. Then everyone knows exactly what has to be done and within what time frame. Writing *measurable* objectives makes a tremendous difference in the success of your planning.

Planning means thinking ahead. You look ahead toward the desired end product and then decide on all the intermediate actions necessary to meet that goal. Sometimes an objective itself describes the intermediate actions. At other times you may wish to break down an objective further into several activities. For example, with objective 4, the nurse first explained the procedures, then demonstrated how they were done, and then helped each family member try them. Their ability to practice was dependent on this sequence of activities. Good planning requires this kind of detail.

Decision making is an important part of planning. Decisions must be made while establishing priorities. Selecting goals and, from a variety of possible solutions, the best courses of action to meet the goals requires decisions. Further decision making is involved in selecting objectives and, when indicated, the specific actions to accomplish the objectives.

To facilitate planning and decision making, the community health nurse involves other people. Clients, of course, must be included at every step. They, after all, are the ones for whom the planning is being done and without whose insights and cooperation the plan may not succeed. At times other nurses are important to involve. Team meetings, nurse-supervisor conferences, or nurse-expert consultant sessions are all useful resources for planning. In addition, the community health nurse will frequently wish to confer with members of other health disciplines. Interdisciplinary team conferences are valuable for gaining a broader perspective and enlisting wider support for the evolving plan.

RECORDING THE PLAN

Recording the plan comes next. Until now, the planning phase has been a series of intellectual exercises done jointly with the client and perhaps with other health team members. You have probably written notes on the decisions made about priorities, goals, objectives, and actions. Now you can spell these out clearly in a format that meets the needs of your particular practice setting (see Fig. 5-5 for an example). Regardless of the type of care plan form(s) you use, certain items should be addressed:

1. *Data base* is all the subjective and objective information—physical, psychological, social, and environmental—collected about clients. It includes background health information (past and present); individual, family, group, and community assessment; and health history or system's review. The data base is usually kept on separate forms that allow space for ongoing entries and analysis.
2. *Needs* are the specific areas related to the client's health that have been identified for intervention. Preferably, they are areas that both client and nurse agree require action. In some settings, they are called problems, problem list, or nursing diagnoses. Goals are statements that describe the

NURSING CARE PLAN

Client _____ Jones Family _____

Date	No.	Need/Goal	Expected Outcomes	Planned Actions	Progress/Evaluation	Date
2/20	1.	Parents and 14-year-old daughter rarely have time to talk to each other. Goal: To increase amount and quality of communication between parents and daughter.	a. Family will eat together at least once a day on weekdays for 3 months.	a. Determine which meal will be eaten together and select appetizing menus.	a. Have eaten all but 2 dinners together since 2/26. Had breakfasts together instead on 4/6 and 4/13. Family feels objective has been accomplished. Plan to continue frequent meals together.	5/28
			b. Family conversation during meals will include discussion of everyone's activities.	b. Parents will show interest in daughter by asking questions and decreasing amount of discussion between themselves. Daughter will ask parents questions about their days.	b. Family states meal conversation is much more satisfying. All say they are learning much about each other. Conversation is free-flowing. Family interaction in front of nurse is relaxed, open. Objective accomplished.	5/28
			c. Family will have one activity together each month for next 3 months.	c. Family will go to a movie in March, eat dinner out in April, have a picnic in May.	c. Watched TV movie instead. Made popcorn. Had a good time.	3/24
					Ate at nice restaurant. Enjoyed being together.	4/21
					Daughter invited friend to picnic on 5/19. All played games together. Family is satisfied that communication goal is met and plans to continue monthly family activities.	5/28
				d. Family will meet with nurse monthly to evaluate progress.		

Figure 5-5. Partial sample of nursing care plan.

resolution of the need. For clarity in planning, both a written need statement and goal statement are helpful.

3. *Expected outcomes* are the objectives. They are specific statements that describe what you hope to accomplish. To achieve comprehensive results, it is often necessary to construct two or three expected outcomes (objectives) for each need/goal. These objectives provide the nurse planner with specific targets to aim at and to design actions around.

4. *Planned actions* are the activities or methods of accomplishing the expected outcomes. They are specific, planned interventions to meet the objectives. Plans should include appropriate actions by nurse and client.

5. *Progress and evaluation* describe the actual outcomes or results and what they mean. What happened? How was each objective met and when, and if not, why not? It is essential to include evaluation in the written care plan. Too often, progress notes become a substitute for evaluation. Progress notes are useful, periodic summaries; evaluation requires analysis and conclusions. Progress notes and evaluation may be combined if space is allowed on the care plan. Generally, it is best to enter progress notes on a separate page.

One way to record the plan is to list items 2–5 in columns with space for the nurse to record specifics (Fig. 5-5). An increasing number of nurses find it helpful to give a copy of the plan to clients. In many instances, having a copy promotes a client's sense of being an equal partner in the responsibility of meeting goals.

IMPLEMENTATION

Implementation is putting the plan into action. It means that the activities delineated in the plan are carried out, some by the nurse, and some by the client. In community health nursing, this is a point of particular emphasis. It is not just nursing action or nursing intervention but *collaborative* implementation. Certainly, as the health professional, the nurse's professional expertise and judgment provide a necessary resource to the client. The nurse is also a catalyst and facilitator in planning and activating the nurse-client action plan. But a primary goal in community health is to help people learn to help themselves toward their optimal level of health. To realize this goal, we must constantly involve clients in the deliberative process and encourage their sense of responsibility and autonomy. Other health team members, too, may participate in carrying out the plan. Therefore, we are all partners in implementation.

PREPARATION

The actual course of implementation, outlined in the plan, should be fairly easy to follow if goals, expected outcomes, and planned actions have been designed carefully. Nurse and clients should have a clear idea of the who, what, why, when, where, and how. Who will be involved in carrying out the plan? What is each person's responsibilities? Do they all understand why and how to do it? Do they know when and where activities will occur? As implementation begins, nurses should review these questions for themselves as well as clients. This is the time to clarify any doubtful areas and thus facilitate a smooth implementation phase.

Even the best planning, though, may require adjustments. For example, the Jones family ran into a snag when they discovered that the three of them could not agree on what constituted an appetizing menu. To solve this unexpected conflict, they elected to take turns planning the menu so that each had a regular opportunity to eat favorite foods. This solution, they decided, would contribute to feelings of good will and enhance mealtime conversation. Thus implementation requires flexibility and adaptation to unanticipated events.

ACTIVITIES

Sometimes implementation is referred to as the action phase of the nursing process. In one sense, this is true because action is finally taken to solve the problem or meet the need. Up to this point, the nursing process has been largely background work. The early steps of the nursing process are much like preparing to build a bridge. Bridge construction requires initial negotiation (interaction); research on bridge construction, environmental considerations, and traffic use (assessment); and bridge design (planning). Implementation is actually building the bridge and seeing its completion.

The process of implementation requires a series of nursing actions. First, the nurse applies appropriate theories to the actions being performed. For the Jones family, the community health nurse used theories of communication and of adolescent behavior, among other theories, to guide the implementation process. Second, the nurse provides an environment that is conducive for carrying out the plan, such as a quiet room in which to hold a teaching session. Third, the nurse prepares the client for the care to be received. This step means building on the interaction established earlier so that there is open communication and trust. Client knowledge, understanding, and attitudes are assessed. The plan is carefully interpreted. Nurse and client form a contractual agreement about the content of the plan and how it is to be carried out. Fourth, the plan is carried out or modified, or both, by the nurse and client. Modification requires constant observation and interchange during implementation since these actions determine the success of the plan and the nature of needed changes. Finally, the nurse documents the implementation process through progress notes.

EVALUATION

Evaluation, the final component of the nursing process, is the last in a sequence of actions leading to the resolution of client health needs. The nursing process, as a professional tool for goal attainment, is not complete without measuring and judging the effectiveness of that goal attainment. Too often emphasis is placed primarily on assessing client needs and planning and implementing care. But how effective was the care? Were client needs truly met? As professional practitioners, we owe it to our clients, ourselves, and to other health service providers to evaluate.

Evaluation is an act of appraisal. When we evaluate something, we judge its value in relation to a standard and a set of criteria. For example, when eating dinner in a restaurant, you evaluate the dinner in terms of the standard of a satisfying meal. The criteria for your standard may include qualities such as a wide variety of choices on the menu, reasonable price, tasty food, nice atmosphere, and good service. You also evaluate the meal for a purpose. Was your money and time well spent and will you want to eat there again? Evaluation requires a purpose, standards and criteria, and judgment skills.

PURPOSE

The ultimate purpose of evaluating care in community health nursing is to determine whether planned actions met client needs, how well they were met, and if not, why not. In the pressure of daily practice, nurses are frequently limited to writing a quick progress note and a short final summary. This substitute for evaluation describes what occurred but does not judge its value. Evaluation is a critical component in the nursing process; without it, there is no basis for knowing whether previous actions were worthwhile and no evidence on which to base future plans. Therefore, we need evaluation to complete the series of activities that help us reach our goal, client health.

STANDARDS AND CRITERIA

Evaluation utilizes standards and criteria. In community health nursing, the standards are the intended results of the nursing care plan—the goals. The criteria for these standards are the specific, expected client behaviors that will demonstrate accomplishment of goals—the objectives. The Jones family had a standard which was their goal to increase the amount and quality of communication between parents and daughter (Fig. 5-5). How did they and the nurse know when the goal was met? The expected outcomes (objectives) were written as specific behaviors; these became criteria for evaluation. When all of the conditions or criteria were met, they knew the goal had been accomplished.

Consider another example. Several diabetic women attending a clinic had a problem with obesity. A community health nurse working in the clinic helped them form a weight loss group. Each woman set a goal of a specific number of pounds to lose in a year and then developed objectives (expected outcomes) to help her reach that goal. One of them, Mrs. Sander, planned the following.

Goal (Standard)
    Lose 50 pounds by the end of the year (target date).
Objectives (Criteria)
    1. Lose 2 pounds a week for the first 10 weeks.
    2. Lose 1 pound a week for the next 30 weeks.
    3. Maintain weight loss for 12 weeks.

The women planned ways to meet each of their objectives such as a specific daily calorie limit and regular exercise program. Some added hobbies or a series of personal rewards (a new dress after losing 15 pounds) to serve as motivators and pleasure substitutes. Mrs. Sanders evaluated the completion of her goal by using the standard (50 pounds a year) and the criteria spelled out in her objectives. To maximize group support and encourage healthy behavior patterns during weight loss, the nurse suggested having a group goal. This became their standard for measuring group success.

Group Standard
    The group will stay healthy while accomplishing 90 percent of the weight loss goals.
Group Criteria
    1. By the end of the year the group will lose a total of at least 90 percent of the sum of the expected individual weight losses.
    2. The group will have no diabetes-related infections during the year.
    3. All of the group members will be exercising at least once a week by the end of the year.
    4. No more than 10 percent of the group will have had an illness that kept them in bed more than one day during the year.

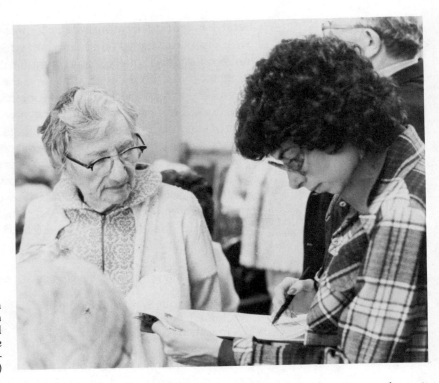

Figure 5-6. Elderly clients in a community health education program are being interviewed to evaluate the outcomes of the program. (Courtesy of Beth Israel Hospital, Boston.)

The prepared standard and set of criteria helped the group evaluate its success.

The above examples emphasize the relationship of good planning to evaluation. When nurse and client prepare clear, specific goals and objectives, there is then no question about how or what to evaluate. It will be obvious that the goal is either met or not met (Fig. 5-6).

JUDGMENT SKILLS

Evaluation requires judgment skills. The nurse compares real outcomes with expected outcomes and looks for discrepancies. When actual client behavior matches the desired behavior, then the goal, if well planned, is met. If it is not met, why not? The nurse will need to examine several possible explanations for the failure. Data collection may have been inadequate, the diagnosis incorrect, the plan unrealistic, or implementation ineffective. Circumstances or client motivation, or both, may have changed. There may not have been enough client participation in one or more parts of the process. After determining the cause of the failure, the nurse can reassess, plan, and initiate corrective action.

QUALITY ASSURANCE

In community health nursing, evaluation is also done to measure the quality of client care, nurse performance, and programs and services [4]. These measurements reflect nursing's increasing concern with quality assurance. An ideal quality assurance system includes [5]:

1. An organizational entity created for assessing quality
2. Establishment of standards or criteria against which quality is assessed
3. A routine system for gathering information
4. Assurance that such information is based on the total population or representative sample of patients or potential patients
5. A process that provides the results of review to patients, the public, providers, and sponsoring organizations, as well as methods to institute corrective actions

With the burgeoning emphasis on accountability in health care, community health nursing is being challenged to devise better ways of documenting service effectiveness and cost efficiency. A variety of methodologies and tools exist and are constantly being developed to facilitate these evaluative processes. One method is the nursing audit which evaluates quality of nursing care by analyzing client records. Some instruments, such as Wandelt's Quality Patient Care Scale, evaluate care while it is being given [10]. All of these methods, however, operate on the same basic principle discussed earlier, that is, that evaluation requires a clear purpose, and a standard and specific criteria against which outcomes are measured.

CHARACTERISTICS

The nursing process provides a framework or structure upon which community health nursing actions are based. Application of the process varies with each situation, but the nature of the process remains the same. Certain elements of that nature are important for community health nurses to emphasize in their practice (see Fig. 5-7).

The process is *deliberative* [11]. That is, it is purposefully, rationally, and carefully thought out. It requires the use of judgment. Community health nurses frequently practice in situations that demand independent thinking and difficult decision making. The nursing process is a tool to facilitate these determinations.

The process is *adaptable* [13]. Its dynamic nature enables the community health nurse to adjust appropriately to each situation, to be flexible in applying the process to client needs. The nurse adapts and individualizes service for each community client.

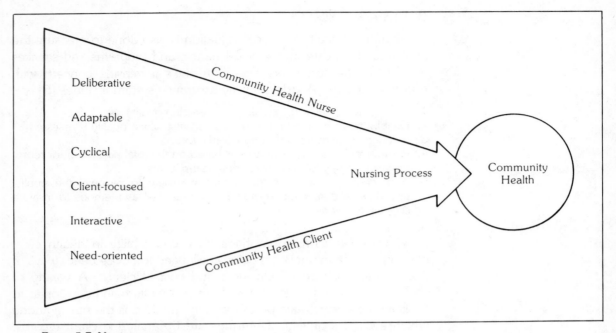

Deliberative

Adaptable

Cyclical

Client-focused

Interactive

Need-oriented

Community Health Nurse

Community Health Client

Nursing Process

Community Health

Figure 5-7. Nursing process characteristics emphasized in community health nursing practice.

The process is *cyclical*. Although a sequence of actions constitutes the framework of the nursing process, these actions are in constant progression [7]. The nurse in any given situation engages in continual interaction, data collection, analysis, intervention, and evaluation. Steps are never unrepeated in the nurse-client relationship. And as interactions between nurse and client continue, various steps in the process are used simultaneously.

The process, because it is used for and with clients, is *client-focused*. Clients are nursing's *raison d'être,* our reason for being. We use the nursing process for the express purpose of helping clients, directly or indirectly, to achieve and maintain health. The client as a total system, whether a family, group, or community, is the target of the nursing process.

The process is *interactive*. Nurse and client are engaged in a process of ongoing interpersonal communication, "a communicative interaction process" [3, p. 512]. Giving and receiving accurate information are necessary to promote understanding between nurse and client and foster effective use of the nursing process. Furthermore, as the consumer movement, patient's rights, and the self-care concept have gained emphasis, client and nurse have increasingly jointly assumed responsibility for promoting client health. The client-nurse relationship can and should be a partnership [13]. Called "peer practice" by some [1], the nursing process is shared by nurse and client.

Finally, the nursing process, as applied in community health, is *need-oriented*. Long association with problem solving has tended to limit the nursing process's focus to the correction of problems. While problem solution is certainly an appropriate use of the nursing process, its application in community health to anticipation of needs and prevention of problems assumes additional significance. This focus is needed if we are to realize the goals of community health, "to protect, promote, and restore the people's health" [9, p. 3].

SUMMARY

The effectiveness of community health nursing practice depends on how well the nursing process is used. The nursing process means appropriately applying a systematic series of actions toward helping clients achieve their optimal level of health. These actions or components of the process include interaction, assessment, planning, implementation, and evaluation.

Interaction is the first component because nurse and client must establish a relationship of reciprocal influence and exchange. It requires effective communication to assess needs and establish trust between nurse and client as partners in the process.

Assessment is a process of appraising client health status to determine existing or possible future needs. Community health nursing is not limited to identifying problems. Rather, there is a strong emphasis on exploring ways to maximize client health potential. Assessment provides the basis for future nursing action. It involves collecting and interpreting data, and diagnosing client needs.

Planning means designing a specific course of action to meet identified client needs. To plan, one must set priorities to client needs, establish goals and objectives, design activities to meet the objectives, and write the care plan. The plan should include a data base, statements describing client needs and goals to be achieved, specific objectives, progress notes, and finally, an evaluation of each objective.

Implementation is activating the plan and seeing it through to completion. During implementation, the nurse applies appropriate theory; provides a facilitative environment; prepares the client for care; with the client, carries out and/or modifies the plan; and documents the implementation.

Evaluation measures and judges the effectiveness of the plan. Were client needs met? If not, why not? To evaluate, we need to understand clearly why we are evaluating. What is our purpose? We also need a standard (goal) and a specific set of criteria (objectives) for each goal to use in measuring the outcomes. There is an important relationship between good planning and evaluation since well-prepared goals and objectives are essential for adequate evaluation. If goals are not met, the failure may result from inadequate assessment or planning. Determining the cause of the failure can lead to corrective action. Evaluation does not end the nursing process; rather, it documents what has been accomplished and what yet needs to be done in order that the process, a continuing cycle, can start again.

Certain characteristics of the nursing process should be emphasized by community health nurses in their practice. The process is *deliberative,* requiring and aiding the exercise of judgment in decision making. It is *adaptable,* encouraging flexibility in practice. It is *cyclical,* fostering a constant, ongoing use of the process. It is *client-focused,* helping the nurse to keep the proper target of client health in view. It is *interactive,* promoting nurse-client communication and client participation. Finally, it is *need-oriented,* encouraging identification of ways to maximize client health potential.

The purpose of this chapter has been to review the nursing process as it applies to community health nursing practice. Many excellent references, listed in the bibliography, give more detailed information about various aspects of the nursing process; the interested reader is encouraged to study these.

REFERENCES

1. Bayer, M., and Brandner, P.   Nurse/patient peer practice. *Am. J. Nurs.* 77:86, 1977.
2. Brill, N. I.   *Working with People: The Helping Process.* Philadelphia: Lippincott, 1973.
3. Daubenmire, M. J., and King, I. M.   Nursing process models: A system approach. *Nurs. Outlook* 21:512, 1973.
4. Decker, F., Stevens, L., Vancini, M., and Wedeking, L.   Using patient outcomes to evaluate community health nursing. *Nurs. Outlook* 27:278, 1979.
5. *Assessing Quality in Health Care: An Evaluation* (final report). Washington, D.C.: Institute of Medicine, National Academy of Sciences, November 1976.
6. Langford, T.   Establishing a nursing contract. *Nurs. Outlook* 26:386, 1978.
7. Marriner, A.   *The Nursing Process* (2nd ed.). St. Louis: Mosby, 1979. P. 4.

8. Mauksch, I. G., and David, M. L. Prescription for survival. *Am. J. Nurs.* 72:2189, 1972.

9. Sheps, C. G. (Chrm.) *Higher Education for Public Health: Report of the Milbank Memorial Fund Commission.* New York: Neale, Watson, 1976. P. 3.

10. Wandelt, M., and Ager, J. *Quality Patient Care Scale.* New York: Appleton-Century-Crofts, 1974.

11. Weidenbach, E. *Clinical Nursing: A Helping Art.* New York: Springer, 1964. P. 41.

12. Williams, C. A. Community health nursing—What is it? *Nurs. Outlook* 25:250, 1977.

13. Yura, H., and Walsh, M. B. *The Nursing Process: Assessing, Planning, Implementing, Evaluating.* New York: Appleton-Century-Crofts, 1973. P. 68.

SELECTED READINGS

Assessing Quality in Health Care: An Evaluation (final report). Washington, D.C.: Institute of Medicine, National Academy of Sciences, November 1976.

Bayer, M., and Brandner, P. Nurse/patient peer practice. *Am. J. Nurs.* 77:86, 1977.

Bloch, D. Evaluating of nursing care in terms of process and outcome: Issues in research and quality assurance. *Nurs. Res.* 24:256, 1975.

Brill, N. I. *Working with People: The Helping Process.* Philadelphia: Lippincott, 1973.

Browning, M. H. *The Nursing Process in Practice.* New York: American Journal of Nursing, 1974.

Daubenmire, M. J., and King, I. M. Nursing process models: A system approach. *Nurs. Outlook* 21:512, 1973.

Davidson, S. V. Community nursing care evaluation. *Fam. Community Health* 1:37, 1978.

Decker, F., Stevens, L., Vancini, M., and Wedeking, L. Using patient outcomes to evaluate community health nursing. *Nurs. Outlook* 27:278, 1979.

Evaluation of Quality of Public Health Nursing. Washington, D.C.: American Public Health Association, Public Health Nursing Section, February 1976.

Hadley, R. D. Nurses develop quality assurance program in community health setting. *Am. Nurse* 10:3, 1978.

Keeler, J. D. The process of program evaluation. *Nurs. Outlook* 20:316, 1972.

Kleffel, D. A Utilization Review Program for Home Health Agencies. Washington, D.C.: Government Printing Office, U.S. Department of Health, Education, and Welfare, HSMHA, Community Health Service (No. HSM 72-6502), 1972.

Knight, J. Applying nursing process in the community. *Nurs. Outlook* 22:708, 1974.

Langford, T. Establishing a nursing contract. *Nurs. Outlook* 26:386, 1978.

Lewis, T. This I believe . . . about the nursing process—Key to care. *Nurs. Outlook* 16:26, 1968.

Marram, G. Patients' evaluation of their care—Importance to the nurse. *Nurs. Outlook* 21:322, 1973.

Marriner, A. *The Nursing Process* (2nd ed.). St. Louis: Mosby, 1979.

Mauksch, I. G., and David, M. L. Prescription for survival. *Am. J. Nurs.* 72:2189, 1972.

Mayers, M. G. A search for assessment criteria. *Nurs. Outlook* 20:323, 1972.

Mayers, M. G. *A Systematic Approach to the Nursing Care Plan.* New York: Appleton-Century-Crofts, 1972.

National League for Nursing. *Accreditation of Home Health Agencies and Community Nursing Services.* New York: National League for Nursing (No. 21–1306), 1975.

National League for Nursing, Division of Community Planning. *Quality Assessment and Patient Care.* New York: National League for Nursing, 1975.

Parzick, J., and Nolan, M., Sr. POMR at work in a home health agency. *Fam. Community Health* 1:101, 1978.

Phaneuf, M., and Wandelt, M. Quality assurance in nursing. *Nurs. Forum* 4:328, 1974.

Ramphal, M. Peer review. *Am. J. Nurs.* 74:63, 1974.

Shaffer, M. K., and Pfeiffer, I. L. Home visit: A gray zone in evaluation. *Am. J. Nurs.* 78:239, 1978.

Wandelt, M., and Ager, J. *Quality Patient Care Scale.* New York: Appleton-Century-Crofts, 1974.

Wray, J. G. Problem-oriented recording in community nursing—A new experience in education. *J. Nurs. Educ.* 16:12, 1977.

Yura, H., and Walsh, M. B. *The Nursing Process: Assessing, Planning, Implementing, Evaluating.* New York: Appleton-Century-Corfts, 1973.

Zimmer, M. Quality Assurance for Outcomes of Patient Care. *Nurs. Clin. North Am.* June:305, 1974.

Six

The Helping Relationship and Contracting

The helping relationship is a primary tool for community health nurses. It contributes to both the prevention of illness and the promotion of client health. In order to use the helping relationship skillfully in community health practice, we must understand the meaning and value of a therapeutic relationship. Unlike ordinary social relationships, it is based on mutual participation in establishing and carrying out goals. The client and the nurse enter into a working agreement to meet specific client needs. The concept of contracting is closely tied to use of the helping relationship. This chapter examines both these tools and discusses their integration into community health nursing practice.

THE HELPING RELATIONSHIP: A DEFINITION

The concept of a helping relationship has undergone a change in recent years. Traditionally, the term *helping* has implied that one individual gives help, and the other individual receives help. Viewed in this manner, the helping relationship inadvertently created a dependency relationship. Given our current consumer needs and our understanding of health care practice, this traditional model is no longer appropriate. Its weakness came from the fact that it made clients dependent on the nurse, undermined their self-confidence, and undercut their self-respect. In short, it reduced the very characteristics that the nurse hoped to foster. This traditional view of the helping relationship reduced clients' motivation to participate in the health care process and detracted from their sense of responsibility for maintaining their health.

This traditional definition has another inherent problem. It implies that the helping relationship occurs only between two individuals, the nurse and a single patient or client. Even the community health nurse working with a family, for example, may think in terms of establishing a helping relationship only with the mother or some other individual, rather than with the family as a whole. In community health nursing, the client will range from a single individual to an entire community. In the course of working, a single community health nurse might develop helping relationships with the following range of clients: (1) an elderly widower living alone in his own home; (2) an extended family of Cuban immigrants; (3) a parenting class of 15 women with preschool children; (4) a lumber company with 95 employees seeking to develop a wellness program; (5) a cluster of elementary schools seeking to improve nutrition among students; and (6) an entire community conducting a self-survey about health practices. Throughout this book, the term *client* refers to this broad range of individuals and groups. In order to maximize the effectiveness of the helping relationship in promoting client health, we need to redefine the meaning of this tool.

The helping relationship means *purposeful interaction between nurse and client based on mutual participation.* This definition highlights only two basic features of the helping relationship; it has a goal and it involves both parties in setting and achieving that goal. In order to explore more fully the meaning of this relationship in the context of community health nursing, we shall examine five characteristics that distinguish it from other types of interaction which will be referred to as simply "social relationships."

CHARACTERISTICS OF THE HELPING RELATIONSHIP

EMPHASIS ON GOALS

First, the helping relationship in community health nursing is goal-directed. The nurse and client recognize specific reasons why they enter into the relationship. For example, a large Thai family who are recent immigrants want to learn about nutrition; the community health nurse can provide them with information. The client group and the nurse enter into the relationship with stated needs to be met and goals to accomplish. Other forms of social interaction, such as encounters between friends, often lack recognized goals.

UNILATERAL BENEFITS

Second, in community health the helping relationship is unilateral, that is, it exists for the benefit of the clients. In developing a helping relationship with the Thai immigrant family concerned about nutrition, shopping for food, and eating in a new cultural setting, the direct benefits accrue to the family. Certainly the nurse gains satisfaction from the interaction, but the relationship is established to meet the needs of the clients. The nurse's satisfaction and growth are a side effect, not a stated objective. Many other social relationships, as among friends, business acquaintances, or professional colleagues, are bilateral. Both parties come to the relationship with an expectation of almost equivalent benefits.

EXPLICIT MUTUAL AGREEMENT

Third, in community health the helping relationship involves explicit mutual agreement. When you interact with a friend, relative, salesperson, or neighbor, the relationship operates with tacit rules; you probably do not talk about the relationship or direct your energy toward seeking an explicit consensus. The helping relationship, on the other hand, involves a reciprocal exchange in which both parties discuss what their interaction will involve. The mother, father, and grandparents in the Thai family may express their desire to provide their children with the right food; they may be concerned about loss of traditional foods and feel overwhelmed when shopping in supermarkets. They want the nurse to assist them to achieve their goals. The nurse discusses her role in giving this assistance. The relationship arises from an explicit, mutual agreement. This discussion of the goals and the nature of the relationship provides a channel within which the work of the relationship takes place.

SET RESPONSIBILITIES

Fourth, the helping relationship in community health nursing assigns set responsibilities to each party. A well-defined relationship clearly states what the client will do and what the nurse will do to accomplish the goals. The nurse, for example, might agree to take several members of the Thai family on a shopping trip, help them prepare a balanced meal, and provide reading materials on infant nutrition. The family would agree to study the materials (perhaps through an older child who can interpret for the adults), ask questions, and follow the example and instructions of the nurse. Each party to the helping relationship develops an understanding of their responsibilities based on realistic and honest expectations. This understanding may not come with the first visit, but as the relationship develops, the nurse works toward this division of responsibilities; together with the client, the nurse explores necessary resources, assesses the capabilities of clients, and discovers their willingness to assume tasks. This structure of recognized responsibilities is often absent in other social relationships. Two friends can enjoy long years of companionship without ever saying, "You do this and I will do these other things." A local church committee, set up to help an immigrant family, may assume all the responsibility for helping provide food for the family rather than dividing the responsibility.

SET BOUNDARIES

Fifth, the helping relationship in community health practice has set boundaries. Nearly every therapeutic relationship has a beginning and an end. A crucial part of defining the helping relationship is determining when and under what conditions to terminate it. The temporal boundaries are determined sometimes by progress toward the goal, sometimes by the number of nurse-client contacts, and often by setting a time limit. A nurse might set up eight sessions to help the Thai family with nutrition problems, or they might meet together weekly until the goal of adequate knowledge and skill was met. Other social relationships, in contrast, are generally open-ended in length. A friendship may end because of misunderstanding, or a business relationship may stop when a partner moves to another city. Table 6-1 summarizes the characteristics that distinguish the helping relationship from other social relationships.

Table 6-1. Comparison Between Helping and Social Relationships

Helping Relationship	Social Relationship
Goal-directed	No specific goals
Unilateral, benefits client	Bilateral, benefits both parties
Explicit mutual agreement	No consensus; casual interaction
Set responsibilities	Unstructured
Time-limited, set boundaries	Open-ended in length and frequency of contacts

CLIENT PARTICIPATION

We have stressed that the helping relationship is based on mutual participation. The extent of that participation, however, varies depending on the client's readiness and ability to participate. The level of wellness at the time of initial nurse-client encounter directly influences participation. Some people are not physically or emotionally well enough to assume an active role in the relationship. A woman recently discharged from the hospital following a mastectomy, for example, has many physical and emotional adjustments with which to cope. Her family, too, must expend additional energies to provide needed support and to cope with the loss of the woman's usual role in the family. They may find it difficult to engage actively in identifying their needs and goals at the start of the relationship. The nurse may have to take stronger initial leadership; however, the goals of a helping relationship are not abandoned. Eventually, as the family level of wellness improves, the nurse can encourage more active participation.

Sometimes clients' previous experiences with health personnel limit participation in the helping relationship. Clients from poverty areas, from different cultural backgrounds, or with little education may need extensive encouragement to participate actively in the helping relationship. Working with a Thai family, recently immigrated to the United States, will be quite different from helping a group of suburban women with infant nutrition. Clients previously regarded by health professionals as incapable of managing their own lives will also take a more passive role in the helping relationship. Even well-educated people with comfortable incomes have often learned to behave passively when dealing with physicians, nurses, or other health professionals. With all these people, unless the nurse persists in efforts to reduce the dependence of clients, the relationship can fall far short of the therapeutic goals.

The nurse's own view of the helping relationship will also influence the degree of client participation. Those accustomed to relating to clients in an adult-to-child manner will restrict client involvement. If the nurse sees her position as more informed and the client's position as one of complete ignorance and need, a paternalistic relationship may develop. All clients have resources on which to build, and the community health nurse helps clients discover them.

Clients who initiate care, such as postpartum mothers who ask for home visits or families who request follow-up care after hospitalization, are frequently best able to assume an active participant role. They have already demonstrated a sense of responsibility for their health by identifying a need and asking for asssistance. The nurse will still have to work carefully to build mutual participation, but its development is more likely to occur.

SKILLS NEEDED IN THE HELPING RELATIONSHIP

Communication is the lifeblood of the helping relationship. It provides the vitality and nourishment necessary to foster a healthy nurse-client relationship. For communication to take place, the client and nurse send and receive messages. As participants in the communication process, community health nurses play both roles, sender and receiver. The nurse working with an alcoholic housewife must learn to "read" the messages this woman sends; the nurse will also have to speak and act in ways that communicate effectively. Community health nursing requires two sets of communication skills—sending skills and receiving skills.

SENDING SKILLS

Sending skills enable us to communicate messages effectively. Through these skills we convey thoughts and feelings to the client. Two important considerations will influence clarity and effectiveness of message sending. First, the extent of our self-awareness will affect the communication. Do we feel anxious, angry, impatient, or concerned? Are we tired? Do certain clients irritate us? What motives and interests do we have for wanting to communicate with the client? Second, our awareness of the receiver will influence the sending of messages. What does the client seem to want or need? Is the message suited to the client's cultural background and level of understanding? Does the message have significance for the client? How does the client respond as we send the message?

We use two main channels to send messages: verbal and nonverbal. Nonverbal messages, those conveyed without words, constitute nearly two-thirds of the messages transmitted in normal communication [2]. We send messages nonverbally in many ways. Our personal appearance, dress, posture, and cleanliness all communicate messages about us. They may enhance or discredit what we say. Body language often speaks louder than words. Facial expressions convey acceptance or rejection, interest or boredom, and apprehension or confidence. Gestures and bodily movements such as hand clenching, finger tapping, or foot swinging all communicate strong messages to our clients. Eye contact or lack of it carries additional meaning. Your tone of voice and use of silence will also send nonverbal messages. Accepting food may communicate acceptance, while getting a chair for a client may say, "I'm interested in your welfare."

Verbal messages communicate ideas, but they also convey attitudes and feelings. We cannot assume that the intent of our words is always understood by our clients. Effective sending skills depend on asking for feedback to make certain that the receiver understood the verbal message's intent. Communication can improve if we avoid jargon. Like all occupations, nursing has its own vocabulary. Often unfamiliar to clients, this jargon may carry different meanings or make the client feel inferior because he cannot speak that language. Mr. Jones did not know what to answer when the nurse asked if he had "voided." Mrs. Wendt felt confused when asked if she had noticed any expressions of "sibling rivalry" by her three-year-old child. When nursing jargon becomes part of our everyday speech, only special effort will enable us to set it aside when interacting with clients. We can summarize the basic rules for effective sending in this manner: keep the message honest and uncomplicated; use as few words as possible to state it; and ask for reactions to make certain that it is understood.

RECEIVING SKILLS

Receiving skills are as important to communication as sending skills. They enable us to receive accurate and complete messages. Receiving skills involve not only listening to what people say but also observing their behavior. If a client says, "I haven't been feeling well," we need to discover the context of this statement. What tone of voice did the client use? What was the meaning of the client's facial expressions? What gestures accompanied the statement? Where did the client tell us about these feelings? Effective receiving skills require training ourselves to observe these kinds of details.

The other main source of receiving is active listening, the skill of assuming responsibility for understanding the meaning of the client's message [14]. Instead of requiring the client to make us understand, we actively work to discover what a client means. Understanding the message from the client's perspective demands careful attention. It arises from a genuine interest in what the speaker has to say. Active listeners demonstrate their interest, perhaps by sitting forward, sustaining eye contact, nodding the head, and asking occasional questions for clarification. They concentrate in order to avoid daydreaming or the pretense of listening, both of which block communication.

We can also listen actively by asking reflective questions. Such questions restate what the client has said:

Client: "Quitting smoking is impossible."
Nurse: "You feel you can't quit smoking?"

Reflective questions have a twofold purpose: to show your sincere attempt to understand accurately the client's message, and to make clear that the client's message and the client are important to you.

Active listening will communicate acceptance and increase trust, especially when we withhold a negative evaluation of the message or the way it is delivered. A critical response to the message cuts off communication. Active listening enables us to encourage the client to deliberate carefully and develop problem-solving skills; it avoids the pitfall of telling the client what to do.

Effective communication, both sending and receiving, is strongly influenced by three factors. First, the previous experiences of both sender and receiver influence their perceptions and the meanings they attach to messages. Requests for clarification will help verify that messages are being received as intended. Second, the respective cultures of sender and receiver influence our understanding and acceptance of messages. A nervous laugh, appropriate as an outlet in one culture, may appear rude and disrespectful to someone from another culture. Silence may indicate patience and thoughtfulness to one group of people but weakness or indifference to another. With many clients, the nurse will have to communicate cross-culturally, which requires patience and constant effort to insure accurate and inoffensive messages. Third, the relationships among participants during communication can significantly influence its effectiveness. Since much of community health nursing involves families and groups, communication patterns become quite complex. When a large number of people are involved, interaction requires skill in eliciting feedback from all members and in generating a common understanding among the group.

INTERPERSONAL SKILLS

In addition to effective communication, the helping relationship also requires three other interpersonal skills—showing respect, empathizing, and developing trust. Each of these skills depends on effective communication but surpasses the mere exchange of messages.

SHOWING RESPECT

Showing respect means conveying the attitude that the client has importance, dignity, and worth. We can express respect by helping the client feel that he has valuable ideas. We can let him know that we want to understand the situation from his point of view. We show respect by the manner in which we address clients; for instance, by using the courtesy titles of "Mr." or "Mrs." until we have permission to use first names. On a more subtle level, the tone of voice can either show respect or make people feel inferior and insignificant. Clients need to feel respected if they are to enter fully into the mutual exchange necessary for a true helping relationship.

EMPATHIZING

Empathizing is another important interpersonal skill. Empathy means the "ability to borrow another person's feelings . . . [and] to understand them while maintaining one's own identity" [5, p. 1548]. We empathize by reflecting the client's feelings, that is, by showing our attempt to understand the source and meanings of those feelings. Empathy is best expressed in the client's language. The same terms and, if possible, the same tone of voice as the clients' should be used. For example, the nurse can reflect sadness if the client seems sad. Empathy is best expressed provisionally, showing that we are still attempting to ascertain the client's true feelings while allowing the client to validate our expression. Empathy conveys the message, "This is the way it seems to me. Is that right?" It focuses attention on clients and their feelings; it shows that the nurse shares their concerns and it makes clients feel important.

DEVELOPING TRUST

Developing trust is necessary for an effective helping relationship. Clients will not express their true feelings if they do not fully trust the nurse. Many times clients will say what they think the nurse wants to hear. They may agree to a plan of action simply because they do not want to displease the nurse. They may hide true feelings because they think that the nurse is eager for a decision. We develop trust by showing that we truly accept clients, that we believe in them as people. Trust generates trust; as the nurse shows confidence in clients, they will respond in kind. Treating them as fully participating partners in the relationship shows that you entrust clients with responsibilities. Trust is also developed through an open, honest, and patient approach with clients. Candid discussion in a flexible time frame encourages clients to share their real feelings and to move at their own pace. As trust develops, the relationship becomes a truly helping one, focused on client needs (Fig. 6-1).

STRUCTURE OF THE HELPING RELATIONSHIP

The skills that lead to an effective helping relationship are used within a particular structure. Awareness of this structure can greatly increase your ability to help clients. Because the relationship is bound by time, the structure involves several phases. The way you use your skills during the first and last phases of the helping relationship may contrast. It is useful to think of the helping relationship's following sequential

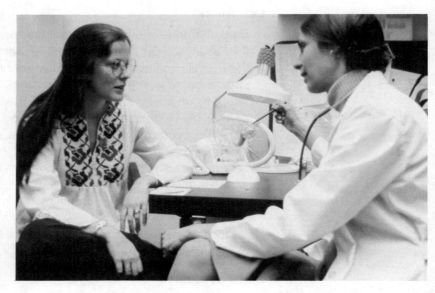

Figure 6-1. Development of trust is crucial to an effective helping relationship. (Courtesy of the Harvard Community Health Plan, Boston.)

structure: (1) a beginning phase when the relationship is just being established; (2) a middle, working phase; and (3) a termination phase when the relationship ends [2]. In the context of this process, the work of identifying and meeting client needs takes place.

The first phase is a period of establishing and defining the relationship. The nurse and client are getting to know each other; they seek to establish communication patterns and develop trust. From these bases, they identify the client's needs and determine the goals toward which they will work.

The middle phase occurs when nurse and client start working together to accomplish the goals of the relationship. Their work may include assessment and planning as well as implementation and evaluation. The cycle of the nursing process will be repeated as needed during this working phase until goals are accomplished and no further goals identified.

The termination phase occurs when the need for nurse and client to work together has ended. In many instances, clients can function on their own. When client and nurse have grown close in the relationship, termination can be difficult. It often requires careful advance preparation to make certain that both parties understand when and why it is taking place. Termination helps to insure a clear-cut end to the relationship. One nurse had made home visits to a refugee family for nearly a year. As their multiple needs declined, she decided to taper off her assistance. Two months before ending the relationship, she discussed termination with the family. At first they were frightened at the loss of help, but slowly they came to accept it and assumed more and more responsibility for their health needs. Had she announced the end of her visits more abruptly, the family might have easily felt confused or rejected.

THE CONCEPT OF CONTRACTING

The primary goal of community health nursing is to promote community health through identifying and meeting client needs. Success demands active participation of the client. The helping relationship is "helping" only in the sense that we assist people in this process. Without mutual participation, the client cannot develop ability in self-care. Contracting makes this goal of self-care explicit.

The concept of self-care has a long history in community health nursing. Public health nursing, as Norris has shown, was founded on self-care concepts and originated self-care practice [9]. More recently, self-care has come into its own through the growth of independent nursing practice. Kinlein, for example, bases her independent practice squarely on this concept. She found that clients had far more capability than was believed in achieving self-care. She believes that nursing means helping clients choose the self-care practices best for them [6]. Like the shopkeeper who expects his customers to make their own selections, the nurse treats clients as independent consumers, saying, "I believe in your ability to assume responsibility for your own health." By making self-care more explicit, contracting can become a powerful tool in community health nursing.

Contracting means negotiating a working agreement between two or more parties. They come to a shared understanding and then give consent to the purposes and terms of the transaction. Some kinds of contracts are familiar, for example, buying a car. Other, less obvious agreements, such as paying tuition for an education, still involve a form of contracting. As a student, you agree with an educational institution on purposes (their financial reimbursement, your degree) and terms of the contract (regular tuition payments, regular learning opportunities), even though a formal document is not signed.

In contrast to legal contracts which are written, binding agreements, the contract in a helping relationship is flexible and based on mutual understanding and trust. Sloan and Schommer define the community nursing contract as "any working agreement, continuously renegotiable" between client and nurse [13, p. 222]. When viewed from this perspective, contracting becomes a valuable tool for community health nurses.

FEATURES OF CONTRACTING

PARTNERSHIP

The concept of contracting as used in the helping relationship incorporates four distinctive features. The first is partnership. All aspects of contracting involve shared participation and agreement between client and nurse; they become partners in the relationship. For example, the Ericksons, an older couple who requested community health nursing visits at home, entered into a partnership with the nurse after the husband was discharged from the hospital with a colostomy. They came to an agreement on what the couple needed and what the nurse could provide. Together they developed goals, outlined methods to meet those goals, and explored resources to help achieve them. They defined the time limits for the contract as well as their separate responsibilities. The contract involved reciprocal negotiation and shared evaluation. A partnership means that both parties are responsible for setting up and carrying out the service.

COMMITMENT

Second, every contract implies a commitment. Both parties make a decision that binds them to fulfilling the purpose of the contract. In the helping relationship, contracting does not mean a binding agreement in the legal sense; rather, it is a pledge of trust and dedication. Accompanying that sense of dedication is a strong motivation to see the contract through to completion. Both parties feel responsible for keeping promises; both want to achieve the intended outcomes. When the nurse and the Ericksons identified their separate tasks, they committed themselves. "Yes, we will do thus and so . . . ."

FORMAT

Format is the third distinctive feature of the concept of contracting. Unlike many nurse-client interactions, contracting defines the terms of the relationship. Thus both client and nurse obtain a clear idea of the purpose of the relationship, of their respective responsibilities, and of the specific limits within which they will work (Fig. 6-2). In other words, contracting provides a framework for the relationship. Once the terms of the contract have been spelled out, there is no question about what has to be done, who is to do it, or within what time frame it is to be

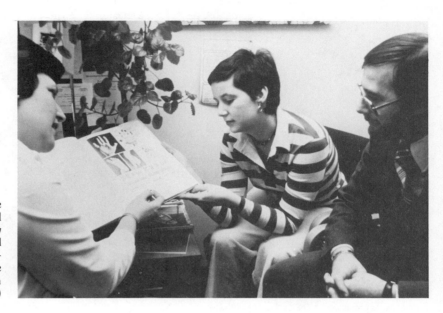

Figure 6-2. An important feature of contracting involves mutual agreement between the family and the nurse on the material they want to cover in their sessions together. (Courtesy of the Harvard Community Health Plan, Boston.)

done. This format helps to prevent a frequently recurring problem in community health nursing, the difficulty of termination of a long-term relationship. It also helps to prevent a dependency relationship from developing.

NEGOTIATION

Finally, contracting always involves negotiation. The nurse proposes to accept certain responsibilities, and then asks if the clients agree. The nurse might ask, "What do you feel you can do to achieve this goal?" A period of give and take occurs in which ideas are discussed and conclusions, which often represent compromises, are reached. A few weeks later, nurse and clients may find that terms they had agreed upon need modification. Perhaps clients have assumed more responsibility than they can realistically handle at that point in time. Perhaps the nurse does not feel comfortable teaching a complex technique and needs to utilize an outside resource. Negotiation during contracting allows for changes that facilitate the ultimate achievement of goals. It provides contracting with built-in flexibility and encourages ongoing communication between clients and nurse. Negotiation gives contracting a dynamic quality (see Fig. 6-3). It becomes a complex process that moves through eight stages, each negotiated between the nurse and clients. This process will be considered later in the chapter.

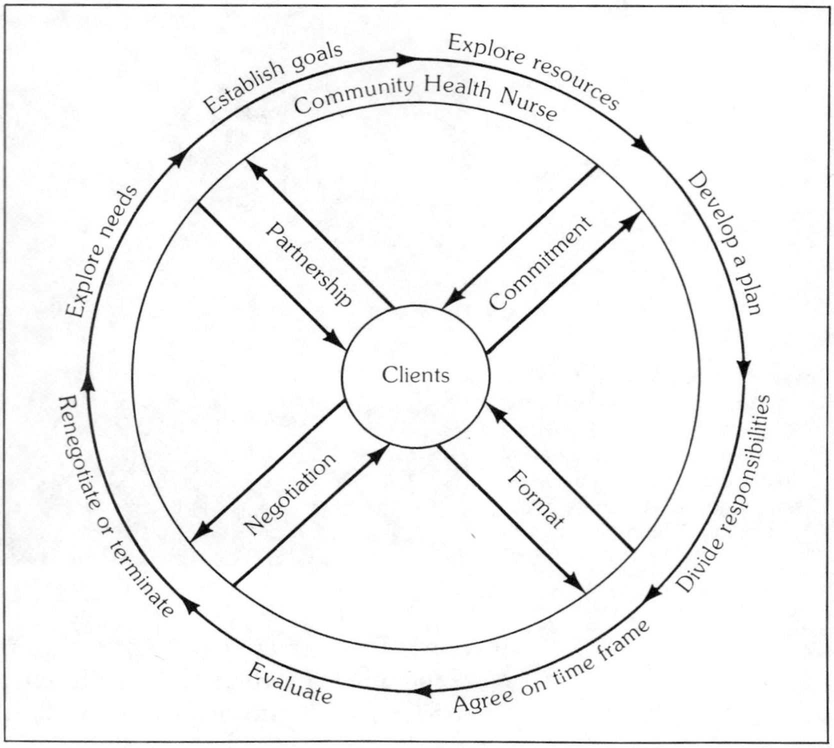

Figure 6-3. The concept and process of contracting. Contracting is based on four distinctive features shown here as spokes that support a wheel. These features form the basis for a reciprocal relationship between nurse and clients. This relationship is not static; it is a dynamic process that moves through phases, represented here as the outer rim of the wheel. The relationship moves forward, focused on meeting clients' needs, and enables the nurse to facilitate ultimate achievement of clients' goals.

VALUE OF CONTRACTING

The value of contracting has been demonstrated in many settings. Contracts have been used for many years in psychiatric nursing settings to promote client self-respect, problem-solving skills, autonomy, and motivation [3, 10]. Other disciplines, such as social work, use contracting as a tool in the helping relationship to enhance realistic planning and emphasize partnership [11]. Educational contracts between students and instructors have proven valuable for facilitating learning [8]. Community health nursing has also used the concept of contracting for many years. Without always labelling it as such, community health nurses have contracted with clients who wanted to lose weight, mutually agreeing to certain exercise and eating patterns for the client and teaching and support responsibilities for the nurse. Often they have set a time limit, such as six months, to achieve the intended weight loss. Community health nurses have entered into contractual relationships with postpartum mothers, new diabetics, postsurgical patients, prenatal groups, and many others. In each case, a partnership developed with agreement as to the purpose of the relationship and the conditions under which it would be carried out. They were, in effect, contracting.

Recognition of contracting as a tool has come more recently. Blair has described her developing awareness of the need to encourage clients to act for themselves rather than place them in a passive, dependent role. Using transactional analysis theory, she developed a professional treatment contract which she defined as "a mutual understanding of the reason for the service and the problems or areas that will be discussed during the [community nursing] visits" [1, p. 588]. Others have worked with the concept and refined it further. In one nursing education setting, students contracted with families and found that reaching a mutual agreement about the goals of service was beneficial to both clients and nurses [12]. Nurses in many settings recognize the value of the mutual participation model and use it to involve clients in the helping relationship and in use of the nursing process. Some suggest that contracting should be treated as a specific step in the helping process [2, 7]. As more and more nurses seek to promote client autonomy and self-care, contracting's wide applicability to nursing practice is being increasingly recognized.

Emphasis on contracting as a *method* rather than a *concept* can create problems. If one's experiences with contracts have all been business agreements, it is possible to carry the stereotype of a cold, formal arrangement into the nursing practice setting. Some nurses fear that asking clients to negotiate a contract will place clients under stress, impede the development of trust, and negatively influence the helping relationship. Others have found that some clients, who prefer to have the nurse make decisions for them, are not ready to enter into any kind of negotiation.

The concept of contracting, however, has much broader application than as simple methodology. As a concept, contracting applies basic principles of adult education—self-direction, mutual negotiation, and mutual evaluation [4]. These principles become both the means and the ends of contracting. To varying degrees, all clients are able to assess, plan, implement, and evaluate in contracting; yet the concept can be applied in a variety of ways. Sloan and Schommer demonstrate that contracting can be formal or informal, written or verbal, simple or detailed, and signed or unsigned by client and nurse [13]. Like all nursing tools, contracting will enhance client health only if adapted to each situation.

The advantages of contracting in community health nursing can now be summarized:

1. It involves clients in their own care.
2. It motivates clients to perform necessary tasks.
3. It individualizes care by focusing on a client's unique needs, whether the client is an individual or a group.
4. It increases the possibility of achieving health goals identified by both client and nurse.
5. It develops problem-solving skills of both nurse and client.
6. It fosters client participation in the decision-making process.
7. It promotes clients' autonomy and self-esteem as they learn self-care.
8. It makes nursing service more efficient and cost-effective.

THE PROCESS OF CONTRACTING

Because contracting is rather complex, some stages will occur before others. Without some kind of sequence, negotiation of a contract can become overwhelming. Consider the fact that this working agreement depends on knowing what the client wants, agreeing on goals, identifying methods to achieve these goals, knowing the resources that the nurse and client bring to the relationship, utilizing appropriate outside resources, setting limits, deciding on responsibilities, and providing for periodic reviews. Each of these tasks requires discussion between, and decision making by, nurse and client.

These tasks are incorporated into the process of contracting in a sequence which provides a guide for the nurse and client. Sloan and Schommer describe eight phases in the process [13]:

1. *Exploration of needs* Assessment of client's health, problems, and needs by client and nurse.
2. *Establishment of goals* Discussion and agreement between client and nurse on goals and objectives.
3. *Exploration of resources* Defining what client and nurse each have to offer to and expect from each other; identifying appropriate resources such as significant others, agencies, and other professionals.
4. *Development of a plan* Identifying methods and activities for achieving the goals.
5. *Division of responsibilities* Negotiating the activities for which client and nurse will each be responsible.
6. *Agreement on time frame* Setting limits for the contract in terms of length of time or number of visits.
7. *Evaluation* Periodic and final assessment of progress toward goals occurring at agreed-upon intervals.
8. *Renegotiation or termination* Agreement to modify, renegotiate, or terminate the contract.

As community health nurses use this process to negotiate a contract, they must adapt it to each situation. The exact sequence of phases may change and some steps may overlap. Nevertheless, the basic elements remain important considerations for successful contracting (see Fig. 6-3).

Consider the way one community health nurse used the contractual process. Eileen met the Nelsons through the agency's well-child clinic. Mrs. Nelson had been bringing sixteen-month-old Thor in for regular checkups and immunizations since they had moved to the city a year earlier. After becoming pregnant again, she approached Eileen about prenatal home visits to learn more about pregnancy and delivery. They made an appointment for Eileen's first visit.

EIGHT PHASES OF CONTRACTING

EXPLORATION OF NEEDS

Eileen explained the importance of focusing the visits on Mrs. Nelson's wants. She questioned Mrs. Nelson about her previous pregnancy, concerns, and interests, and suggested possible topics for discussion. In Eileen's agency, the supervisor and staff had developed a prenatal catalogue, a scrapbook of topics helpful to prospective mothers which was illustrated with pictures from magazines. It was, in effect, a sales catalogue that depicted many of the services the nurses could offer. Activities shown included teaching nutrition, demonstrating exercises, discussing growth and development of the fetus, changes in the mother's body, the process of labor and delivery, postpartum developments, and care of the newborn. Eileen had found the catalogue useful for helping clients to become aware of their choices and to select topics to cover in the contractual relationship. She offered to bring it on the second visit and, at that time, they would make some definite decisions about what Mrs. Nelson wanted.

ESTABLISHMENT OF GOALS

After examining and discussing the catalogue items and exploring other potential health needs, Eileen and Mrs. Nelson agreed to focus on pregnancy, labor, and delivery. They agreed upon the goals of a comfortable pregnancy and a modified natural childbirth for Mrs. Nelson. To make these goals more workable, they broke them down into objectives. One, for example, was to use Lamaze breathing techniques during childbirth. Another was to eat a well-balanced diet that would make Mrs. Nelson feel energetic and still keep her weight gain under twenty pounds.

EXPLORATION OF RESOURCES

Eileen questioned further about the amount of time and energy Mrs. Nelson wanted to commit to this project. Could she spend half an hour a day, for instance, on exercises? They discussed what Mrs. Nelson was willing to do and what Eileen, given her time schedule, could realistically do. Mr. Nelson wanted to be present during teaching sessions. They also agreed that Mrs. Nelson would consult her obstetrician.

DEVELOPMENT OF A PLAN

By the end of the second visit, Eileen and Mrs. Nelson had made a list of the specific, goal-related topics to cover in each session. Beside each topic they wrote down methods and activities. For example, on the next visit, Eileen would bring teaching tools and pamphlets and explain components of a well-balanced diet during pregnancy. Mrs. Nelson, then, would prepare a sample menu for her family that included a proper balance of the foods she needed. Since Mr. Nelson was to be part of the contract, they decided to have him look over the plan, make suggestions, and meet with them on the subsequent visits. The Nelsons both agreed to be present for each appointment. They changed the visit time to late afternoon when Mr. Nelson arrived home from work.

DIVISION OF RESPONSIBILITIES

Eileen encouraged the Nelsons to take an active role in each visit. Mrs. Nelson agreed to practice the exercises half an hour daily and to keep a record of her diet. Mr. Nelson's responsibilities were to encourage his wife to stick to the diet and exercises and to practice them with her when feasible. They agreed that Eileen would be responsible for presenting new material, demonstrating exercises and other techniques, and indicating whether or not the Nelsons were performing new activities correctly.

AGREEMENT ON TIME FRAME

Their list of topics helped Eileen and the Nelsons decide on the number of visits needed. They agreed on a schedule that spread visits throughout the pregnancy and six weeks postpartum. From the start, then, all parties agreed on a tentative termination date for the relationship.

EVALUATION

A part of their plan was to do monthly evaluations to determine the satisfaction each felt with the plan and the progress being made. This built in the possibility of renegotiation; anyone could suggest needed changes at those times. At the conclusion of the contract period (six weeks postpartum), they agreed to discuss how well all the goals had been met.

RENEGOTIATION OR TERMINATION

The Nelsons and Eileen agreed to renegotiate the time frame of the contract if new needs arose. Otherwise, they would terminate the service at the six weeks postpartum date.

LEVELS OF CONTRACTING

Community health nurses conduct the contracting process at levels which range from formal to informal. The degree of formality depends in large measure on the nurse's comfort in using this tool and clients' readiness to assume responsibility for self-care. At the most formal level, the parties usually negotiate a written contract. Drawn up by mutual agreement, each person signs it and a third party sometimes witnesses the signing. This form of contract is sometimes used in mental health settings where the seriousness of the working agreement and the need to involve the client actively are important aspects of therapy [3]. Less formal contracts, such as that with the Nelsons, are more commonly used. The nursing care plan becomes the written contract; thus no additional paper work is required. In one suburban health department, community health nurses contract with clients of a hypertension clinic. Part of their written care plan is a list of the client's goals and methods for achieving them (see Fig. 6-4). Under the column entitled responsibility, the nurse or client is listed as responsible for carrying out the activity.

Some situations lend themselves best to a more modified use of contracting. For example, one nurse had been making regular visits to a man dying of cancer. After his death, she contracted informally with his wife to continue visits for the purpose of helping her work through the grieving process. They discussed and agreed on the goals, methods, and responsibilities each would have, but did not negotiate a formal contract. Another community mental health nurse formed a therapy group composed of her individual clients. She used modified contracting by discussing with clients the purpose of the group and the

CLIENT-NURSE CONTRACT

Date accomplished	Goals	Date begun	Date ended	Methods	Responsibility
	1. To understand hypertension			a. Explain physiology of hypertension	N
				b. Interpret pamphlet on hypertension	C
				c. List risk factors associated with hypertension	C
	2. To decrease stress at work			a. Identify coping skills	N-C
				b. Explore possibility of job change	C
				c. List ways to relieve stress on job	N-C
				d. Design plan to relieve stress at work	C
				e. Implement plan until blood pressure is down to 115/75	C
	3. To lose 10 lb within 2 months			a. Explain nutritional factors influencing hypertension	N
				b. Design a diet plan	N-C
				c. Prepare exercise plan	C
				d. Implement plans until weight goal achieved	C

Length of contract:

Fee determination:

Signatures: Client _____ Date _____

Nurse _____ Date _____

Figure 6-4. Part of a contract developed between a client (C) and a nurse (N) in a community hypertension clinic.

number of sessions needed, and by obtaining their agreement to attend all sessions.

Informal contracting does involve some form of verbal agreement about relatively uncomplicated tasks. "You take your pills every day as prescribed, and I will get a homemaker for you." "You come to the clinic each week, and I will show you how to plan your diabetic diet." Sometimes nurses use contracting informally without realizing it. They conclude a home visit by agreeing with the family about the purpose and time of the next appointment. Conscious use of the tool, however, is a more effective way to provide structure for the relationship and foster client involvement, regardless of the level at which it is applied.

The level of contracting may also change during the development of a helping relationship. Clients often need education about their options. Initially they may have difficulty in identifying needs and making choices. The nurse can work to promote their self-confidence and help them assume increasing responsibility for their own health. Through these efforts, contracting becomes a consciously recognized part of the relationship. Clients can then become fully participating partners.

SUMMARY

The helping relationship is a tool for promoting client health and the ability to engage in self-care. It is goal-directed, unilateral in that it exists for the benefit of the client, and limited by time; it encourages mutual participation and involves clearly defined responsibilities.

Successful development of a helping relationship depends on the community health nurse's effective use of communication and interpersonal skills. To send and receive verbal or nonverbal messages well requires awareness of ourselves as well as of the client. It involves recognition of variables that might influence a message's interpretation. Nurses can cultivate the following skills: active listening, seeking feedback, showing respect, empathizing, and developing trust.

The helping relationship moves through three phases. During the beginning phase, the relationship is established and defined. The middle phase is a working period focused on meeting identified goals. The termination phase occurs when client and nurse no longer need to work together.

Contracting has four distinctive features. First, it involves partnership. Contracting utilizes shared participation and two-way agreement between client and nurse. Second, it involves commitment, a promise to carry out certain responsibilities. Third, contracting's format defines goals, methods, responsibilities, and time limits. Fourth, contracting involves negotiation between client and nurse.

The process of contracting utilizes eight phases which may sometimes vary in sequence or overlap: (1) exploration of needs; (2) establishment of goals; (3) exploration of resources; (4) development of a plan; (5) division of responsibilities; (6) agreement on time frame; (7) evaluation; and (8) renegotiation or termination.

Community health nurses practice contracting at levels ranging from formal to informal. Choice of level depends on the nurse's skill, client readiness, and demands of the situation. Clients may need assistance and instruction before they can assume the responsibilities of partners in contracting.

REFERENCES

1. Blair, K. K. It's the patient's problem and decision. *Nurs. Outlook* 19: 588, 1971.
2. Brill, N. *Working with People: The Helping Process.* Philadelphia: Lippincott, 1973. Pp. 36, 54, 72.
3. Davis, R. C., and Woodcock, E. The nursing contract: An alternative in care. *J. Psychiatr. Nurs.* 9:26, 1971.
4. Gustafson, M. B. Let's broaden our horizons about the use of contracts. *Intern. Nurs. Rev.* 24(1):19, 1977.
5. Kalisch, B. What is empathy? *Am. J. Nurs.* 73:1548, 1973.
6. Kinlein, L. M. *Independent Nursing Practice with Clients.* Philadelphia: Lippincott, 1977. P. 23.
7. Langford, T. Establishing a nursing contract. *Nurs. Outlook* 26(6):386, 1978.
8. Lindberg, J., and Simms, L. Contract grading: Incentives and rewards. *Image* 7(1):20, 1974.
9. Norris, C. M. Self-Care. *Am. J. Nurs.* 79:489, 1979.
10. Rosen, B. Contract therapy. *Nurs. Times* 74:119, 1978.
11. Sauer, J. K. The process of contracting in the helping relationship. *Minnesota Welfare* Summer:12, 1973.
12. Sheridan, A., and Smith, R. Student-family contracts. *Nurs. Outlook* 23(2):114, 1975.
13. Sloan, M., and Schommer, B. T. The Process of Contracting in Community Nursing. In B. Spradley [Ed.], *Contemporary Community Nursing.* Boston: Little, Brown, 1975. Pp. 221–229.
14. Wismer, J. Communication Effectiveness: Active Listening and Sending Feeling Messages. In J. W. Pfeiffer and J. Jones (Eds.), *The 1978 Annual Handbook for Group Facilitators.* La Jolla, Calif.: University Associates, 1978. P. 120.

SELECTED READINGS

Aiken, L., and Aiken, J.   A systematic approach to the evaluation of interpersonal relationships. *Am. J. Nurs.* 73:863, 1973.

Almore, M. G.   Dyadic communication. *Am. J. Nurs.* 79:1076, 1979.

Avila, D., Combs, A. W., and Purskey, W.   *The Helping Relationship Sourcebook.* Boston: Allyn and Bacon, 1971.

Blair, K. K.   It's the patient's problem and decision. *Nurs. Outlook* 19:588, 1971.

Brammer, L. M.   *The Helping Relationship, Process and Skills.* Englewood Cliffs, N.J.: Prentice-Hall, 1973.

Brill, N. I.   *Working with People: The Helping Process.* Philadelphia: Lippincott, 1973.

Combs, A. W., et al.   *Helping Relationship—Basic Concepts for the Helping Professions.* Boston: Allyn and Bacon, 1971.

Davis, R. C., and Woodcock, E.   The nursing contract: An alternative in care. *J. Psychiatr. Nurs.* 9:26, 1971.

Delaney, C., et al.   Promoting autonomy: Clinical contracts. *J. Nurs. Educ.* 16:22, 1977.

Gustafson, M. B.   Let's broaden our horizons about the use of contracts. *Intern. Nurs. Rev.* 24(1):18, 1977.

Hein, E. C.   *Communication in Nursing Practice.* Boston: Little, Brown, 1973.

Kalisch, B.   What is empathy? *Am. J. Nurs.* 73:1548, 1973.

Kinlein, M. L.   *Independent Nursing Practice with Clients.* Philadelphia: Lippincott, 1977.

Kron, T. T.   *Communication in Nursing.* Philadelphia: Saunders, 1972.

La Monica, E. L., et al.   Empathy: Educating nurses in professional practice. *J. Nurs. Educ.* 17(2):3, 1978.

Langford, T.   Establishing a nursing contract. *Nurs. Outlook* 26:386, 1978.

Levin, L. S., et al.   *Self-Care: Lay Initiatives in Health.* New York: Neale, Watson, 1976.

Lindberg, J. B., and Simms, L. M.   Contract grading: Incentives and rewards. *Image* 7(1):20, 1974.

Loomis, M.   The Health Care Contract. In M. Loomis, *Group Process for Nurses.* St. Louis: Mosby, 1979. Chap. 5.

Milio, N.   Self-care in urban settings. *Health Educ. Monogr.* 5:136, 1977.

Murphy, S.   Mutuality and the message: A conceptual model for nurse-client communication. *Oregon Nurse* 42:10, 1977.

Norris, C. M.   Self-care. *Am. J. Nurs.* 79:486, 1979.

O'Brien, M.   *Communications and Relationships in Nursing.* St. Louis: Mosby, 1978.

Orlando, I. J.   *The Dynamic Nurse-Patient Relationship.* New York: Putnam, 1961.

Peplau, H. E. *Interpersonal Relations in Nursing.* New York: Putnam, 1952.

Price, J. and Braden, C. The reality in home visits. *Am. J. Nurs.* 78:1536, 1978.

Rosen, B. Contract therapy. *Nurs. Times* 74:119, 1978.

Rowen, K., and Waring, B. The teaching contract. *Nurs. Outlook* 20:594, 1972.

Sauer, J. K. The Process of Contracting in the Helping Relationship. *Minnesota Welfare* Summer:12, 1973.

Seeger, P. A. Self-awareness and nursing. *J. Psychiatr. Nurs.* 15:24, 1977.

Sheridan, A., and Smith, R. A. Student-family contracts. *Nurs. Outlook* 23:114, 1975.

Sloan, M., and Schommer, B. T. The Process of Contracting in Community Nursing. In B. W. Spradley (Ed.), *Contemporary Community Nursing.* Boston: Little, Brown, 1975.

Stuart, R. B. Behavioral contracting within the families of delinquents. *J. Behav. Ther. Exp. Psychiatr.* 2:1, 1971.

Ulschak, F. L. Contracting: A Process and a Tool. In J. W. Pfeiffer and J. Jones (Eds.), *The 1978 Annual Handbook for Group Facilitators.* La Jolla, Calif.: University Associates, 1978.

Van Dersal, W. R. How to be a good communicator—And a better nurse. *Nursing '74* 4(12):57, 1974.

Wang, R. Y., et al. Contracting for weight reduction—Making the sacrifices worthwhile. *Matern. Child Nurs. J.* 3(1):46, 1978.

Wismer, J. Communication Effectiveness: Active Listening and Sending Feeling Messages. In J. W. Pfeiffer and J. Jones (Eds.), *The 1978 Annual Handbook for Group Facilitators.* La Jolla, Calif.: University Associates, 1978.

Zangari, M., and Duffy, P. Contracting with Patients in Day-to-Day Practice. *Am. J. Nurs.* 80:451, 1980.

SEVEN

HEALTH TEACHING

Clients in community health have many educational needs. A family with a newly diagnosed diabetic member needs to understand and regulate the diabetic regimen. A young couple with their first baby want to learn all the aspects of infant care, such as bathing, feeding, diapering, and formula preparation. Parents of young children form a group because they need to learn about parenting. A women's self-help group seeks to develop understanding of the female role and to acquire skills in assertiveness. Senior citizens adjusting to retirement and the aging process search for increased understanding and meaningful activities. Such situations all present community health nurses with the opportunity and challenge to meet client needs through health teaching.

Teaching represents a fundamental task in the nursing profession: "All nurses function as teachers. Nurses teach patients, families, ancillary personnel, and each other. Teaching is inherent in the nurse's role whether or not the nurse consciously cultivates and exhibits teacher behaviors" [2]. Identifying a need that is best met through teaching raises a series of questions. How can we teach effectively? What content should we cover? What method of presentation will communicate most effectively? What pamphlets or other visual aids can we use as teaching devices? How do we know when the client has grasped the information or mastered the skills? In other words, what makes teaching effective and how are teaching skills acquired? This chapter answers these questions and discusses the application of teaching as a tool in community health nursing practice.

THE NATURE OF LEARNING

The goal of all teaching is learning. Learning involves far more than the simple sharing of information. We have all been presented with information that was not interesting, relevant to our needs, or comprehensible. In such situations, we found it difficult to learn. The nurse as teacher seeks to relate information in such a way that the learner understands and some behavior change results. Effective teaching is a cause; learning becomes the effect. We cannot assume that imparting knowledge will guarantee understanding or change client health practices. To teach effectively in community health, we must understand the nature of learning. We want to consider three forms of learning—cognitive, affective, and psychomotor [1]. Then the teaching strategies that produce these kinds of learning can be examined.

COGNITIVE LEARNING

Cognitive learning involves the mind and thinking processes. It is mental knowledge. When we grasp the meaning and relationship of a series of facts, we experience cognitive learning. For example, acquisition of the following facts and relationships involves cognition: community groups have health needs; learning can meet some of those needs; community health nurses can foster learning among client populations; and effective teaching results in learning. The cognitive domain deals with "the recall or recognition of knowledge and the development of intellectual abilities and skills" [1]. It is useful to consider six major categories or levels in the cognitive domain [3].

KNOWLEDGE

Knowledge, the lowest level of learning, involves recall. If you can remember material previously learned, you have acquired knowledge. Nurses purposely aim for this level in teaching with some clients, particularly those who have limited ability to grasp the rationale behind prescribed health measures. For example, it is entirely appropriate to teach elderly patients the symptoms of stroke. Your goal may be for them to recall the facts about this illness rather than to understand underlying causes or treatment procedures. Clients may then remember that medication should be taken daily, that regular exercise will restore function, and that complete abstinence from alcohol is necessary, even though they may not grasp the reasons behind these measures.

COMPREHENSION

The second level of cognitive learning, comprehension, combines remembering with understanding. When possible, teaching aims at instilling at least minimum understanding. We want clients to grasp the meaning and to recognize the importance of suggested health behaviors. At the first level of cognitive learning, we can teach a hypertensive person to take medication daily. But comprehension will occur when we help this individual and her family to understand how her medication and lifestyle affect blood pressure, and how control of each factor can reduce the risk of stroke. We can teach pregnant women the relationship between nutrition and fetal development to help them realize the importance of a healthy diet.

APPLICATION

Application is the third level of cognitive learning. Here the learner takes understood material and applies it to new and actual situations. A more desirable level than the first two, application approaches the possibility of self-care, in which clients use their knowledge. To encourage application, the nurse can design teaching plans that show clients how to put knowledge into practice. One nurse suggested that the diabetic write down his Clinitest readings on a sheet of paper to show her at the next visit. Another, after instructing adolescents in a weight loss group about nutrition, asked each to keep a diet record for a week, draw up a diet plan, and share this plan with the group at the next meeting.

It is one thing to show a new mother how to bathe her infant; it is quite another to observe a return demonstration. The test of application is a transfer of understanding into practice. The pregnant woman who understands that her physical health and eating habits directly influence the health of her baby has not reached this level if she continues smoking and eating unbalanced foods. The diabetic who recognizes the high risk of infection has not applied this knowledge if he is careless with foot care. The construction worker who understands on-the-job hazards but seldom wears a protective hat in the work area has yet to transfer comprehension into practice.

ANALYSIS

The fourth level of cognitive learning is analysis. At this level, the learner breaks material down into parts, distinguishes between elements, and understands the relationships among the parts. A mother, for example, analyzes when she seeks to determine the cause of an infant's crying. After viewing the total situation, she then breaks it down into variables such as hunger, pain, loneliness, type of crying, and intensity of crying. She examines these parts and draws conclusions about their relationships. Analysis precedes problem solution in the same way that diagnosis precedes treatment. The learner carefully scrutinizes all the variables or elements and their relationships to each other in order to explain the situation. Similarly, analysis precedes identification of needs since we must first study all the assessment variables before we can draw conclusions about client needs. A family that studies its own communication patterns for the purpose of identifying sources of conflict is using analysis. This level of learning becomes a preliminary step toward problem solving. In our health teaching we foster clients' analytic skills by showing them how to isolate the parts in a situation and then encouraging them to do so themselves.

SYNTHESIS

Synthesis, a fifth level of cognitive learning, is the ability to form elements into a new whole. At this level of intellectual functioning, learners go beyond analyzing material to create something unique from it. Clients who achieve learning at this level will not only analyze their problems but also find solutions for them. For example, a nurse/teacher may assist mental health clients in a therapy group to analyze their frequent depression and then to generate their own plan for alleviating it. Synthesis combines all the earlier levels of cognitive learning to culminate in the production of a unique plan. A young couple who want to toilet train their two-year-old child learn the physiologic and psychological dimensions of toilet training, analyze their own situation, and then develop strategies (their own unique plan) for training the child. As health teachers, we facilitate synthesis by assisting and encouraging clients to develop their own solutions with specific plans. When someone identifies a problem, we can ask, "What are some possible causes? Do you see anything we have overlooked about the problem?" But when the client asks for a solution after such analysis, the nurse can encourage synthesis by asking, "What are some possible solutions to this problem that you might carry out?"

EVALUATION

The highest level of cognitive learning is evaluation. For the learner, to evaluate means to judge the usefulness of new material compared to a stated purpose [3]. Such a judgment requires specific criteria. Clients can learn to judge, for example, the consistency of their health behavior by comparing it to standards such as abstinence from smoking, maintenance of normal weight, or regular exercise. These are criteria established by others; however, clients may establish their own criteria. Parents may evaluate their parenting effectiveness when their parenting group sets up specific objectives as desired outcomes. The group, for example, could design activities to enhance parent-child communication, and members could then judge their performances by using the desired outcomes as evaluation criteria. When we, as nurse/teachers, aim for this level of client learning, we have made self-care a concrete objective. Evaluation, because it goes beyond attempts at problem solving, enables the client to judge the adequacy of solutions, to critique lifestyle and health-related behavior, and to anticipate needed improvements.

Cognitive learning at any of the levels we have described can be measured easily in terms of learner behaviors. We know, for instance, that clients have achieved our teaching objectives for application of knowledge when their behavior demonstrates actual use of the information we have taught. Client roles in cognitive learning range from relatively passive (at the knowledge level) to active (at the evaluation level). Conversely, as the client becomes more active, the nurse/teacher role becomes less directive. Table 7-1 illustrates client and nurse behaviors for each level.

AFFECTIVE LEARNING

The second domain in which learning occurs involves emotion, feeling, or affect. This kind of learning deals with "changes in interest, attitudes, and values" [1]. Here, as teachers, we face the task of trying to influence what clients value and feel. We want them to develop an ability to accept ideas that promote healthier behavior patterns but may conflict with their own values.

Attitudes and values are learned [6]. They develop gradually over time as the way in which an individual feels and responds is molded by family, peers, experiences, and societal influences. These feelings and responses are the result of imitation and conditioning. In this way, clients acquire their health-related beliefs and practices. Because attitudes and values become part of the person, they are difficult to change unless the nurse/teacher is aware of how they develop.

Affective learning occurs on several levels as the learner responds with varying degrees of involvement and commitment. At the first level, the learner is simply receptive. He is willing to listen, show

Table 7-1. Cognitive Learning

Level	Illustrative Client Behavior	Illustrative Nurse Behavior
Knowledge (recalls, knows)	States that insulin, if taken, will control own diabetes	Gives information
Comprehension (understands)	Describes insulin action and purpose	Explains information
Application (uses learning)	Adjusts insulin dosage daily to maintain proper blood sugar level	Suggests how to use learning
Analysis (examines, explains)	Discusses relationships between insulin, diet, activity, and diabetic control	Demonstrates and encourages analysis
Synthesis (integrates with other learning, generates new ideas)	Develops a plan for controlling own diabetes which incorporates above learning	Promotes client formulation of own plan
Evaluation (judges according to a standard)	Compares degree of diabetic control (outcomes) with desired control (objectives)	Facilitates evaluation

awareness, and be attentive. The teacher aims at acquiring and focusing the student's attention [3]. This limited goal may be all the client is ready for at the early stages of the nurse-client relationship.

At the second level, the learner becomes an active participant by responding to the information in some way. At this level, clients show willingness to read educational material that we give them, participate in discussion, complete assignments such as keeping a diet record, or voluntarily seek out more information on their own.

At the third level, the learner attaches value to the information. Valuing ranges from simple acceptance through appreciation to commitment. For example, a nurse taught members of a therapy group a number of principles concerning group effectiveness. She explained the importance of a democratic group process and ways to improve group skills. Members showed acceptance when they acknowledged the importance of these ideas. They showed appreciation by starting to practice the ideas. Commitment came when they assumed responsibility for having their group function well.

The final level of affective learning occurs when the learner internalizes an idea or value. The value system now controls learner behavior. Consistent practice is a crucial test at this level. The client who knows and respects the value of exercise, but only occasionally plays tennis or does calisthenics, has not internalized the value. Even several weeks of enthusiastic jogging is not evidence of an internalized value. If the jogging continues for six months, a year, and longer, learning is probably internalized.

Affective learning often remains elusive, difficult to measure. Indeed, this quality may influence community health nurses to concentrate their efforts on cognitive learning goals. Yet client attitudes and values have a major effect on the outcome of cognitive learning, desired behavior changes. For this reason, the two domains must remain linked in teaching; otherwise, results may quickly fade.

Attitudes and values can change in the same way they were first learned, that is, through imitation and conditioning [6]. Role models, particularly those from the client's peer group, who practice the desired health behaviors can be a strong influence. The use of groups like mastectomy clubs or chemical dependency support groups can have a powerful effect. Attitudes often change when you provide the client with a satisfying experience during the learning process. The nurse who recognizes the client's participation in a group, praises a client for completing an assignment, or commends a person for sticking to a diet plan will have more success than the nurse who only criticizes failures. Table 7-2 shows client and nurse behaviors for each level of affective learning.

To influence affective learning requires patience. Values and attitudes will seldom change overnight. Keep in mind that other forces will continue to reinforce former values. For example, a middle-aged housewife may value pursuing a career for self-fulfillment but cannot because her husband opposes an independent activity. Promoting cognitive learning by helping the client understand and try out positive health practices is also useful for influencing attitude change.

PSYCHOMOTOR LEARNING

The psychomotor domain includes visible, demonstrable performance skills that require some kind of neuromuscular coordination. Community health clients need to learn skills such as bathing an infant, doing range-of-motion exercises, irrigating a catheter, walking on crutches, examining breasts, taking a temperature, preparing special diets, and doing prenatal breathing exercises.

For psychomotor learning to take place, three conditions must be met. First, the learner must be capable of the skill. If you attempt to

Table 7-2. Affective Learning

Level	Illustrative Client Behavior	Illustrative Nurse Behavior
Receptive (listens, pays attention)	Attentive to family planning instruction	Directs client's attention
Responsive (participates, reacts)	Discusses pros and cons of various methods	Encourages client involvement
Valuing (accepts, appreciates, commits)	Selects a method for use	Respects client's right to decide
Internal consistency (organizes values to fit together)	Understands and accepts responsibility for limiting number of children	Brings client into contact with role models
Adoption (incorporates new values into lifestyle)	Consistently practices birth control	Positively reinforces healthy behaviors

teach an elderly diabetic man with tremulous hands and fading vision to give his own insulin injections, it could frustrate and possibly harm him. Some other person more physically capable should probably be enlisted and taught the skill. Clients' intellectual and emotional capabilities also influence their capacity to learn motor skills. We should not expect a person of limited intelligence to learn complex skills. Match the degree of complexity to the learner's level of functioning. Developmental stage is another point to consider in determining whether a skill is appropriate to teach. For example, most children can put on some article of clothing at two years of age but are not ready to learn to fasten buttons until well past their third birthday.

The learner must also have a sensory image of how to perform the skill. This is a second condition for psychomotor learning. Through sight, hearing, touch, and sometimes taste or smell, clients gain a picture of the skill. They acquire this sensory image by means of demonstration. Our first image of how to drive a car, for instance, comes from watching someone else drive. We observe their eyes, hands, and feet, the coordination between clutch and gear shift, auto speed, and road conditions. Verbal explanations enhance our understanding of the mechanics of driving. In order to teach clients motor skills effectively, we have to provide them with an adequate sensory image. We must demonstrate and explain slowly, one point at a time, and repeatedly if needed, until they understand the proper sequence of actions necessary to achieve the skill.

The third necessary condition for psychomotor learning is practice.

Table 7-3. Nurse Behaviors in Psychomotor Learning

Determining Capability	Providing Sensory Image	Encouraging Practice
Nurse assesses client's physical, intellectual, and emotional ability	Nurse demonstrates and explains	Nurse uses guidance and positive reinforcement

After acquiring a sensory image, the learner can start to perform the skill. Mastery will come over time as the learner repeats the performance until it is smooth, coordinated, and unhesitating. During this process the teacher should be available to provide guidance and encouragement. In the early stages of practice the teacher may need to use "hands on" guidance to give the learner a sense of how the performance should feel. Similarly, a nurse demonstrates passive range-of-motion exercises on a client's wife to show her how they should feel before she learns to do them for her husband. During practice, feedback from the nurse will enable the learner to know if the skill is being performed correctly. When the client gives a return demonstration, the teacher can make suggestions, give encouragement, and thereby maximize learning effectiveness.

The psychomotor domain, like the cognitive and affective domains, ranges from simple to complex levels of functioning. It is necessary to exercise judgment in assessing clients' ability to perform the skill. Even clients with limited ability can often move on to higher levels once they have mastered simple skills. Nurse behaviors that influence psychomotor learning are shown in Table 7-3.

TEACHING

A sixth grade teacher recently announced to her class, "My job here is to teach; your job is to learn. I don't care whether you learn or not, but if you want to learn, that's your responsibility. I'm being paid to teach." This kind of noncaring message only creates confusion and consternation among students. Yet, without meaning to, nurses may convey a similar message to clients. "I'm here to teach you how to get healthy and stay healthy," we say in so many words. "Whether you do or not is up to you." It is almost as though, having carried out our teaching responsibility, we can wash our hands of the whole business. How often do nurses chart "patient taught colostomy care," "diabetic teaching done," "explained medication dosage and side effects," and "baby bath and formula preparation demonstrated" with little awareness of whether and how much learning occurred?

Teaching lies at one end of a process. At the other end is learning. Without learning, teaching becomes useless in much the same way that communication does not occur unless a message is both sent and received. The sixth grade teacher was trying to point this out to her students when she pushed the entire responsibility for learning on their shoulders. While we can question the effectiveness of her approach, her point remains valid. Learners must take responsibility for their own learning [4]. We obstruct that process if we assume complete responsibility for bringing about changed behavior. Without a thirst for health information, our clients can be led to water but still will not participate in the learning process. Teaching, then, becomes a matter of facilitating both the thirst and the best conditions for satisfying it. Teaching in community health nursing means to influence, motivate, and act as catalysts in the learning process. We "bring knowledge and learner together and stimulate a reaction" [2]. We facilitate learning when we make it as easy as possible for clients to change. To do this, we need to know basic principles underlying the teaching-learning process. Teaching also requires the use of appropriate tools to influence learning.

TEACHING-LEARNING PRINCIPLES

CLIENT READINESS

Clients' readiness to learn influences teaching effectiveness. A young primipara was not ready for prenatal teaching on fetal growth and development. She had strong fears, the nurse discovered, that "losing her figure" would make her sexually unattractive to her husband. Until these anxieties had subsided, the teaching would remain ineffective. Clients' needs, interests, and concerns determine their readiness for learning. Another factor that influences readiness is educational background. If a group of women who never completed grade school meet to learn how to care for a sick person in the home, sessions should present material simply, factually, and in terms that they understand. To discuss complex concepts of health, illness, and scientific research would be above their level of readiness.

Maturational level also affects readiness. A one-year-old child is not ready to share his toys but a five-year-old child has reached a level that makes him ready to learn these social skills. An adolescent mother who is still working on normal developmental tasks of her age group may not be ready to learn parenting skills. Readiness of the client will determine the amount of material presented in each teaching session (Fig. 7-1). The pace or speed with which you present information must be manageable. A moderate amount of anxiety will often increase

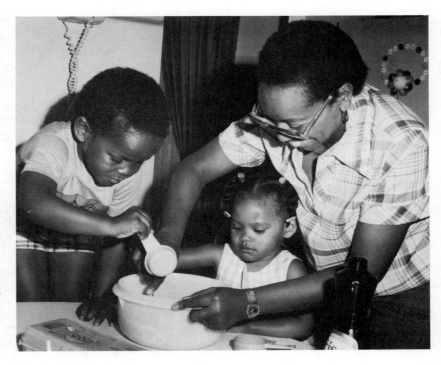

Figure 7-1. The boy in this family is old enough to help measure the ingredients for the cake. His younger sister helps to stir. Their maturational level influences their readiness to learn new tasks. (From C. Schuster and S. Ashburn, *The Process of Human Development: A Holistic Approach.* Boston: Little, Brown, 1980. Photograph by Glenn Jackson.)

client receptivity to learning; however, high or low levels of anxiety can have the opposite effect.

CLIENT PERCEPTION

Clients' perceptions affect their learning. People's perceptions, the way they see the world, act like a screening device through which all new information must pass [5]. Our perceptions help us to interpret and attach meaning to things. For example, one person views a piece of sculpture and exclaims over its beauty. Another person, seeing the same object, remarks on its ugliness and lack of coherence. These two people have different perceptions. In community health nursing, one client may view the notion of parenting as a positive, growth-producing relationship; another may see it as a conflict-ridden, unhappy experience to avoid. Each kind of perception has a different consequence for learning.

A wide range of variables affect human perception. These variables include values, past experiences, culture, religion, personality, developmental stage, educational and economic level, surrounding social forces, and the physical environment (Fig. 7-2). An adolescent boy

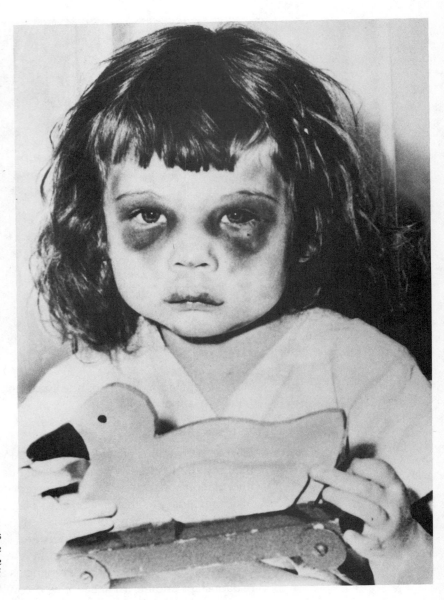

Figure 7-2. The abused child's
experience will strongly influence
her future perceptions of the
parenting role. (Courtesy of
United Press International.)

who has been told to stop taking drugs will resist if he perceives this instruction as an affront to his identity and independence. He wants to make decisions for himself. The nurse/teacher, recognizing the forces at work, will try to work within the boy's frame of reference by presenting information in a way that still gives the boy options to make his own choices. Otherwise, his perception of the situation will limit his learning.

Frequently clients use selective perception. They screen out some of our statements and pay attention to those that fit their values or personal desires. A nurse was teaching a client the various risk factors in coronary disease; the individual screened out smoking and obesity, paying attention only to factors that would not require a drastic change in lifestyle. We must know our clients, understand their backgrounds and values, and learn what their perceptions are before our teaching can influence their learning potential.

CLIENT PARTICIPATION

The degree of client participation in the educational process directly influences the amount of client learning. One nurse discovered this principle when working with a group of people nearing retirement. After talking to them about the changes and needs they would face met with little response, she shifted to a different method of teaching. She distributed pamphlets and asked everyone to read each week and come prepared for discussion. Slowly the group began to participate in their own learning to a greater degree. Whenever the nurse works with clients in a learning context, one of the first questions to discuss is "What does the client want to learn?" As Carl Rogers has said [7]:

learning is facilitated when the student participates responsibly in the learning process. When he chooses his own directions, helps to discover his own learning resources, formulates his own problems, decides his own course of action, lives with the consequences of each of these choices, then significant learning is maximized.

The amount of learning is directly proportional to the learners' involvement. A group of senior citizens attended a class on nutrition and aging, yet still made almost no changes in their diet or eating patterns. It was not until the members became actively involved in the class, encouraged by the nurse to present problems and solutions for food purchasing and preparation on limited budgets, that any significant behavior changes occurred.

Contracting, discussed in Chapter Six, can contribute to the nurse's teaching goals. It directly involves the client in a partnership to determine goals, content, and time for learning. Contracting in the context of teaching can develop a great sense of accountability in clients for their own learning.

SUBJECT'S RELEVANCE TO CLIENT

Subject matter that is relevant to the client is learned more readily and retained longer than information that is not meaningful. Learners gain the most from subject matter immediately useful to their own purposes. Consider two middle management level men taking a physical fitness course offered by their employer. One, a father of a cub scout, has agreed to co-lead his son's troop on a two-week backpacking trip in the mountains. He wants to get in shape. The second man is taking the course because it is required by the company. Its only relevance to his own purposes is that it keeps him from gaining his boss's disfavor. There can be little question as to which man will learn and retain the most. The course has considerable relevance and meaning to the first man, almost none to the second.

Relevance influences the speed of learning. When a two-year-old child sees his little friend from down the street riding a tricycle, he quickly learns to peddle his own. It becomes very important to him to learn; therefore, he learns quickly. The diabetic who must give herself daily injections of insulin learns that skill very quickly (Fig. 7-3). A housewife and mother with a broken leg rapidly learns to manage crutch-walking. Each client sees considerable relevance in the learning and thus accomplishes it with great speed. "There is evidence that the time for learning various subjects would be cut to a fraction of the time currently allotted if the material were perceived by the learner as related to his own purposes. Probably one-third to one-fifth of the present time allotment would be sufficient" [7].

When subject matter is relevant to the learner, there is also greater retention of knowledge. The learner, upon seeing the usefulness of the material, develops a strong motivation to acquire and utilize it, and will be less likely to forget it. Even in instances when a previously learned motor skill has not been used for many years, it is often quickly recaptured under such conditions.

CLIENT SATISFACTION

The client must derive satisfaction from learning to maintain motivation and increase self-direction [6]. Learners need to feel a sense of steady

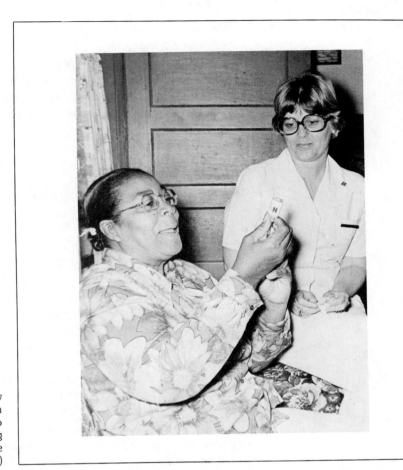

Figure 7-3. This client quickly learns to give herself daily insulin injections because she is eager to return to as normal functioning as possible. (Courtesy of Lake Charles Lousiana Press.)

progress in the learning process. Obstacles, frustrations, and failures along the way discourage and impede learning. Many stroke patients with potential for rehabilitation give up trying to regain speech or use of paralyzed limbs because they become too frustrated and dissatisfied in the process. On the other hand, clients who experience satisfaction and progress in their speech and muscle retraining maintain their motivation and work on exercises without prompting.

Realistic goals contribute to learner satisfaction. Objectives should be set within the learner's ability, thereby avoiding the frustration that comes from a too difficult task and the loss of interest that results from one too easy. Setting objectives requires agreement on goals, periodic reviews, and revision of goals if they become too easy or too difficult.

We further promote clients' learning satisfaction by designing tasks with rewards. One nurse led a class for obese adolescents and together they set the goal of a three pound weight loss each week. The school nurse helped the group design a plan which included counting calories and a "buddy system" as ways to help bring about a behavior change. If each member in the group achieved the three pound goal, the group went on a field trip or excursion of their choice as a reward. These students found this learning experience satisfying because goals were attainable and their progress was rewarded. Instead of competing with one another, the group set out to help each member achieve the goal. As a result, most kept the weight off after the class had finished.

CLIENT APPLICATION

Learning is reinforced through application. The students in the weight loss group began immediately to count calories. They could begin to apply their knowledge. The learner needs as many opportunities as possible to apply the learning in daily life. If they arise during the teaching-learning process, the client can try out new knowledge and skills under supervision. The learner is given an opportunity to start integrating the learning into his daily life at a time when the teacher is there to help reinforce that pattern.

Take a prenatal class as an example. The learning only begins with explanations of proper diet, exercise, breathing techniques, hygiene, avoidance of alcohol and tobacco, and so on. More learning occurs as the group discusses these issues and applies them intellectually, exploring ways they could practice them at home. Additional reinforcement comes by demonstrating how to do these activities; sample diets, demonstrations of exercises, display of posters, pamphlets, or models may be used. The group can begin application in the classroom by making diet plans, doing exercises, role playing parenting behavior, or engaging in group problem solving. Then the members can be encouraged to apply these activities on a daily basis at home and prepare to share their results at future sessions.

Frequent use of newly acquired information fosters transfer of learning to other situations. Our major goal of prevention and health promotion depends on such a transfer. For instance, mothers who learn and practice a well-balanced diet, free of non-nutritious snacks, can be encouraged to offer more nourishing foods to their whole families. The family that practices asepsis and good hand-washing techniques when caring for a postsurgical wound can learn to transfer this same principle to prevention of infection in daily living.

TEACHING PROCESS

The process of teaching in community health nursing follows steps similar to the nursing process:

1. *Interaction*   Establish basic communication patterns between client and nurse.
2. *Assessment*   Determine clients' present status and identify needs for teaching.
3. *Goal Setting*   Identify needed changes and prepare objectives that describe the desired learning outcomes.
4. *Planning*   Design a plan for the learning experience that meets the objectives; include the content to be covered, sequence of topics, best conditions for learning (place, kind of environment), methods, and tools (visual aids, exercises, etc.). A written plan is best; it may or may not be part of the written nursing care plan.
5. *Teaching*   Implement the learning experience by carrying out the planned activities.
6. *Evaluation*   Determine whether learning objectives were met and if not, why not. Evaluation measures progress toward goals and can indicate future learning needs.

Teaching occurs on many levels and incorporates various types of activities. It can be formal or informal, planned or unplanned. Formal presentations, such as lectures, are generally planned and fairly structured. Some teaching is less formal but still planned and relatively structured, as in group discussions where questions stimulate exploration of ideas and guide thinking. Informal levels of teaching, such as counseling or anticipatory guidance, require background preparation but often no definite plan of presentation. The teaching process is guided by the client's concerns. Teaching often occurs in casual conversations, spontaneously in situations where clients raise unexpected questions, or when a crisis arises. In these instances, nurses draw on their background of knowledge and exercise professional judgment in their teaching. Finally, we teach by example: actions usually speak louder than words. If we teach the importance of asepsis in the home care of a wound, then fail to wash our hands before changing the dressing, the message of our actions will carry more impact than our words. The healthy nurse who exhibits healthy practices serves as a role model as well as a health teacher.

TEACHING METHODS AND TOOLS

LECTURE

There are times when the community health nurse will present information to a large group, such as a PTA meeting, a women's club luncheon, or a county board of commissioners. Under such circumstances, the lecture method, a formal kind of presentation, may be the most efficient means of communicating health information. However, lectures tend to create a passive learning atmosphere for the audience unless accompanied by strategies devised to involve the learners. Many individuals are visual rather than auditory learners. To capture their attention, slides, overhead projections, films, or videotapes can supplement the lecture. Allowing time for questions and discussion after a lecture will also involve the learners more actively.

DISCUSSION

Two-way communication is an important feature of the learning process. Learners need an opportunity to raise questions, make comments, reason out loud, and receive feedback in order to develop understanding. Discussion, used in conjunction with other teaching methods such as demonstration, lecture, and role playing, will improve their effectiveness. In group teaching, discussion enables clients to learn from one another as well as from the nurse. One difficulty that can arise is monopolization of the discussion by one person while others seldom express themselves. The nurse/teacher must exercise leadership in controlling and guiding the discussion so that learning opportunities are maximized. Prepared objectives and discussion organized around specific questions or topics make the discussion most fruitful.

DEMONSTRATION

The demonstration method is often used for teaching motor skills and is best accompanied by explanation and discussion. It can give the client a clear sensory image of how to perform the skill. Because a demonstration should be within easy visual and auditory range of the learner, it is best to demonstrate in front of small groups. Use the same kind of equipment that the client will use in order to show exactly how the skill should be performed, and provide the client with ample opportunity to practice until the skill is perfected. Again, objectives, content, and sequence of learning activities should all be planned ahead of time.

ROLE PLAYING

There are times when having clients assume and act out roles maximizes learning. A parenting group, for example, found it helpful to place themselves in the role of their children; their feelings about various ways to respond became more apparent. Reversing roles can effectively teach a married couple in conflict about better ways to communicate. In order to prevent role playing from becoming a game with little learning, plan the proposed drama with clear objectives in mind. What behavioral outcomes do you hope to achieve? Define the context, the "stage," clearly so that everyone shares in the situation. Then define each role ahead of time, making sure everyone understands their performance. Emphasize that no wrong or right performance exists, merely the way they see people behaving in everyday life. Avoid having people play themselves; it can be both embarrassing and difficult to achieve objectivity. After the drama has concluded, elicit discussion with carefully prepared questions.

Many different tools, often used in combination, are useful during the teaching process. Visual images—pictures, slides, films, posters, chalkboards, videotapes, bulletin boards, flash cards, pamphlets, and even gestures—can enhance almost any learning. Some tools such as sound films, record players, or tape recorders provide an auditory stimulus. Other tools, for example, models or objects, allow clients both visual and tactile learning (Fig. 7-4). Still others, such as programmed instruction or games, involve learners actively through reading and activity.

SUMMARY

A large part of community health nursing practice involves teaching. Far more than to simply give health information to clients, the purpose of teaching is to change client behavior to healthier practices.

Understanding the nature of learning contributes to the effectiveness of teaching in community health. Learning occurs in three domains—cognitive, affective, and psychomotor. The cognitive domain refers to learning that takes place intellectually, through the mind. It ranges in levels of learner functioning from simple recall to complex evaluation. As the learner moves up the scale of cognitive learning, he becomes more self-directed; the nurse/teacher assumes a more facilitative role.

Affective learning means the changing of attitudes and values. The learner may experience several levels of affective involvement from simple listening to adopting the new value. Again, as the client/learner involvement increases, the nurse/teacher becomes less directive.

Psychomotor learning involves the acquisition of motor skills. Clients who need to learn psychomotor skills must meet three conditions: they must be capable of the skill; they must develop a sensory image of the skill; and they must practice the skill.

Teaching in community health nursing is the facilitation of learning

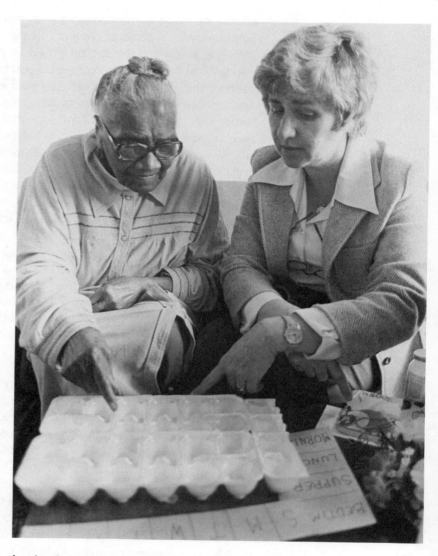

Figure 7-4. Teaching methods and tools vary with clients' learning needs. On this home visit the nurse uses an egg container with labels to help an elderly woman with limited vision devise a plan for taking her medications. (Courtesy of Beth Israel Hospital, Boston. Photograph by Michael Lutch.)

that leads to behavior change in the client. Thus teaching is a catalytic process based on the following teaching-learning principles:

1. Client readiness for learning influences teaching effectiveness.
2. Clients' perceptions affect their learning.
3. The degree of client participation in the educational process directly influences the amount of client learning.
4. Subject matter that is relevant to the client is learned more readily and retained longer than information that is not meaningful.

5. The client must derive satisfaction from the learning to maintain motivation and increase self-direction.
6. Learning is reinforced through application.

The teaching process in community health nursing is similar to the steps of the nursing process. It includes interaction, assessment, goal setting, planning, teaching, and evaluation. The actual teaching may be formal or informal, planned or unplanned. Methods may range from structured lecture presentations to demonstration and role playing. Selection of a tool depends on how well it suits the client/learner and helps to meet the desired objectives.

REFERENCES

1. Bloom, B. (Ed.). *Taxonomy of Educational Objectives: The Classification of Educational Goals. Handbook I: Cognitive Domain.* New York: Longman, 1956.
2. Douglass, L. M., and Bevis, E. O. *Nursing Leadership in Action— Principles and Application to Staff Situations.* St. Louis: Mosby, 1974. Pp. 30, 31.
3. Gronlund, N. E. *Stating Behavioral Objectives for Classroom Instruction.* New York: Macmillan, 1970. Pp. 20, 22.
4. Levin, L. S. Patient education and self-care: How do they differ? *Nurs. Outlook* 26:170, 1978.
5. Marriner, A. Health Teaching. In A. Marriner, *The Nursing Process* (2nd ed.). St. Louis: Mosby, 1979. P. 137.
6. Redman, B. K. *The Process of Patient Teaching in Nursing* (3rd ed.). St. Louis: Mosby, 1976. Pp. 62–67.
7. Rogers, C. *Freedom to Learn.* Columbus, Ohio: Merrill, 1969. Pp. 158–162.

SELECTED READINGS

Bigge, M. L. *Learning Theories for Teachers.* New York: Harper and Row, 1971.

Bloom, B. (Ed.). *Taxonomy of Educational Objectives: The Classification of Educational Goals. Handbook I: Cognitive Domain.* New York: Longman, 1956.

Borgman, M. F. Exercise and health maintenance. *J. Nurs. Educ.* 16(1):6, 1977.

Bryan, N. E. Every nurse a teacher. *Austral. Nurses J.* 4(1):31, 1974.

Buford, L. M. Group education to reduce overweight: Classes for mentally handicapped children. *Am. J. Nurs.* 75:1194, 1975.

Crow, M., Bradshaw, B., and Guest, F. True to life: A relevant approach to patient education. *Am. J. Public Health* 62:1328, 1972.

Douglass, L. M., and Bevis, E. O. *Nursing Leadership in Action—Principles and Application to Staff Situations.* St. Louis: Mosby, 1974.

Flowers, L. K. The development of a program for treating obesity. *Hosp. Community Psychiatry* 27(5):342, 1976.

Green, L. W. Evaluation and measurement: Some dilemmas for health education. *Am. J. Public Health* 67:155, 1977.

Gronlund, N. E. *Stating behavioral objectives for classroom instruction.* New York: Macmillan, 1970.

Haskin, J., Hawley, N., and Weinberger, J. Project teen concern: An educational approach to the prevention of venereal disease and premature parenthood. *J. Sch. Health* 46(4):231, 1976.

Hein, E. C. Teaching psychosocial wellness in family and community health nursing. *Nurse Educator* 3:22, 1978.

Heit, P. Educating the nurse–community health educator to educate. *J. Nurs. Educ.* 17(1):21, 1978.

Hill, W. F. *Learning—A Survey of Psychological Interpretations.* Scranton, Pa.: Chandler, 1971.

Jones, P., and Oertel, W. Developing patient teaching objectives + techniques: A self-instructional program. *Nurse Educator* 2(5):3, 1977.

Knowles, M. *The Modern Practice of Adult Education.* New York: Associated Press, 1970.

Knowles, M. *Self-Directed Learning: A Guide for Learners and Teachers.* New York: Associated Press, 1975.

Kopelke, C. E. Group education to reduce overweight . . . in a blue-collar community. *Am. J. Nurs.* 75:1993, 1975.

Kyle, J. R., and Savino, A. B. Teaching parents behavior modification. *Nurs. Outlook* 21:717, 1973.

Leahy, K. M., and Bell, A. T. *Teaching Methods in Public Health Nursing.* Philadelphia: Saunders, 1952.

Levin, L. S. Patient education and self-care: How do they differ? *Nurs. Outlook* 26:170, 1978.

Marriner, A. The role of the school nurse in health education. *Am. J. Public Health* 61:2155, 1971.

Marriner, A. Health Teaching. In A. Marriner, *The Nursing Process* (2nd ed.). St. Louis: Mosby, 1979. P. 133.

Milio, N. A broad perspective on health: A teaching-learning tool. *Nurs. Outlook* 24:160, 1976.

Milio, N. A framework for prevention: Changing health-damaging to health-generating life patterns. *Am. J. Public Health* 66:435, 1976.

Mohammed, M. F. Patients' understanding of written health information. *Nurs. Res.* 13:100, 1964.

Murray, R., and Zentner, J. Guidelines for more effective health teaching. *Nursing '76* 6(2):44, 1976.

Narrow, B. *Patient teaching in nursing practice: A patient and family-centered approach.* Somerset, N.J.: Wiley, 1979.

Neeman, R. L., and Neeman, M. Complexities of smoking education. *J. Sch. Health* 45(1):17, 1975.

Pohl, M. *The Teaching Function of the Nursing Practitioner* (2nd ed.). Dubuque, Iowa: Brown, 1973.

Redman, B. K. *The Process of Patient Teaching in Nursing* (4th ed.). St. Louis: Mosby, 1980.

Reilly, D. E. (Ed.). *Teaching and Evaluating the Affective Domain in Nursing Programs.* Thorofare, N.J.: Charles B. Slack, 1978.

Richie, N. D. Some guidelines for conducting a health fair. *Public Health Rep.* 91:261, 1976.

Robinson, G., and Filkins, M. Group teaching with outpatients. *Am. J. Nurs.* 64:110, 1964.

Rogers, C. R. *Freedom to Learn.* Columbus, Ohio: Merrill, 1969.

Schweer, J. E., and Gebbie, K. M. *Creative Teaching in Clinical Nursing.* St. Louis: Mosby, 1976.

Simmons, J. (Ed.). Making health education work. *Am. J. Public Health* (Oct. Suppl.) 65:1–49, 1975.

Stewart, R. F. Education for health maintenance. *Occup. Health Nurs.* 22(6):14, 1974.

Thompson, W. Health education: II. How do we communicate? *Nurs. Times* 74:1561, 1978.

Tinch, J. For sickness or for health? *Nurs. Mirror* 140(17):71, 1975.

Valadez, A. M., and Heusinkveld, K. B. Teaching nursing students to teach patients. *J. Nurs. Educ.* 16(4):10, 1977.

EIGHT

CRISIS INTERVENTION AND PREVENTION

All human beings, individually and collectively, experience periods of upset, trouble, even danger. A teenager discovers she is pregnant. The father and breadwinner in a family loses his job. A beloved leader dies. A man faces retirement. An accident at a nuclear power plant threatens a community. A woman has her first baby. These life experiences produce stress and anxiety. Each event causes changes in peoples' behavior; each requires days, weeks, even months of adjustment and coping. These are times of crisis.

People respond differently to crisis. Some see the event as a challenge; others see it as adversity. What one person defines as crisis, another treats as a normal occurrence. Some seek out the help they need and come through the experience unscathed, perhaps even stronger than before. Others, unable to cope, incur severe, sometimes permanent, damage.

Regardless of their responses, people in a crisis need help. Equally important, they are receptive to help. Community health practitioners have a unique opportunity to provide that assistance because we can see clients frequently and in a broad environmental context. Not only can we give assistance during a time of crisis, but we can also help people equip themselves with the tools needed in crisis management and prevention. Furthermore, community health practitioners are concerned about crises at the aggregate level. When the Three Mile Island nuclear power plant accident occurred, for example, it created a crisis for families, groups, communities, and, indeed, our whole society. Major professional challenges in community health are to prevent crises and to help people in crisis. This chapter examines how we can sharpen our knowledge and skills in the practice of crisis prevention and intervention.

CRISIS THEORY

Our understanding about crises has grown considerably. At one time, we equated crisis only with disaster; it might have been natural (a flood), economic (a stock market crash), political (a presidential assassination), environmental (water polluted with chemicals), personal (death of a loved one), or another form of disaster. Researchers have studied the nature of crisis and have now developed a body of knowledge called crisis theory. Initially limited to the field of mental health, crisis theory now influences every field of health care. We know, for example, that a crisis is not an event per se, but rather people's perception of the event. We know that different kinds of crises occur; we can explain why people respond the way they do in a crisis; we can predict the phases that people go through in a crisis of any kind. These are important aspects to understand before we can prevent, manage, or intervene in crises.

DYNAMICS OF CRISIS

How does a crisis occur? People as living systems behave in certain ways, which are generally unconscious, in order to maintain relative equilibrium within themselves and in their relations with others. When some internal or external force disrupts the system's balance and alters its functioning, loss of homeostasis occurs. To restore equilibrium, people attempt to cope. They develop problem-solving behaviors that become habitual through repeated, although not always successful, use. Caplan points out that during the brief period before a problem is resolved, the person experiences tension [3]. But the tension is manageable because the person knows from previous problem-solving successes that the outcomes will be positive. He has also learned techniques for handling the tension. For example, John has a blowout while driving his car. This event creates a brief period of tension. But as John locates the spare and begins to change the flat tire, his anxiety subsides. He uses his knowledge to solve the problem.

In a crisis, the dynamics change. The problem is unfamiliar and greater than usual. It calls for a dramatic alteration of the person's accustomed role or responsibilities, or both. Tension develops. The individual tries his customary problem-solving responses only to find them inadequate. It becomes impossible to restore equilibrium; anxiety mounts. If, instead of a flat tire, John's car has a head-on collision with a truck, pinning him underneath the wreckage, he cannot use his past knowledge to solve the problem. His anxiety rises and a crisis ensues.

The problem persists and tension grows more apparent. The person continues to apply his usual problem-solving techniques or directs his efforts toward handling his tension. John, for example, may call loudly for help or tell himself, "Don't worry, someone will get you out." If these efforts fail to solve the problem, the feelings of anxiety and inadequacy will increase. "A person in this situation feels helpless—he is caught in a state of great emotional upset and feels unable to take action *on his own* to solve the problem" [1, p. 1].

Increased stress caused by further rise in tension and anxiety serves as a catalyst for some people to resolve the problem. Realizing that they cannot solve it on their own with their usual coping mechanisms, they mobilize new internal resources, seek outside help, and define the problem in a new way that makes it manageable.

For others, the problem remains. Stimulated by the same tension, they may seek new solutions without success. The help they receive may not redefine their problem in a realistic and workable manner. They may choose to avoid the problem by resigning themselves to it or minimizing its importance. Tension and anxiety mount rapidly or gradually, but ultimately people reach a point beyond which they can no longer function. Drastic results can follow, such as suicide, mass hysteria, myocardial infarction, psychotic breaks, ulcers, and family or group disintegration.

Caplan has summarized in four stages the effect of rising tension on the functioning of the person in crisis [3]:

1. Tension develops (as a result of precipitating event)	People use customary problem-solving responses in order to restore equilibrium.
2. Tension increases	Failure to cope leads to feeling upset and ineffectual.
3. Tension rises further	Increased tension acts as a stimulus to mobilize internal and external resources. People try to redefine the situation and may solve the problem, in which case tension abates.
4. Tension reaches threshold	If problem continues unsolved (or avoided), the breaking point is reached, causing major disorganization both socially and individually.

Thus, in a crisis, a certain amount of tension or stress may promote problem resolution and restoration of equilibrium. However, stress that becomes too intense and is unrelieved will ultimately lead to system breakdown.

DEFINITION OF CRISIS

Crisis is a temporary state of severe disequilibrium for persons who face a situation they find threatening and which they can neither escape from nor solve with their usual coping abilities [3, 4].

Let us look at several key characteristics of this definition in the context of a family in which the father is killed unexpectedly in a plane crash [3]. Crisis begins with a sense that things are *out of balance*. It causes the awareness of being upset, a state of considerable disequilibrium with resulting tension. Crises create "sudden discontinuities in the functioning pattern" [3, p. 39]. The man's wife and three children feel shattered by the news. The rhythm of their family life comes to a halt. Bills go unpaid; someone else must prepare meals. The family has been pushed out of balance.

Crisis is a *temporary condition.* A system's strong need to regain homeostasis means that the disequilibrium of a crisis does not go on indefinitely. Most crises last from four to six weeks [1]. In this family, as shocking as the loss might seem, life begins to return to a more regular pattern in a few weeks. Although the members will feel the loss of husband and father for years, the crisis will soon disappear.

A crisis involves *cognitive uncertainty.* Much stress comes from not understanding the situation and not knowing its outcome. Immediate questions about notifying friends and planning the funeral raise uncertainty for the family that has lost a father. Long-range questions can plague every family member.

A crisis situation is *hazardous.* For the persons involved, crisis represents an actual loss (the death of a loved one), the threat of a loss (terminal illness), or an overwhelming challenge (the offer of an important job). With her husband dead, the wife faces sudden financial insecurity. She has also lost her major source of emotional support.

Crisis brings on *psychophysiologic symptoms.* People react somatically to the stress. They may experience appetite fluctuations, sleeplessness, body aches, nausea, muscle tension, perspiration, rapid pulse, and other signs of anxiety, as well as fear, shame, guilt, or excitement. The specific reaction depends on the nature of the situation, how it is perceived, and inherited tendencies. The children who have lost their father become irritable, cry, and may feel sick. The wife and mother may experience shortness of breath and exhaustion.

A crisis situation is *inescapable*. People face an unavoidable demand for change. The experience cannot be reversed or ignored. It requires some kind of action or response. When the head of a household dies suddenly, the other family members cannot escape the loss. Death brings inevitable changes for each of the remaining individuals.

Crisis often reveals *inadequate coping skills*. Habitual problem-solving resources do not work in this situation. The children have all known times when their father was absent from the family and have developed ways to cope with such temporary loss. But in this crisis situation, their father's death means permanent loss. They cannot deal with it in the same way.

Crisis creates a feeling of *helplessness*. The person feels over-whelmed, paralyzed, and unable to think or take action on his or her own. It is a time when the family members may ask others what to do. Sometimes helplessness takes the form of immobility; the wife may be unable to make even the simplest decisions.

Crisis elicits *exaggerated defense mechanisms*. Behaviors such as rationalizing excessively, compensating for losses, and blaming others are often evident. The wife may blame her husband's boss for over-working him and making him take the business trip that ended fatally.

Each crisis presents a unique problem, one too difficult for the person to solve alone with his normal coping mechanisms yet one too important to ignore. The problem represents a threat to the satisfaction of some basic need. An imbalance exists between supply and demand: the resources of the person are insufficient under the circumstances.

Every crisis constitutes a turning point. It presents people with an opportunity for growth toward a healthier state; it also brings the danger of increased vulnerability to illness. Growth occurs when we mature in the crisis and develop more effective problem-solving skills. Some persons, drawing on new resources, redefine the crisis of divorce, for instance, as a challenge to make a new life, to discover themselves and their potential, and to learn to establish healthier relationships with others. Those who engage in healthy adaptation during a crisis will emerge unharmed, even strengthened. They have become prepared to cope with similar events in the future.

Crises, however, present dangers as well as provide opportunities. The loss of homeostasis increases the person's vulnerability to illness, mental or physical, and regression [11]. Some divorced persons, for instance, may not handle the crisis well; they may receive inadequate help from others and become bitter, withdrawn, and resentful. These individuals have moved toward an unhealthy outcome as a result of maladaptive behavior. Ways in which the nurse can help the person or group handle crisis adaptively will be examined later.

KINDS OF CRISES

When disease struck Philadelphia following an American Legion convention, panic and fear spread quickly. Who would contract the rapidly developing symptoms next and perhaps die? The situation threatened the very lives of the city's residents. An overwhelming feeling of helplessness arose as public health authorities and city officials struggled in vain to control the disease and identify its cause. For many people it was clearly a crisis.

Other less dramatic and less threatening events can still create anxiety and stress. They also require coping skills beyond those practiced by the persons involved. A young couple is overwhelmed at the responsibility of becoming parents. An elderly woman panics at the thought of moving to a nursing home. A boy entering puberty feels confused and anxious. Like the Legionnaires' disease outbreak, these too are crises, but of a different type.

There are two kinds of crises. The Legionnaires' disease event exemplifies a situational (or accidental) crisis. The other kind is a maturational (or developmental) crisis.

MATURATIONAL CRISES

Maturational crises are periods of disruption that occur at transition points in normal growth and development. The people involved feel threatened by the demands placed on them; they have difficulty making the changes necessary to fit the new stage of development.

During the process of normal biopsychosocial growth, we go through a succession of life cycle stages. These begin with birth and continue through old age, each stage quite different from the previous one. As we leave one stage and enter a new one, we experience a transitional period characterized by changes in role expectations and behavior. It is a period of upset and disequilibrium. In recent years popular writers like Sheehy, Levinson, and Goodman have called these periods "passages," "transitions," and "turning points" [5, 9, 12]. They are the times when maturational crises occur (Fig. 8-1).

Most maturational crises begin with a gradual onset. The change is evolutionary rather than revolutionary. We can anticipate and even

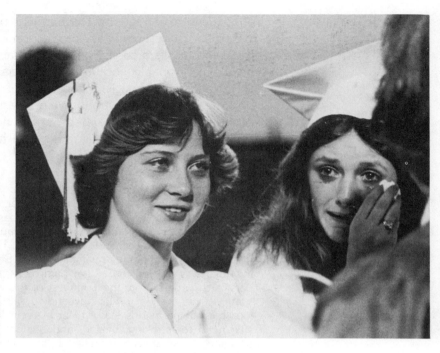

Figure 8-1. Graduation, like any maturational transition, is a time of mixed feelings. Some individuals can take it in stride. For others, it may become a time of crisis. (Courtesy *Mt. Vernon News.*)

prepare to start school, enter adolescence, leave home, get married, have a baby, retire, or die. People move into and through each transitional period knowing in advance that some kind of change will be required. In many instances, we have already seen other people experience these transitions. As a result, maturational crises have a degree of predictability. They offer the possibility of a period of time for anticipation and adjustment.

Maturational crises arise from both physical and social changes. Each new life stage confronts us with changed relationships, responsibilities, and roles. Consider the transition to parenthood, for example. It demands a change in role from caring for oneself and one's mate to include nurturing, caring for, and protecting a completely helpless child. Relationships with other adults, other children, and even one's own parents also change. Parenthood becomes an entrance into a previously unexperienced part of the adult world. New parents may fear the unknown. Will this infant develop normally? Can I give adequate care? Parents often feel anxiety over the responsibility of shaping this new person's life and satisfying society's expectations for their child's proper education and training. They may worry about the increased financial burden and struggle with mixed feelings about giving up a large measure of freedom. This transition places considerable stress on the person, which contributes to tension buildup, feelings of helplessness, and resultant crisis. Some individuals adapt quickly; others cannot cope, probably because earlier maturational crises went unresolved. If a person lacks a repertoire of adaptive skills, a crisis can become major and disastrous. We can easily see how abused children become abusive parents when most, if not all, of their maturational crises have been detrimental rather than healthy.

CASE EXAMPLE

Marcia Sand is 39 years old. Married for 22 years, she has been a capable homemaker and mother of 4 children. Her husband Lou, a construction worker for the past 20 years, thinks Marcia does a "super job at home." In the past, Marcia's time was filled with cooking, laundry, cleaning, shopping, and meeting the endless demands of the family. Their limited income prompted her to adopt many money-saving strategies. She made most of her own and the children's clothes, did all her own baking, and raised vegetables in her backyard garden. Now the youngest of the children, Tommy, has just left home to join the Navy. Her husband spends much of his spare time at the local bar with his friends, leaving Marcia alone. With a nearly empty house and little need for cooking, baking, and sewing, Marcia has lost her sense of usefulness. She thinks of taking a job, but knows her choices are limited since she has only a high school education. Marcia has not slept well in weeks; she wakes up tired and drags through the day barely able to manage the simplest task. She cries frequently but does not know why. Her hair, always neat and attractive in the past, looks bedraggled, and her shoulders slump. "I just can't seem to get on top of things anymore," she complains.

Marcia has entered a maturational crisis that is sometimes called the "empty nest" syndrome. She faces a turning point in her life, a time when parenting has ended. Leaving her satisfying homemaker role, she faces a new life stage filled with unknowns, changes, and a seeming lack of purpose. The transition came about gradually, almost imperceptibly, but now she must deal with it. Yet she feels unable to cope and wishes to turn to someone who would understand and lend her strength. She needs crisis intervention.

SITUATIONAL CRISES

A situational crisis is an acute state of disequilibrium precipitated by an unexpected external event perceived as hazardous. It requires behavioral changes and coping mechanisms beyond the abilities of the people involved.

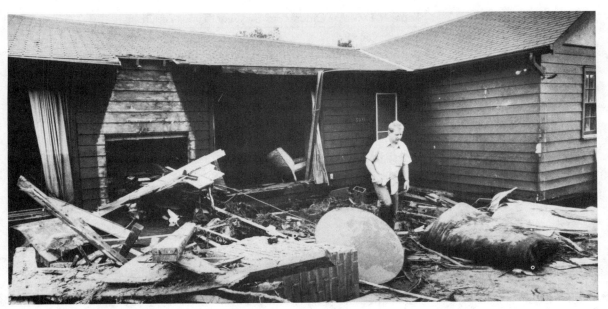

Figure 8-2. Unexpected events like the flood that ravaged this home can suddenly create a situational crisis. (Photograph by Heinz Kluetmier. © Time, Inc.)

Sudden events over which we have little or no control come in many forms (Fig. 8-2). A tornado destroys a family's home and all their possessions. Another family loses its young mother through cancer. A middle-aged man, caught in a company merger, loses his job. After 25 years of marriage, a couple gets divorced. Epilepsy strikes a young man. These kinds of events, which involve loss or the threat of loss, represent life hazards to those affected. Some crisis-precipitating events can be positive, such as a significant job promotion or news of a large inheritance; however, they still make increased demands on individuals [3]. Integrity is threatened and equilibrium disrupted during these situational or accidental crises.

Situational crises arise from external sources, that is, events or conditions generally outside of the person's normal life process. They are extraordinary experiences; they create life changes and disrupt equilibrium by imposing stresses that are usually foreign to ordinary living. The result is overwhelming tension and incapacitation. Natural disasters, for example, are clearly an external cause of a situational crisis. Said one client, "I shall never forget my feelings when one of my high school classmates was killed instantly by lightning. A popular boy, Mel's death threw us all into crisis."

Community health nurses see an almost infinite variety of situational

Table 8-1. Major Differences Between Types of Crises

Maturational Crisis	Situational Crisis
Part of normal growth and development	Unexpected period of upset in normalcy
Precipitated by a life transition point	Precipitated by a hazardous event
Gradual onset	Sudden onset
Response to maturational demands and society's expectations	Externally imposed "accident"

crises; included are debilitating disease, economic misfortune, unemployment, physical abuse, divorce, unwanted pregnancy, chemical abuse, sudden death of a loved one, and many others. In each situation, people feel overwhelmed and need help to cope. Skilled intervention can make the difference between a healthy or unhealthy outcome.

CASE EXAMPLE

The Cooper family eagerly anticipated the birth of their first child. When they first learned that Danny had a harelip and cleft palate, Jan and Frank were numb. They were immediately overwhelmed by the shock of seeing their disfigured baby and worrying about the possibility of other defects. Then came the first painful days adjusting to Danny's appearance and trying to feed and care for him. Jan and Frank alternated between feelings of guilt ("Perhaps we didn't do something right during pregnancy!") and resentment ("Why did this have to happen to us?"). Added to these anxieties was the specter of several corrective surgeries. Each operation threatened them with the risk to Danny, the stress of hospitalization, the struggle to stay with Danny while juggling jobs, the consequences to home life, and the impossible financial costs. How could they handle it all? They felt unable to cope.

As with most situational crises, this one took the Coopers completely by surprise. It upset their normal pattern of living and disrupted their equilibrium. The onset was sudden, precipitated by an event that they perceived as threatening to their well-being. Unlike maturational crises which are brought on by normal demands of growth, their child's congenital defect was externally imposed. And it required behavior changes and adjustments that the Coopers' usual coping abilities were not equipped to handle. These abilities needed help too.

Maturational and situational crises share the characteristics of crises in general described earlier. Their major differences are summarized in Table 8-1. These two kinds of crises overlap in actual experience. The Coopers, for example, experienced a maturational crisis (birth) and a situational crisis (birth defect) simultaneously; thus their stress was compounded. A maturational crisis of midlife may become complicated by situational crises such as divorce and job change occurring at

Table 8-2. Phases of Crisis

Phase	1. Shock	2. Defensive Retreat	3. Acknowledgment	4. Adaptation
Duration	Hours	Days	Weeks	Months
Perception of reality	Momentarily clear, then clouded	Avoids or denies reality	Gradually faces reality	Tests reality
Emotional response	Numb, then anxious, helpless, over-whelmed	Indifferent, euphoric, or angry	Depressed (agitated, apathetic, or bitter)	Diminished anxiety, positive, hopeful
Cognitive ability	Unable to plan, reason, or comprehend situation	Rigid, narrow focus, re-sistant to change	Disorganized, begins redefinition and problem solving	Reorganized, effective reconstruction
Behavior	Disoriented, unable to cope	Fight or flight	Reoriented toward coping, purposeful	Mastery and stabilizing efforts

Source: Adapted from S. L. Fink, Crisis and motivation: A theoretical model. *Arch. Phys. Med. Rehabil.* 48:592, 1967.

the same time. The transition a child faces entering school may occur at the same time the family moves to a new neighborhood and a new infant joins the family. The child must share his parents' attention and affection with a new sibling at a time when all the resources the child can muster are needed. Overlapping crises are not uncommon, and they compound the stress felt by the persons involved. Those who might normally work through one crisis in a healthy way may find that compound events overwhelm them and create intense crisis.

PHASES OF A CRISIS

Regardless of the kind of crisis, people follow a fairly predictable pattern when they respond to the event and seek to regain equilibrium. This pattern progresses in four phases—shock, withdrawal, acknowledgment, and resolution [3, 4, 11] (see Table 8-2).

SHOCK

The shock, or impact, phase occurs when the client encounters the crisis situation. For the first few moments or even hours, one is primarily aware of the event itself. A loved one has died; a job has ended; retirement has begun. However, the significance of that knowledge has not yet been absorbed. The impact of the shock leaves the individual feeling numb or indifferent, possibly even momentarily euphoric. Then a period of realization follows when panic sets in. The client feels overwhelmed, anxious, and helpless. One's perception of reality becomes clouded, and it becomes difficult to make plans, think logically, or understand the situation. During the shock phase, the client may try usual problem-solving means but without success. Self-esteem is threatened, and behavior is disorganized and disoriented. Clients at this point are usually receptive to suggestions and assistance (Fig. 8-3). The entire shock phase generally lasts only a few hours, although in some instances it may extend into days.

DEFENSIVE RETREAT

As the client moves into Phase 2, his chief efforts are aimed at reducing the stress of the moment. At first, he may directly confront the problem with previously effective strategies. The retiree may say, "This is tough, but I've handled tough problems before. I can do it again." However, the demands of the situation are such that stress remains. He may unrealistically try to redefine the problem by saying, "I can always get another job." Because the person has not dealt with reality or his sense of loss and anxiety, the stress continues unabated. Out of necessity, like an organism under attack, his response becomes one of "fight or flight." The fight response often expresses itself in attacking and blaming others for the situation. Avoidance of reality, wishful thinking, and denial represent typical attempts by people in this phase to escape the situation. The bereaved person may refuse to believe that the loved one is dead; the patient with a new diagnosis of cancer will ignore it and avoid treatment. Emotional expressions in this phase fluctuate between indifference, apathy, euphoria, and anger. As though the person wore blinders, there is a narrowing of focus, a progressive rigidity in thinking and a strong resistance to viewing the situation in any other way.

Some individuals find it difficult to leave the defensive retreat phase of crisis. Denial temporarily provides security behind which they can hide; they can avoid the harshness of reality. It also offers a brief respite, a time for recouping energy needed to regain equilibrium. In this sense, denial may be useful as a stepping stone toward healthy adaptation. But extended denial, a maladaptive response, leads to poor physical, mental, spiritual, and psychological health.

ACKNOWLEDGMENT

The time comes when individuals working through crisis must face reality. Phase 3 begins when the facts of the situation force themselves on the person. Gradual recognition and acceptance occur with concomitant efforts to resolve the crisis. The person who has lost a job, for example, can no longer deny that it has happened. There is recognition and gradual, albeit painful, acceptance of the loss. Assessment of

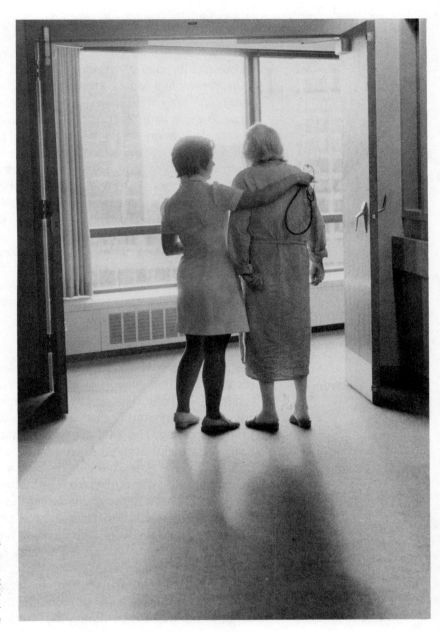

Figure 8-3. Hearing bad news may send people into shock, the first phase of crisis. Support and assistance are greatly needed at this time. (Courtesy of Beth Israel Hospital, Boston. Photograph by Michael Lutch.)

the situation's significance and planning for its management can now begin.

However, the harshness of reality frequently leads to depression expressed in apathy, agitation, remorse, or bitterness. The divorced person may feel at fault or, conversely, that he has been treated unfairly. The pain of rejection, loss of the relationship, and anxiety about how to cope with the present and future can all combine to create severe depression. The acknowledgment phase is a time of mourning, self-depreciation, and emotional decline. From these feelings, however, and with outside help, a restructuring of coping abilities begins. The person moves from disorganized thinking to redefining and attempting to solve the problem. His behavior becomes more purposeful, his planning more realistic. Tension, though still felt, is converted into a constructive energy force.

Again, maladaptive responses can occur when individuals retreat from this phase and continue to deny the problem. Some choose long-term nonreality or the more drastic escape of suicide. Most people, however, discover that the acknowledgment phase is often completed within a few weeks.

ADAPTATION

The final phase of crisis occurs as people engage in successful problem resolution and adaptation to a new life. They not only face reality but test it by restructuring their lives to make them workable. The adaptation phase is marked by feelings of hope and a positive approach to problem solving. The level of anxiety diminishes as people gain a new sense of identity and self-worth. They can talk about the situation openly. They reorganize their thinking toward effective reconstruction, making the best use of their own and other available resources. Their behavior is directed toward mastering the situation and stabilizing the change. People who successfully complete the adaptation phase, which may last for weeks or months, have developed new coping abilities. They have grown stronger, more mature, and better equipped to deal with future crises.

It is helpful for the therapist to recognize the pattern that emotions follow throughout the crisis sequence. Emotions are initially high, then begin to decline rapidly during the shock phase as people feel overwhelmed and increasingly anxious. If it is a crisis for a group, anxiety seems to spread from one person to another. Emotional decline's lowest point occurs at the end of the defensive retreat phase, resulting in depression and exhaustion. In the acknowledgment phase, the

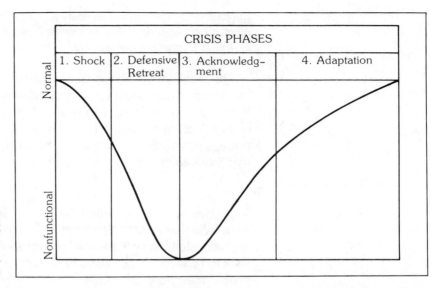

Figure 8-4. Varying emotional levels during crisis. (Adapted from R. G. Hirschowitz, Crisis/ Transition Sequence. *Levinson Letter.* Cambridge, Mass.: Levinson Institutes.)

emotional level begins to climb as people start to face and cope with reality. Finally, emotions are back to a normal level of functioning by the end of the adaptation phase [6].

In the crisis sequence, each succeeding phase lasts longer than the previous one; thus, an increasing amount of adaptive energy is required. Effective professional intervention may significantly reduce the length of time spent in each phase. Figure 8-4 depicts the emotional curve in relation to the varying lengths of each phase. These phases parallel the Kubler-Ross stages of dying—shock, denial, anger, bargaining, depression, and acceptance [8]. They have also been expressed as (1) Who, me?; (2) Not me!; (3) Why me?; and (4) Yes, me. The latter sequence provides a colloquial but useful description of the crisis stages.

CRISIS INTERVENTION

People in crisis need help. They often desperately want help. The crisis and its associated disequilibrium has a two-fold effect on the individuals involved. It renders them temporarily helpless, unable to cope on their own, and thus makes them especially receptive to outside influence. Secondly, this very desire for assistance triggers a helping response from the people nearby. Caplan explains [3, p. 48]:

in crisis . . . , as the individual's tension rises to a climax, he begins not only to mobilize his own resources, but also to solicit help from others. The signs of his increasing tension appear to have a significant effect on others, so that they are stimulated to come to his assistance. This reciprocal pattern of seeking and offering help appears to have primitive biosocial roots; similar phenomena can be found in many social animals.

The significance of this phenomenon cannot be overemphasized. People in crisis will seek and generally receive some kind of help, but the nature of that help can rule in favor of or against a healthy outcome. A client's desire for assistance gives the helping professional a prime opportunity to intervene; it also presents a challenge to make that intervention as effective as possible.

GOAL

The primary goal of crisis intervention is to reestablish equilibrium. Minimally that goal involves resolving the immediate crisis and restoring clients to their precrisis level of functioning. Ultimately, however, we seek to raise that functioning to a healthier, more mature level that will enable them to cope with and prevent future crises. As we discussed earlier, crises tend to be self-limiting, which causes intervention time to last from four to six weeks [1]. The urgency of the situation and its time limitations require the prompt, focused attention of both client and nurse working together to achieve intervention goals.

METHODS

Crisis intervention in community health may utilize one or both of two approaches, generic and individual. For the majority of crisis encounters, the generic approach is more appropriate.

GENERIC APPROACH

The generic approach designs intervention to fit a particular type of crisis. That is, treatment focuses on the nature and course of the crisis, rather than on the psychodynamics of each client [1]. Crisis intervention using the generic approach is tailored to a specific kind of crisis, situational or maturational, and includes four important elements: (1) direct encouragement of adaptive behavior, (2) general support, (3) environmental manipulation, and (4) anticipatory guidance [7]. For example, the generic approach used with mastectomy clients encourages discussion and analysis of feelings, uses exercises to regain physical functioning, and creates a supportive, caring atmosphere. The nurse helps in fitting and use of prostheses, rebuilding of self-image, and strengthening of self-esteem through positive interpersonal relationships. The community nurse also prepares the client to handle future feelings of depression and anxiety related to bodily disfigurement and possibility of metastasis.

The generic approach does not require advanced professional psychotherapy skills. More important for community health practice, it works well with families, groups, and even communities caught in crisis. The community health nurse may lead a group of cancer patients, grieving spouses, or adolescents struggling with developmental crisis, or an entire community recovering from flood, tornado, or some other disaster. The generic approach allows you to intervene with any group of people who have a crisis in common. It offers them a broader base of support, since such a group can offer resources for the members beyond those brought by the nurse. Whether a family or a group of divorcees, new ostomy patients, or new retirement home residents, the client can benefit from the generic approach in a time of crisis.

INDIVIDUAL APPROACH

The individual approach is used when the client does not respond to the generic approach or needs special therapy. Individual crisis intervention should not be confused with individual psychotherapy. The latter tends to focus on the client's developmental past, although the extent of that focus depends on the type of psychotherapy. Crisis intervention, on the other hand, directs treatment toward the immediate state of disequilibrium, identifying its causes and developing coping mechanisms. Family members or significant others are included during the process of crisis resolution. When this approach is needed, clients are usually referred to a professional with specialized training.

STEPS FOR INTERVENTION

Crisis intervention in community health assumes that clients have resources (Fig. 8-5). If we can tap their potential for managing stress events, people in crisis will need minimal direct assistance. In accordance with the self-care concept, crisis intervention seeks to identify and build on client strengths. Aguilera and Messick outline a series of four steps for intervention during crisis [1].

ASSESSMENT

Initially, we need to assess the nature of the crisis and the clients' response to it. How severe is the problem and what risks do the clients face? Are other people also at risk? Assessment must be rapid but thorough, focusing on some specific areas.

First, concentrate on the immediate problem in order to make an

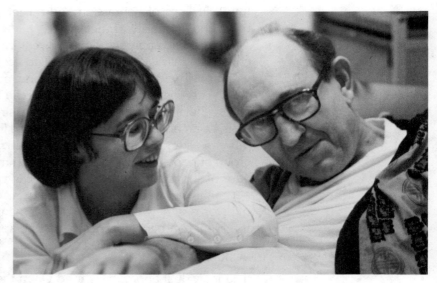

Figure 8-5. Healthy family relationships provide a resource to avert crisis or minimize its effect. This father, sick and missing work, is comforted by his teen-aged daughter. (Courtesy of Beth Israel Hospital, Boston. Photograph by Michael Lutch.)

accurate diagnosis. Why have they asked for help right now? How do they define the problem? What happened to precipitate the crisis? When did it occur? Was it a sudden accidental event or a slower developmental one?

Next, focus on the clients' perception of the event. What does the crisis mean to them and how do they think it will affect their future? Are they viewing the situation realistically? When crisis occurs to a family or group, some members see the situation differently from others. During intervention, all should be encouraged to express themselves, to talk about the crisis and share their feelings about its meaning. Acceptance of the range of feelings is important.

Determine what persons are available for support; consider family, friends, clergy, other professionals, community members, and agencies. Who are clients close to and who do they trust? One advantage of group intervention is that the members provide some of this support for each other. In subsequent sessions, the *quality* of support should be evaluated. Sometimes a well-meaning individual may worsen the situation or deter clients from facing and coping with reality.

Next, assess the clients' coping abilities. Have they had similar kinds of experiences in the past? What techniques have they previously used to relieve tension and anxiety? Which ones have they tried in this situation, and if they have not worked, why not? Clients should be encouraged to think of other stress-relieving techniques, perhaps ones used formerly, and to try them.

Finally, and of crucial importance, find out if there is a possibility of suicide or homicide. Ask directly and specifically about any plans or hints of anyone to kill himself or anyone else. If plans are specific and the threat appears real, psychiatric referral is indicated. Do not discount threats as idle talk.

PLANNING THERAPEUTIC INTERVENTION

Several factors influence the extent of the clients' disequilibrium; try to determine them before making intervention plans. The major balancing factors—clients' perception of the event, situational supports, human resources, and clients' coping skills—have been assessed in the first step [1]. While continuing to explore these, the nurse now also considers clients' general health status, age, past experiences with similar types of situations, sociocultural and religious influences, and the actual assets and liabilities of the situation. This additional assessment helps to clarify the situation and gives the nurse the opportunity to encourage further clients' participation in the resolution process. If clients remain in the defensive retreat phase of crisis, you can give only simple tasks until they face reality and begin problem solving.

The plan is based on the kind of crisis (situational or maturational, acute or chronically recurring), the crisis's effects on the clients (can they still work, go to school, keep house?), the phase of crisis the clients are in, the ways significant others are affected and respond, and the clients' strengths and available resources.

Using the problem-solving process, nurse and clients develop the plan. They review the event that precipitated the crisis, obvious symptoms, and the disruption in the clients' lives. The plan may focus on one or several areas. For instance, clients may need to grasp intellectually the meaning of the crisis or to engage in greater expression of feelings, or both. Part of the plan may be directed toward finding appropriate replacement, such as temporary housing, emergency financial aid, or physical care, for material losses. Another part may focus on assisting clients to identify and use more effective coping techniques or locate supportive agencies and resource persons. The plan will also include the development of realistic goals for the future.

INTERVENTION

During intervention it is important for nurse and clients to continue to communicate. They should discuss what is happening, review the plan and the rationale behind its elements, and make appropriate changes in the plan when indicated. It is helpful to assign definite activities at the end of each session so that clients can try out different solutions and evaluate various coping behaviors.

The intervention step is enhanced by use of the following guidelines [2, 10, 11].

DEMONSTRATE ACCEPTANCE OF CLIENTS

A crisis will often shatter the ego. Clients need to feel the support of a positive, caring person who does not judge their feelings or behavior. Some negative expressions such as anger, withdrawal, and denial are normal aspects of the early phases of crisis. Accept them as normal.

HELP CLIENTS CONFRONT CRISIS

Clients need to face and discuss the situation. Expressing their feelings reduces tension and improves reality perception. Recounting what has actually occurred may be painful but it helps the client confront the crisis. Do not assume that once the client has told you about the event, no further recounting is necessary. Each time the story is told, the client comes closer to dealing realistically with the crisis.

HELP CLIENTS FIND FACTS

Distorted ideas and unknown factors of the situation create additional tension and may lead to maladaptive responses. For instance, it would help the Coopers to know that their son's cleft palate was unpreventable. Facts about surgical treatment and speech training would also be important for them to know.

HELP CLIENTS EXPRESS FEELINGS OPENLY

Suppressed feelings can be harmful. For instance, a widow may feel guilty that she is glad her husband is gone. Expression of these feelings helps reduce tension and gives the client an opportunity to deal with them.

DO NOT OFFER FALSE REASSURANCE

Clients need to face reality, not avoid it. A statement such as "Don't worry, it will all work out" is demeaning and meaningless. Rather, we need to make positive statements about our faith in their ability to cope. "It is a very difficult situation, but I believe you will be able to deal with it."

DISCOURAGE CLIENTS FROM BLAMING OTHERS

Clients often blame others as a way to avoid reality and the responsibility for problem-solving. Withhold judgment when they blame others, but point out other causal factors and avenues for dealing with the situation.

HELP CLIENTS SEEK OUT COPING MECHANISMS

Explore and test old and new techniques to reduce stress and anxiety. Ask questions. What are all the things we might do together to resolve the problem? What are the things that need to be done? What do you think you can do? This assistance gives clients more adaptive energy to work toward resolution.

ENCOURAGE CLIENTS TO ACCEPT HELP

Denial in the early phases of crisis cuts off help. Encouraging clients to acknowledge the problem is a first step toward acceptance of help. Often, however, clients fear the loss of their independence and the invasion of their privacy. A client may state, "I ought to be able to handle this problem." At this point, the community nurse can assure clients that people in a crisis of this sort almost always need help. Preparing clients to accept help will enable them to make the best use of what others have to offer.

PROMOTE DEVELOPMENT OF NEW, POSITIVE RELATIONSHIPS

Clients who have lost a significant person through death or divorce should be encouraged to find new people to fill the void and provide needed supports and satisfactions.

RESOLUTION AND ANTICIPATORY PLANNING

In the final step, we (clients and nurse) evaluate, stabilize, and plan for the future. First, we evaluate the outcome of the intervention. Are clients using effective coping skills and exhibiting appropriate behavior? Are adequate resources and support persons available? Is the diagnosed problem solved, and have the desired results been accomplished? Analysis of these outcomes gives a greater understanding for coping with future crisis.

To stabilize the change, we identify and reinforce all the positive coping mechanisms and behaviors. We discuss why they are effective and how to use them in future stress situations. We can summarize the crisis experience, emphasizing the clients' successes with coping in order to reconfirm progress and reinforce self-confidence. We can point to evidence that they have reached their precrisis, or even higher, level of functioning.

Clients' plans for the future should include setting realistic goals and means for implementing them. We can also review with clients how their handling of the present crisis can help them cope with future crises.

CRISIS PREVENTION

Many people go through crises unnecessarily, ones that might have been prevented. Other crises could be shortened in length or diminished in intensity through preventive measures. Because of the nature and philosophy of community health practice, nurses should engage in crisis prevention as much as, or even more than in mere intervention. Furthermore, community health nurses are in a unique position to prevent or detect crises early. They encounter clients or would-be clients in settings where these individuals are most likely to behave in an unaffected, natural manner. Also, through their participation in communities' communication networks, they can learn about potential family and community problems.

PRIMARY PREVENTION

We shall consider crisis prevention in terms of three levels—primary, secondary, and tertiary. Primary crisis prevention means keeping the crisis from ever happening; we completely obstruct its occurrence. Both maturational and situational crises can, in some cases, be prevented by anticipatory action. Let us examine what this prevention involves.

A primary crisis prevention program in community health has two major goals [3]. The first objective is to make certain that individuals have adequate provision for basic needs. For the community health nurse, this goal involves health promotion. Any activity that fosters healthful practices and counteracts influences detrimental to healthy living can help prevent a crisis. For instance, nurses teach and encourage families to eat well-balanced, nourishing meals. They also discourage the local school, scout groups, churches, or other community groups from serving junk food snacks. Healthy children will have less trouble coping with crises that occur than children in poor health. Health promotion should deal with physical, psychological, sociocultural, and spiritual needs. Like purchasing insurance or depositing money in

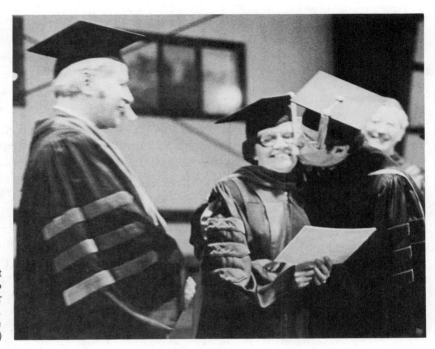

Figure 8-6. Many women avert midlife crisis by returning to school and starting a new career after raising their children. (Courtesy of the *Mt. Vernon News.*)

an account, storing up reserves in these areas safeguards the client against stressful times.

The second goal of primary crisis prevention is anticipatory action. Because maturational crises are often predictable, community nurses can help clients prepare for them. You can discuss the kinds of adjustments and role changes the next transition period will require (Fig. 8-5). Marcia Sands could have avoided an empty nest midlife crisis through anticipatory planning. Knowing that the children would inevitably leave home and that they contributed to her primary satisfactions in life, Marcia could have made plans to start developing new relationships and new work outlets. Placing an aging parent in a nursing home is often a crisis for the entire family, one that anticipatory planning can make less intense. Even situational crises, like many "accidents," are often predictable. There may be a family history of myocardial infarctions, for example, that family members can prevent. Making changes in diet, exercise patterns, and job choices, as well as learning stress-coping skills may greatly reduce the risks.

Anticipatory work means experiencing some of the feelings of loss, tension, or anxiety before the crisis-precipitating event occurs (Fig. 8-6). It is much easier to do this at a time when energy and intellectual processes are at a high level of functioning. Anticipatory work dissipates the impact of the crisis event. Grief work, for example, can begin before the terminally ill family member actually dies. A crisis of large proportions can thus be prevented.

SECONDARY PREVENTION

Secondary crisis prevention focuses on early detection and treatment. It seeks to reduce the intensity and duration of a crisis and to promote adaptive behavior. Community health nurses often encounter clients in the early stages of a crisis. A newly pregnant woman, for example, can be assisted to work through the phases of transition in a relatively short period of time.

During the course of normal practice, community health nurses can watch for signs that a person may be entering a crisis. By considering suspect any event that might potentially provoke crisis, the nurse can monitor clients' responses. Several simultaneous or rapidly succeeding stress events may forecast impending crisis. One family appeared to handle a job loss well; they coped adequately with the death of a grandparent a few weeks later. However, their crisis became full-blown when the mother of the family learned she must have surgery. Nursing intervention at an early stage could have prevented the crisis from reaching major proportions and enabled the family to regain equilibrium sooner.

TERTIARY PREVENTION

Tertiary crisis prevention involves reducing the amount and degree of disability or damage resulting from crisis. Although it involves rehabilitative work, it can help a client's recovery and reduce the risk of future crises. In this sense, it is a preventive measure. Clients can easily become caught in a web of maladaptive responses. For instance, a divorced person does not recover from the experience, remains bitter and hostile, and begins to drink heavily, which leads to a new crisis of alcoholism. A grieving spouse continues for months or years to deny his wife's death, withdraws socially, and develops chronic physical problems. A person in the crisis of old age cannot accept her aging and adopts bizarre and offensive dress and mannerisms. Tertiary crisis prevention involves helping these clients to face the reality of their present situation and to develop improved coping skills. Working with these individuals in groups is a particularly effective means of providing support, reality orientation, and the prevention of further disability.

SUMMARY

Crisis is a temporary state of severe disequilibrium for persons who face a threatening situation. It is a state that they can neither avoid nor solve with their usual coping abilities. A crisis occurs when some force disrupts the functioning of an individual or group and thus causes a loss of homeostasis. A crisis creates tension; subsequently, efforts are made to solve the problem and reduce the tension. When such efforts meet with failure, people feel upset, redefine the situation, try other solutions, and, if failure continues, eventually reach the breaking point.

There are two kinds of crises, situational and maturational. Maturational crises are disruptions that occur during transitional periods in normal growth and development. They usually have a gradual onset and are often predictable. Situational crises, on the other hand, are precipitated by an unexpected external event. They have a sudden onset.

Crises tend to progress through four stages—shock, defensive retreat, acknowledgment, and adaptation. The individual's perception of the crisis changes through these four stages, as does emotional response, cognitive ability, and behavior.

People in crisis both need and seek help. Crisis intervention builds on these two phenomena to achieve its primary goal, reestablishment of equilibrium. The two major methods for crisis intervention are the generic and individual approaches. The generic approach deals with a single type of crisis, such as rape, and often works with groups of people caught in the same crisis. The individual approach is used when the client does not respond to the generic approach or needs additional therapy. Crisis intervention begins with assessment of the situation; then a therapeutic intervention is planned. Next, the nurse carries out the intervention, building on the strengths and self-care ability of the client. Finally, resolution and anticipatory planning for possible future crises occur.

The frequency and intensity of crises can be diminished. Primary crisis prevention seeks to obstruct occurrence of crisis through promoting a high level of wellness and teaching people to anticipate and thus avoid possible crises. Secondary crisis prevention focuses on early detection and treatment. Tertiary crisis prevention seeks to reduce the degree of disability resulting from crisis.

REFERENCES

1. Aguilera, D. C., and Messick, J. M. *Crisis Intervention: Theory and Methodology* (3rd ed.). St. Louis: Mosby, 1978. Pp. 1, 21, 22, 62, 70.

2. Cadden, V.   Crisis in the Family. In G. Caplan, *Principles of Preventive Psychiatry.* New York: Basic Books, 1964. Pp. 288–296.
3. Caplan, G.   *Principles of Preventive Psychiatry.* New York: Basic Books, 1964. Pp. 35, 39, 40, 48, 53, 56.
4. Fink, S. L.   Crisis and motivation: A theoretical model. *Arch. Phys. Med. Rehabil.* 48:592, 1967.
5. Goodman, E.   *Turning Points.* New York: Doubleday, 1979.
6. Hirschowitz, R. G.   Crisis/Transition Sequence. *Levinson Letter.* Cambridge, Mass.: Levinson Institute. P. 4.
7. Jacobson, G., Strickler, M., and Morely, W.   Generic and individual approaches to crisis intervention. *Am. J. Public Health* 58:339, 1968.
8. Kubler-Ross, E.   *On Death and Dying.* New York: Macmillan, 1969.
9. Levinson, D. J.   *The Seasons of a Man's Life.* New York: Knopf, 1978.
10. Morely, W. E., Messick, J. M., and Aguilera, D. C.   Crisis: Paradigms of intervention. *J Psychiatr. Nurs.* 5:537, 1967.
11. Murray, R., and Zentner, J.   *Nursing Concepts for Health Promotion.* Englewood Cliffs, N.J.: Prentice-Hall, 1975. P. 208, 211, 219.
12. Sheehy, G.   *Passages: Predictable Crises of Adult Life.* New York: Dutton, 1976.

SELECTED READINGS

Aguilera, D. C., and Messick, J. M.   *Crisis Intervention: Theory and Methodology* (3rd ed.). St. Louis: Mosby, 1978.
Brandon, S.   Crisis theory and possibilities of therapeutic intervention. *Br. J. Psychiatry* 117:541, 1970.
Brose, C.   Theories of Family Crisis. In D. Hymovich and M. Barnard (Eds.), *Family Health Care.* New York: McGraw-Hill, 1973.
Cadden, V.   Crisis in the Family. In G. Caplan, *Principles of Preventive Psychiatry.* New York: Basic Books, 1964.
Caplan, G.   *Principles of Preventive Psychiatry.* New York: Basic Books, 1964.
Chandler, H. M.   Family crisis intervention: Point and counterpoint in the psychosocial revolution. *J. Natl. Med. Assoc.* 64:211, 1972.
Christ, J.   The adolescent crisis syndrome: Its clinical significance in the outpatient service. *Psychiatr. Forum* 3(1):25, 1972.
Clark, T.   Counseling victims of rape. *Am. J. Nurs.* 76:1964, 1976.
Clark, T., and Jaffe, D. T.   Change within youth crisis centers. *Am. J. Orthopsychiatry* 42:675, 1972.
Collins, M.   *Communication in Health Care: Understanding and Implementing Effective Human Relations.* St. Louis: Mosby, 1977.
Comstock, B., and McDermott, M.   Group therapy for patients who attempt suicide. *Int. J. Group Psychother.* 25(1):44, 1975.
Donner, G. J.   Parenthood as a crisis. *Perspect. Psychiatr. Care* 10(2):84, 1972.

Dzik, R. S.   Transactional analysis in crisis intervention. *J. Gynecol. Nurs.* 5(1):31, 1976.

Ebersole, P. P.   Crisis Intervention with the Aged. In I. M. Burnside, *Nursing and the Aged.* New York: McGraw-Hill, 1976.

Eisler, R., and Hersen, M.   Behavioral techniques in family-oriented crisis intervention. *Arch. Gen. Psychiatry* 28(1):111, 1973.

Fallom, C. W.   Providing relevant brief service to couples in marital crises. *Am. J. Orthopsychiatry* 43(2):235, 1973.

Fink, S. L.   Crisis and motivation: A theoretical model. *Arch. Phys. Med. Rehab.* 48:592, 1967.

Foreman, N. J., and Zerwekh, J. V.   Drug crisis intervention. *Am. J. Nurs.* 71:1736, 1971.

Freudenberger, H. J.   Crisis intervention, individual and group counseling, and the psychology of the counseling staff of a free clinic. *J. Soc. Issues* 30(1):77, 1974.

Golan, N.   When is a client in crisis? *Soc. Casework* 50:389, 1969.

Goldstein, S., and Giddings, J.   Multiple Impact Therapy: An Approach to Crisis Intervention with Families. In G. Specter, *Crisis Intervention* (Behavioral Publications No. 210). New York: Behavioral Publications, 1973.

Hall, J. E., and Weaver, B. (Eds.).   *Nursing of Families in Crisis.* Philadelphia: Lippincott, 1974.

Hitchcock, J. M.   Crisis intervention—The pebble in the pool. *Am. J. Nurs.* 73:1388, 1973.

Hoff, L. *People in Crisis: Understanding and Helping.* New York: Addison-Wesley, 1978.

Holstrom, L., and Burgess, A.   Assessing trauma in the rape victim. *Am. J. Nurs.* 75(8):1288, 1975.

Hott, J. R.   Mobilizing Family Strengths in Health Maintenance and Coping with Illness. In A. Reinhardt, and M. Quinn (Eds.), *Current Practice in Family-Centered Community Nursing.* St. Louis: Mosby, 1977.

Hott, J. R.   The crisis of expectant fatherhood. *Am. J. Nurs.* 76:1436, 1976.

Jacobson, G.   Emergency services in community mental health: Problems and promise. *Am. J. Public Health* 64:124, 1974.

Jacobson, G., Strickler, M., and Morely, W.   Generic and individual approaches to crisis intervention. *Am. J. Public Health* 58:339, 1968.

Kubler-Ross, E.   *On Death and Dying.* New York: Macmillan, 1969.

Lavietes, R. L.   Crisis intervention with ghetto children: Mythology and reality. *Am. J. Orthopsychiatry* 44(2):241, 1974.

Marks, M. J.   The grieving patient and family. *Am. J. Nurs.* 76:1488, 1976.

Marmer, J.   The Crisis of Middle Age. In L. H. Schwartz and J. L. Schwartz, *The Psychodynamics of Patient Care.* Englewood Cliffs, N.J.: Prentice-Hall, 1972.

McClellan, M. S.   Crisis groups in special care areas. *Nurs. Clin. North Am.* 7:363, 1972.

Messick, J. M.   Crisis intervention concepts: Implications for nursing practices. *J. Psychiatr. Nurs.* 10(5):3, 1972.

Morely, W. E., Messick, J. M., and Aguilera, D. C.   Crisis: Paradigms of intervention. *J. Psychiatr. Nurs.* 5:537, 1967.

Nakushian, J.   Restoring parents' equilibrium after sudden infant death. *Am. J. Nurs.* 76:1600, 1976.

O'Brien, M. J.   *Communication and Relationship in Nursing* (2nd ed.). St. Louis: Mosby, 1978.

Parad, H. J. (Ed.).   *Crisis Intervention.* New York: Family Service Assn. of America, 1965.

Price, J. L., and Braden, C.   The reality in home visits. *Am. J. Nurs.* 78(9):1536, 1978.

Rapoport, R.   Normal crises, family structure, and mental health. *Fam. Process* 2:68, 1963.

Selkin, J.   Rape. *Psychol. Today,* pp. 71–76, Jan. 1975.

Specter, G.   *Crisis Intervention* (Behavioral Publications No. 210). New York: Behavioral Publications, 1973.

Strickler, M., and LaSor, B.   The concept of loss in crisis intervention. *Ment. Hyg.* 54:301, 1970.

Van Antwerp, M.   Primary prevention: A challenge to mental health associations. *Ment. Hyg.* 54:453, 1970.

Williams, F.   Intervention in Maturational Crises. *Perspect. Psychiatr. Care* 9:240, 1971.

Woehning, M., and Martinson, I.   Family Nursing During Death and Dying. In B. W. Spradley (Ed.), *Contemporary Community Nursing.* Boston: Little, Brown, 1975.

Zelbach, J. Z.   Crisis in chronic problem families: Psychiatric care of the underprivileged. *Int. Psychiatry Clin.* 8(2):101, 1971.

NINE

EPIDEMIOLOGY

The practice of nursing has traditionally rested on two important cornerstones of scientific knowledge—biophysical and psychosocial study. The biophysical basis involves the study of human anatomy and physiology, etiology and treatment of disease, and processes of physical development. The psychosocial basis includes the study of psychological and social development, psychiatric illness, and social aspects of nursing care.

Community health nursing adds a third cornerstone of scientific knowledge to these two; that is, information on the health and illness characteristics of population groups. For example, a community health nurse wants to develop a plan to prevent an outbreak of rubella, a communicable disease that affects the human fetus with congenital rubella syndrome. In order to develop such a prevention plan, information about population groups is required. Which members of a community have been immunized against rubella? What is the expected number of rubella cases (the morbidity rate)? What members of the community have the highest risk of rubella? Any program of screening, immunization, or health promotion regarding rubella must be based on this kind of information about population groups in order to be effective. This information comes from *epidemiology,* a specialized form of scientific research.

Epidemiology is the study of the distribution and determinants of health and illness states in human population groups. The community health nurse makes use of epidemiology whenever she asks questions such as, "What is the prevalence of a particular illness in a population? What is the incidence of a certain level of physical fitness or wellness in

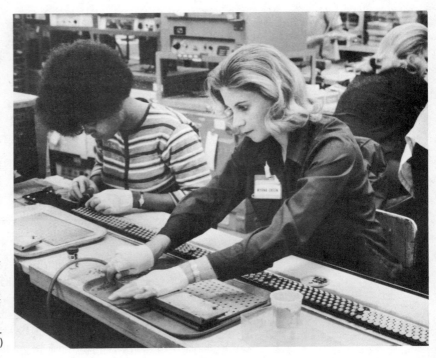

Figure 9-1. Epidemiologic research focuses on the health of population groups. Safety and stress factors for workers on an assembly line make up one of the many areas for study. (Photograph by Ralph Crane for *Life*. © 1972, Time, Inc.)

a community? What characteristics are associated with these states of health and illness? What environmental factors are associated with these states of health and illness? How can we intervene in a community to prevent health problems and promote wellness?

APPLICATION TO COMMUNITY HEALTH NURSING

As long as the nurse focuses on the individual as the client, epidemiology may have little to offer. However, community health nursing and epidemiology have a single theme in common, the health of groups. Epidemiology offers community nurses a specific methodology for assessing the health of families, local groups, and entire communities (Fig. 9-1). Furthermore, it provides a frame of reference for investigating and improving clinical practice in any setting. Whether the community health nurse's goals are aimed at improving a family's nutrition, controlling an outbreak of sexually transmitted diseases, dealing with health problems created by a blizzard, or assisting mothers who choose to have a home birth, epidemiologic data can be useful.

Consider one example. In Cali, Colombia, many potential clients were not using available child health services. In order to discover why some and not others used the services and to develop remedial actions, epidemiologic data was needed. How many children were in the target population? What characterized the mothers and children who did and did not use the services? What illness problems existed? How many children had been immunized for what illnesses? Dr. Beatrice J. Selwyn, a nurse and epidemiologist, selected a single *barrio* with a population of more than 50,000 people for epidemiologic study. Trained assistants interviewed a sample of 529 mothers with children under 5 years of age; among other findings, Selwyn discovered the characteristics of those who did not use the available child health services. This information laid a groundwork for identifying the target population and designing services to reach that population. For example, nonusers did not read newspapers but did listen to the radio, which suggested an effective line of communication about new services. Selwyn summarized the value of this kind of investigation: "Answers obtained in the interview suggest ways to structure delivery systems to the subculture of the population to be served, e.g., taking immunization services to the homes of mothers rather than waiting for them to come to the service" [18, p. 235].

USE OF EXISTING DATA

Before we examine more carefully the nature of epidemiology, three levels for using this approach in community health nursing practice should be considered. The most basic level is use of existing epidemiologic data. Journals, books, official records, and agency records are excellent sources of information for the community health nurse. If a nurse becomes aware that several rubella cases have occurred in the community, existing data will place those cases in perspective. For example, although a vaccine for active immunization offers a means to eliminate congenital rubella syndrome, epidemiologic data reveals that, in 1975, 30 percent of 5- to 9-year-old children in the United States had not been immunized [5]. If the nurse decides, after reviewing such data, to aim an immunization program at susceptible child-bearing adults, existing studies can be of further benefit. For example, Chappell and his associates screened a group of 457 medical, graduate, and physician assistant students and found that 18 percent were estimated at risk for rubella [6]. This kind of information can be of great value in a rubella prevention program.

The health of school populations is of concern to many community health nurses. Existing epidemiologic data can be used to plan parent education programs, health promotion among students, and almost any other type of service. For example, the Division of Nursing of the National Institutes of Health, in cooperation with the Delaware State Department of Education, began a long-term epidemiologic study of school populations as a basis for changing school nursing practice [1]. They found, for example, that parent-nurse contacts were most likely to occur among upper social class parents, both white and nonwhite, who worried about their child's health. They also found that parents varied in the reasons for keeping a child home; a large proportion would send their child to school with symptoms of a communicable disease. This data suggests that community health nurses working with schools, at least in the state of Delaware, might seriously consider a parent education program regarding such parental decisions.

INFORMAL INVESTIGATIONS

The second level for using epidemiology involves informal investigations. Almost every client encountered by the community health nurse can precipitate such a study. If you discover an abused child at a clinic, the records can be screened for possible additional cases of child abuse. If several cases of diabetes come to the attention of a nurse visiting homes on a Navaho reservation, informal inquiries about the incidence and age of onset of this disease among the Indian population might result. A community health nurse working in a clinic may raise the question, "Why don't the people who need our services come to the clinic?" A single day spent collecting epidemiologic data in an informal manner can shed light on this question. Perhaps, as Selwyn found in Colombia, nonusers have less knowledge about health and health services [18]. This information could lead to a change in clinic activities that would increase communication with those who need services.

Consider an example of how one nurse used an informal epidemiologic study to improve health care within a city jail. In dealing with incarcerated habitual intoxicants, Katherine Chavigny observed that neither jail staff nor health professionals addressed chronic alcoholic patients by name. "When names were essential for communication with the latter group, diminutives, nicknames, or at best, first names were used" [7, p. 637]. Chavigny hypothesized that a lack of respect for the patients in the jail threatened their health by creating barriers to services offered. She carried out an informal study by introducing a simple change: she began to say "Mr." when addressing each patient in every nursing contact. Within several months, eye contact with patients, which had been almost nonexistent, increased to an estimated 70 percent. Patients formerly withdrawn began to express needs for the services offered by the health care team. Epidemiology seeks to identify variables that affect the health of groups and larger populations. Although this experimental epidemiologic study was of an informal nature, the nurse was able to identify at least one important factor and introduce a change that affected health care delivery.

SCIENTIFIC STUDIES

The third level for using epidemiology in community health nursing involves carefully designed scientific studies. Nursing, as a profession, has recognized the need to develop a systematic body of knowledge on which to base nursing practice. In the future, systematic research will become an accepted part of the community health nurse's role. We have already noted Selwyn's study to determine the use patterns of health services for mothers with children under 5 years of age. Dozens of other epidemiologic research studies done by nurses could be cited. For example, three nurses in Salt Lake City collaborated on a study of women who chose home birth. They discovered that this group did not differ from the total population in age, marital, and socioeconomic status. However, nearly half of the women had planned to have home births as a result of reported hostility from health professionals [4]. This study provides important information for community nurses working with women who plan to have home delivery. After an outbreak of trichinosis in Illinois, two nurses became involved with other investigators in an epidemiologic study of the epidemic. They concluded that the medical expenses and lost wages from this epidemic could have been prevented by a program to control trichinosis in swine [16]. Systematic studies such as these, as well as informal studies and use of existing data, require an understanding of epidemiology. After a discussion of the nature and history of this discipline, we will examine the investigative process used for collecting epidemiologic data.

THE NATURE OF EPIDEMIOLOGY

The roots of epidemiology can be traced back to Hippocrates (460–377 B.C.). Called by some the first epidemiologist, Hippocrates believed that disease not only affected individuals but was a mass phenomenon. He was one of the first to associate disease occurrence with lifestyle and environmental factors. However, it was not until the late nineteenth century that modern epidemiology actually came into existence. The term derived from the Greek words *epi* (upon), *demos* (the people), and *logos* (knowledge), thus meaning the knowledge or study of what happens to people.

One of the most dramatic things to happen to communities of people was epidemic diseases. Cholera, bubonic plague, and smallpox swept through community after community, killing thousands of people, changing the community structure, and altering the lifestyle of masses of people. Epidemiology became a distinct branch of medical science through its concern with epidemics of infectious diseases. In 1348, the Black Death swept through Europe and England, killing millions of people. In England alone, approximately one-fourth of the population died from the plague, which takes one of two forms. If the plague bacilli infect the lymph glands of armpit or groin, a lump or bubo develops (thus the name *bubonic plague*). If the bacilli lodge in the lungs, pneumonia, or *pneumonic plague,* results. The plague continued in Europe, but with less force, for three centuries and then waned, only to reappear in an epidemic in Hong Kong in 1896.

Kitasato, a Japanese bacteriologist, discovered the plague bacillus during this Hong Kong epidemic; within ten years, epidemiologists had traced its life cycle from rats to fleas to humans. Now intervention was possible and public health officials declared war on rats, seeking to make ships and wharf buildings rat-proof. The first major campaign against rats took place in California after an outbreak of plague in 1900. Although successful, the bacillus appears to have spread to ground squirrels, and cases still occur occasionally in this country [3].

Host, Agent, Environmental Model

Through intensive study of infectious diseases, epidemiologists began to think about disease states in terms of causal agent, susceptible host, and environment. The agent responsible for plague is the plague bacillus; humans are susceptible hosts, along with rats and a few other animals. But fleas that bite both rats and humans must be present in order to transfer the bacillus from rats to the human host. Numerous environmental factors influence these relationships. The black rat, once native to India and a carrier of the plague, came to Europe with the Crusaders and became the source of the Black Death in 1348. Historic records even then indicated that some people were more susceptible to the plague than others. Far more men died from this disease than women and children, who were often not, or only mildly, affected. The host, agent, and environment model, shown in Figure 9-2, offered the epidemiologist a plan for intervention. As soon as the agent was

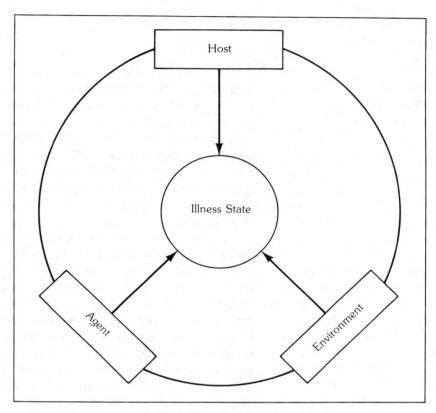

Figure 9-2. Epidemiologic model. Epidemiologists study the causal agent, the susceptible host, and environmental factors that contribute to an illness state (or a wellness state). Intervention may act on any of these three to prevent the spread of illness or to improve health in a population.

identified, measures could be taken to keep the bacillus from contacting human hosts; eradicating rats known to carry the disease was a major preventive measure.

As the threat of the great epidemic diseases declined, epidemiologists began to focus on other infectious diseases such as diphtheria, infant diarrhea, typhoid, tuberculosis, and syphilis. They also sought to discover the host characteristics, agent, and environmental factors in diseases such as scurvy among sailors and the occupational disease of scrotal cancer among chimney sweeps. In recent years, epidemiologists have turned to the study of major causes of death and disability, such as cancer, cardiovascular disorders, mental illness, accidents, arthritis, and congenital defects. Equally important, rather than concentrating only on illness, they have focused on how agent, host, and environment are involved in wellness at various levels. In response to an escalating demand for health promotion, health and health care services have come under the scrutiny of epidemiology.

CAUSAL RELATIONSHIPS

EARLY THEORIES

The purpose of epidemiologic study has been to discover causal relationships in order to offer effective prevention. Over the years, as scientific knowledge of health and disease has expanded, epidemiology has changed. Early causal thinking was dominated by Sydenham's miasma theory. This theory explained that disease was caused by noxious vapors associated with decaying organic matter. Prevention based on this theory attempted to eliminate the sources of the miasma (vapors). Despite its reasoning, this type of prevention has had some positive consequences since we now know that decaying organic matter can be a source of infectious diseases.

A contagion theory of disease had developed by the mid-eighteenth century. This theory inspired various concepts of immunity and even some initial attempts at vaccination against smallpox. Late in the nineteenth century, the germ theory of disease was established. Epidemiologic efforts then began to focus on identifying the microorganisms that caused the disease as a first step in prevention. Once the agent had been identified, measures could be taken to contain its spread. Fumigating ships to kill rats, protecting wharf buildings and human habitations against rats, and removing rat food supplies from easy access were all measures to prevent the spread of the plague bacilli.

Up to this point, epidemiologists viewed disease in terms of a simple cause and effect relationship. Finding a single cause (plague bacilli) and attacking it (eliminating rats) seemed the solution for preventing many diseases. In the case of bubonic plague, this approach appeared quite effective. However, scientific research revealed that disease causation was much more complex than at first suspected. For example, although most members of a group might be exposed to the plague, many did not contract the disease. With bubonic plague, as with many other infectious diseases, the characteristics of the host can determine the spread of the disease. Not everyone in a population is at risk; we now know that, "Untreated bubonic plague has a case fatality rate commonly reported to be about 50 percent; occasionally it is no more than a localized infection of short duration (pestis minor), and fully virulent plague organisms have been recovered from throat cultures of asymptomatic contacts of plague patients" [2, p. 716]. Clearly, such evidence makes it difficult to speak of a single cause for plague and many other disease states.

Furthermore, even the agent and course of transmission can be quite complex. Although it is a flea that carries the bacilli from rat to human in bubonic plague, pneumonic plague can spread directly from one human being to another. The environment must also be considered as part of the cause in nearly every disease and health state. Considering the plague again, evidence suggests that it originated in the high steppes of Asia and spread to other parts of the world. After a rather successful attempt to control the spread of plague in California during the early part of this century, epidemiologists discovered that the ground squirrel also carried the bacillus. But the question arose as to whether the bacillus spread from the rat to the ground squirrel or whether it had always been part of the squirrel's ecology. Although this question has not been answered, we do know that the western United States offers an environment conducive to squirrels, their plague-carrying fleas, and the plague bacillus. Although isolated cases continue to occur, epidemics have not occurred and are quite unlikely since squirrels usually live in an environment somewhat separated from humans.

CHAIN OF CAUSATION

As our thinking about disease causation has grown more complex around the tripartite model of host, agent, and environment, epidemiologists have used the idea of a chain of causation (see Fig. 9-3). The chain begins by identifying the *reservoir,* that is, the usual habitation of the causal agent. In plague, that reservoir may be other humans, rats, squirrels, and a few other animals. In malaria, humans are the major reservoir for the parasitic agents, although recent evidence has shown that certain monkeys also act as a reservoir [3]. Next, the agent must have a portal of exit from the reservoir as well as some mode of transmission. The next link in the chain of causation is the agent itself. Malaria, for example, actually consists of four distinct diseases caused by one of four protozoa, which are tiny microorganisms. These agents spend part of their life cycle in the body of the *Anopheles* mosquito, which acts as a mode of transmission. The mosquito bite provides a portal of exit as well as a portal of entry into the human host.

The circle surrounding this chain of causation in Figure 9-3 represents the environment, which can have a profound influence on almost any point along the chain. Consider the impact of environmental factors in the malaria epidemic of Ceylon in 1934–1935. Two or three million cases occurred, resulting in eighty thousand deaths. Malaria occurred frequently in the dry northern area where sparse vegetation

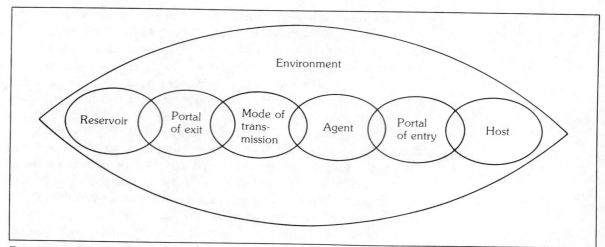

Figure 9-3. Chain of causation in infectious disease.

allowed pools of water to be exposed to the sun and provided an excellent breeding ground for the *Anopheles* mosquito. The more populous southwestern area which had heavy monsoon rains was relatively free from malaria. In 1934 a severe drought changed this environment drastically; rivers almost dried up, leaving stagnant pools of water for mosquito breeding. Widespread crop failure caused the population to become badly undernourished, which added to the conditions that would foster a malaria epidemic. The epidemic hit in October, 1934 with devastating results for the population, and the environment must certainly be seen as a major part of the causal chain [3].

MULTIPLE CAUSATION

Recently, more advanced concepts of multiple causation have emerged to explain the existence of health and illness states and to provide guiding principles for epidemiologic practice. Sometimes discussed as a "web of causation," this view tries to identify all the possible influences on the health and illness processes [11]. Figure 9-4 shows the web of causation for myocardial infarction; such a health problem cannot be explained in single causal terms, even if that cause represents part of a larger chain. Recognizing multiple causes offers many points for prevention, health promotion, and treatment. For example, Figure 9-4 suggests interventions such as directly attacking significant coronary atherosclerosis (bypass surgery), reducing the incidence of obesity, helping people quit smoking, developing an exercise program, and making changes in diet.

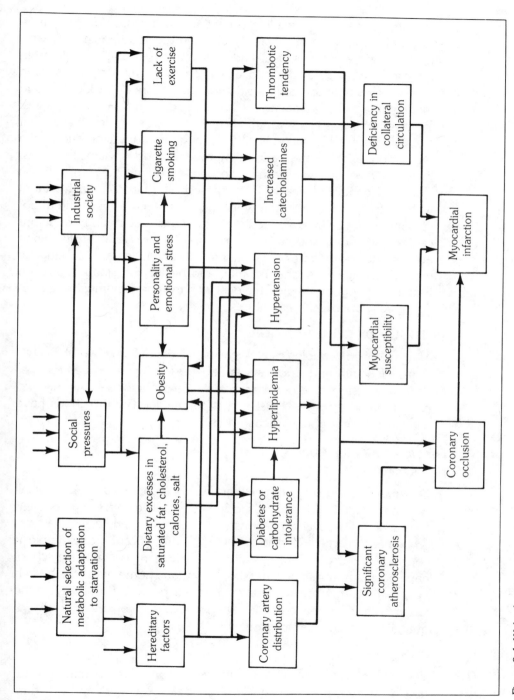

Figure 9-4. Web of causation for myocardial infarction. (From G. D. Friedman, *Primer of Epidemiology.* New York: McGraw-Hill, 1974. Reprinted by permission.)

Contemporary epidemiologists continue to explore new and more comprehensive ways of viewing health and illness. Lifestyle, behavior, environment, and stress of all kinds have an impact on health states. In the model of host, agent, and environment, we can note a shifting emphasis over time. Early epidemiologists worked to identify and manage the causative agent; the focus of concern was disease states. Then emphasis shifted to the host. Who was susceptible? What characteristics led to susceptibility? Through immunization and health promotion, efforts were made to improve the host resistance. Increasingly, however, we have come to recognize the limitations imposed on individual control of health. Even those in the best of health cannot withstand toxic agents in the workplace, nuclear wastes in the atmosphere from power plant accidents, or other debilitating conditions created by modern society. More and more, public health professionals are turning to a study of environmental conditions and looking for ways to change those that contribute to health and illness. But even today we recognize the need to deal with the complex multiple causation involved in health and illness.

METHODS OF EPIDEMIOLOGIC INVESTIGATION

The goal of epidemiologic investigation is to identify the causal mechanisms of health and illness states and to develop measures for preventing illness and promoting health. Epidemiologists employ two basic methods, observational and experimental. Both methods have relevance for community health nursing.

OBSERVATIONAL METHOD

DESCRIPTIVE STUDIES

Observational studies can be either *descriptive* or *analytic*. As we shall see, the analytic studies always include descriptive data but go beyond it to search for specific relationships. Descriptive studies seek to describe health-related conditions as they naturally occur. For example, a community nurse might try to discover how many children in a school have been immunized for measles, how many home births occur each year in the county, or how many cases of syphilis have occurred in the last month. Descriptive studies almost always involve some form of quantification and statistical analysis.

COUNTS

The simplest measure of description is a count. For example, several health professionals did an epidemiologic study of rape to provide data for a rape treatment, detection, and prevention program offered by the City Health Department of Houston, Texas [17]. One of the first steps in their research was to make a simple count of the number of rapes that occurred. They gathered data from the Houston Police Department; for the two years 1974–1975, 875 rapes were reported and 258 rapes attempted. Making a count of this type is always influenced by the definition of what you count. This count, for example, does not represent all rapes occurring, but only those reported to the police. As in most kinds of research, availability of data influenced the items counted in this case. Before making use of any statistics, whether from official state offices, the census bureau, or a health agency, it is necessary to discover what the information represents.

The count of reported rapes and attempted rapes describes two groups in Houston, but it does not describe all rape in the city. Only the number of persons who fall into the groups "reported being raped" and "reported an attempted rape" is known. If we want to use this count as a means of understanding a characteristic about the total city, it must be seen in proportion. That is, we have to divide it by the total number in the population of this city. Consider the different meanings such counts would have if the population of Houston were 50,000 on the one hand, or 500,000 on the other.

RATES

In order to express a count as a proportion, or rate, you first have to decide on the population you want to study. If you consider 875 reported rapes in relation to the total number of inhabitants, you will have one rate; if you consider them in relation to the total female population of Houston, you will be given a different proportion. In epidemiology, the *population* represents the universe of people defined as the objects of your study. Because it is difficult, if not impossible, to study the entire population, most epidemiologic studies draw a sample to represent that group. For example, Beatrice Selwyn wanted to study "mothers with children under 5 years of age" in Cali, Colombia. She selected one barrio with 50,000 residents, and then drew a sample of 529 mothers for interviews [18]. Sometimes, it is important to seek a random sample; at other times, a sample of convenience is sufficient. In many small epidemiologic studies it may be possible to study nearly every person in the population, thus eliminating the need for a sample.

Several proportions have wide use in epidemiology. Those most important for the community health nurse to understand include prevalence rate, period prevalence rate, and incidence rate.

PREVALENCE RATE

The prevalence rate describes a situation at a specific time [11]. If a nurse discovers 50 cases of measles in an elementary school, she has a simple count, if she divides that number by the number of students in the school, she has described the prevalence of measles. For instance, if the school has 500 students, the prevalence of measles on that day would be 10 percent (50 measles/500 population).

$$\text{Prevalence rate} = \frac{\text{Number of persons with a characteristic}}{\text{Total number in population}}$$

PERIOD PREVALENCE RATE

In the study of reported rapes in Houston, the investigators had a count for a two-year period, 1974–1975. Rather than portraying only one day, this number covered an extended period of time. The two-year period prevalence rate was .08 percent of the total population of females in Houston.

$$\text{Period prevalence rate} = \frac{\substack{\text{Number of persons with a characteristic} \\ \text{during a period of time}}}{\text{Total number in population}}$$

INCIDENCE RATE

Not everyone in a population is at risk for developing a disease, being raped, or having some other health–illness characteristic. The incidence rate recognizes this fact; for example, some childhood diseases give lifelong immunity. The children in a school who have had such diseases would be removed from the total in the school population. The incidence rate, after 3 weeks of a measles epidemic in a school, was 15 percent per day. The health literature is not always consistent in the use of the term *incidence;* sometimes this word is used synonymously with prevalence rates and the reader must take this into consideration.

$$\text{Incidence rate} = \frac{\substack{\text{Number of persons} \\ \text{developing a disease}}}{\text{Total number at risk}} \text{ per unit of time}$$

COMPUTING RATES

In order to make comparisons between populations, such as those of San Francisco and Seattle, epidemiologists often use a common base population in computing rates. For example, instead of merely saying that the rate of an illness is 13 percent in one city and 25 percent in another, the comparison is made per 100,000 persons in the population. This population base can vary for different purposes from 1,000 to 100,000. The following are some formulas for computing rates commonly used in community health:

$$\text{Mortality rate} = \frac{\text{Number of reported deaths}}{\begin{array}{c}\text{Estimated population as of}\\ \text{July 1 of same year}\end{array}} \times 100,000$$

$$\text{Infant mortality rate} = \frac{\begin{array}{c}\text{Number of deaths under}\\ \text{1 year of age for given year}\end{array}}{\begin{array}{c}\text{Number of live births}\\ \text{reported for same year}\end{array}} \times 1,000$$

$$\text{Case fatality rate} = \frac{\begin{array}{c}\text{Number of deaths from}\\ \text{a particular disease}\end{array}}{\begin{array}{c}\text{Total number with the}\\ \text{disease}\end{array}}$$

The goal of descriptive studies is to identify the patterns of occurrence of any health-related condition. In a descriptive study of child abuse, for example, the investigator would note the age, sex, race or ethnic group, and physical and emotional conditions of the children affected. In addition, data would be collected that described the economic status and occupation of parents, the location and setting of abusive behavior, and the time and season of the year when abuse occurred. In the study on reported rape in Houston, the investigators described the age, sex, and ethnic background of victims and offenders, and other features such as location and time of the crime. Figure 9-5 shows two temporal characteristics—time of day and day of week—of the pattern of reported rape. Although this pattern does not identify the *cause* of rape, it does describe facets of this health condition and suggest avenues for intervention or prevention.

ANALYTIC STUDIES

The second kind of observational study is *analytic*. It differs from descriptive study only by its attempt to determine causal factors, to explain the described phenomena. Analytic studies tend to be more

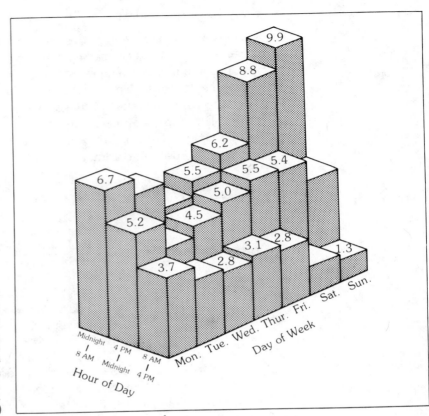

Figure 9-5. Distribution (by percent, scale 0 to 10) of reported rape by hour of day and day of week, in Houston, Texas, 1974–1975. (From J. Sanford et al., Patterns of reported rape in a tri-ethnic population: Houston, Texas, 1974–1975. *Am. J. Public Health* 69(5):483, 1979. Reprinted by permission.)

specific than descriptive studies in their focus. They test hypotheses or seek to answer specific questions. For example, one nurse set out to test the hypothesis that "wife-battering is related to violence in the victim's childhood family of origin" [15]. This study interviewed all the women who applied for legal assistance at a legal aid bureau in Baltimore, Maryland during a five-day period. Fifty women agreed to participate in an in-depth interview. The investigators described many characteristics of these women, 20 of whom were battered wives and 30 of whom were non-battered. No significant differences were found in variables such as age, race, education, and years of marriage. However, the hypothesis that those women beaten by their husbands had come from families where their mothers had been victims of the battered wife syndrome was confirmed. Like many analytic studies, this one gathered a great deal of descriptive data as well.

PREVALENCE STUDIES

Observational studies fall into three types—prevalence studies, case-control studies, and cohort studies. A prevalence study describes the pattern of occurrence, as in the study of reported rapes in Houston. It may examine causal factors, but these are always from the same time frame and the same population. Such causes are based on inferences from a single examination and most likely need further testing for validation.

CASE-CONTROL STUDIES

Case-control studies make a comparison between persons with a health–illness condition (cases) and those who lack this condition (controls). In the study of battered wives, the 20 women who had been beaten by their husbands represented the cases; the 30 who had not experienced violence were the controls. In a case-control study, both groups should share as many characteristics as possible in order to isolate possible causes. Comparison between one group of women in their early twenties with another group in their late seventies would have invalidated the conclusion in the study of the battered wife syndrome.

COHORT STUDIES

Cohort studies, rather than measure the relationship of variables in existing conditions, study the development of a condition over time. A cohort study begins by selecting a group of persons who display certain defined characteristics before the onset of the condition being investigated. In studying a disease, the cohort might include individuals initially free of the disease but known to have been exposed. They would be followed over time to see what variables were associated with the development or nondevelopment of the disease. In one school, several nurses studied two matched cohorts of children. One group received focused public health nursing attention; the other received routine school nursing services. These cohorts were studied over time to see what differences occurred as a result of the different treatment. Decreased absenteeism resulted in the first group [13].

RETROSPECTIVE AND PROSPECTIVE STUDIES

Finally, all the various types of observational studies may be either retrospective or prospective. A retrospective study decides on an investigation, then goes back and reviews existing data. The study of reported rapes in Houston was a retrospective study, utilizing police department data which had been collected earlier. Prospective studies decide on an investigation, identify variables and possible hypotheses, and then collect the data. They deal with current information and provide a direct measure of the variables in question.

In actual practice, the various types of studies just discussed are frequently mixed. A case-control study may include description and analysis with a retrospective focus; a cohort study may be conducted prospectively or retrospectively. Flexibility is essential to allow the investigator as much freedom as possible in choosing the most useful methodology.

EXPERIMENTAL METHOD

Experimental epidemiology, while used much less than the observational method, is valuable; it is used to study epidemics, the etiology of human disease, the value of preventive and therapeutic measures, and the evaluation of health services [12].

Experimental studies are carried out under controlled conditions. The investigator exposes one group (the experimental group) to some condition thought to cause disease, improve health, prevent disease, or influence health in some way. This exposure takes place under carefully controlled conditions and may involve animal or human populations. In human populations, experimental studies should almost always deal with disease prevention or health promotion; for obvious ethical reasons, studies that induce disease usually require an animal population. For instance, while humans can be used to test polio vaccine, experimental studies to test the cause of polio would not be done on humans. In addition to an experimental group, this method uses a similar group to see if any changes occur without the exposure (the control group).

Consider the following example of an experimental study in community health. Hypertension screening has been recognized as a valuable tool for identifying new hypertensive clients in the community. Many different strategies, from media advertising to setting up centers at local fire stations, have been used to motivate community members to have their blood pressure taken. One group of researchers wanted to find out what type of intervention would motivate the largest number of people to participate in the hypertension screening. They selected 5 target areas in an inner city and used a different form of experimental intervention with a sample of 200 households in 4 areas;

the fifth area served as a control group. Intervention took forms such as home visits without warning by health workers offering to take blood pressures, letters inviting people to a clinic for blood pressure checks, and letters that offered gifts if people would come to the clinic. The results showed that the highest yield of new hypertensive clients came from home visits by community members trained to take blood pressure measurements. Even letters announcing the time and nature of the visit did not increase the number of new hypertensive clients [20].

The community health nurse has many opportunities to conduct experimental studies in the course of working with groups. The study need not be elaborate; even without a control group, it can provide important data for future nursing practice. Several investigators associated with the Heart Disease Prevention Program at Stanford University carried out a small but valuable study. It involved a small sample size (eleven persons), used volunteers, and did not use a control group. The researchers reviewed the evidence that smoking by pregnant women significantly increases the incidence of perinatal deaths. Earlier studies had also shown that if women stopped smoking within the first trimester of pregnancy, the risk of perinatal death could be eliminated. A survey revealed that most intervention strategies used in this situation had been of short-term duration, such as admonishments from physicians. It was hypothesized that a longer, more intensive intervention strategy, that is, 6 two-hour classes over 7 weeks, would significantly increase the number of women who quit smoking during pregnancy. A group of eleven women volunteered, went through part or all of the course, and "the absolute level of abstinence achieved—both during the remaining period of pregnancy and postpartum—ranks well above other results reported in the literature" [8, p. 897]. Similar experimental studies could be done with almost any small group that the community health nurse works with.

An expanding area of experimental epidemiology involves the use of computers to simulate epidemics. With mathematical models it is possible to determine the probability of various aspects of disease occurrence. This approach, called "theoretical epidemiology" by Lilienfeld, is making an increased contribution to our knowledge of etiology and prevention [12].

Occasionally, an experiment occurs naturally in which conditions offer the researcher the chance to make important discoveries. John Snow discovered such a "natural experiment" in London in 1854. In studying an epidemic of cholera, he observed one group that contracted the disease and another that did not. Closer inspection revealed that the major difference between these groups was their water supply. Eventually the spread of cholera was traced to the water supply of the group with high mobidity rate (sickness).

THE INVESTIGATIVE PROCESS

The community health nurse who carries out an epidemiologic investigation becomes a detective. You begin with a problem to solve, a puzzle to unravel, a question to answer. Then you begin to search for basic information, clues that might help answer the question. But information is never self-explanatory and, like a detective, the nurse must analyze and interpret every additional clue. Slowly there is a narrowing of possible suspects until you finally identify the causes of a disease, the consequences of a prevention plan, or the results of treatment. On the basis of this investigation, you can then draw further conclusions and make new applications to improve health services.

The investigative process involves six steps. Both an informal study in the course of nursing practice and the most comprehensive epidemiologic research project can be undertaken with these steps. They are:

1. Identify the problem.
2. Review the literature.
3. Design the study.
4. Collect the data.
5. Analyze the findings.
6. Develop conclusions and applications.

We want to consider each of these steps in the context of a single health research project, a comprehensive clinic set up in a high school in St. Paul, Minnesota [10].

IDENTIFY THE PROBLEM

Community health nurses are constantly confronted with threats to the health and well-being of the community. Almost daily, questions are raised, puzzles presented, and problems identified. Pregnant women who smoke threaten the health of unborn children; what can be done to reduce this behavior? Rape is increasing; what can be done to bring aid to victims? Children are injured and die from bicycle accidents; why do these occur and how can they be prevented? Several farmers have been killed in tractor accidents; what can be done to prevent them? Any threat to the health of a group offers a fertile ground for epidemiologic investigation.

Health professionals in St. Paul began with a problem: the delivery of health services to teenagers in the inner city was inadequate. The junior-senior high school population showed evidence of needed health services. The dropout rate was twice as great as the city's average; fertility rates were three to six times higher. The school dropout rate for girls who became pregnant was 45 percent. Testing for venereal disease, advice about contraception, instruction in nutrition, and other forms of health maintenance were needed.

REVIEW THE LITERATURE

All too often, after identifying a problem, health professionals rush to take immediate action. Every investigation should begin with a review of the literature. If you want to reduce the incidence of smoking among pregnant women, some other published study may suggest lines of action and research. If falls from windows have become a health problem in Chicago, the excellent study and prevention program developed in New York would be of great value [19]. Even the discovery that little, if any, research has been done on the problem you select can be valuable information. Conversely, the fact that many studies already exist does not mean you should discard a project, but perhaps only narrow it into channels not previously investigated.

One of the most valuable sources in the literature is the "review article." For example, the team that set up the comprehensive clinic in St. Paul discovered an article in the *American Journal of Obstetrics and Gynecology* entitled "Medical and social factors affecting early teenage pregnancy. A literature review and summary of the findings of the Louisiana Infant Mortality Study" [9]. Although not specifically about the delivery of health care to teenagers, it reviewed many articles that touched on this subject. A review of the literature often suggests hypotheses from discoveries made in other studies. For example, researchers in the clinic project found reports that pregnant students have a better chance of completing their education if they remained in their regular school. This finding became one hypothesis that could be tested by epidemiologic research. Even more important, the health care team used this finding as a basis for formulating a new hypothesis, that is, setting up a comprehensive clinic in the school would encourage pregnant students to complete their education [10].

DESIGN THE STUDY

The first step in designing a study is to formulate some specific question to answer, perhaps a hypothesis to test. Sometimes this hypothesis may emerge from the review of literature, as in the clinic project, but at other times it will have to be developed through your own analysis and hunches. It is a good idea to write out one or more hypotheses to test, questions to answer. We can rephrase the hypothesis implied by the clinic project as follows: The creation of a comprehensive clinic inside a public high school will improve the delivery of health services to teenagers.

In designing the study it is necessary to decide on what type or combination of types will be used. Will an observational study or an experimental study best suit the goals of the research? Will the data be collected retrospectively from existing records or will you collect new data? Who will conduct interviews? What kinds of data will be needed to measure the outcomes of intervention?

Planning for the project in St. Paul began 2 full years before the clinic was established. Through the St. Paul-Ramsey Hospital, the Maternal and Infant Care Project No. 519 came into existence. The St. Paul public schools became involved and a committee with representatives from students, parents, faculty, and other community agencies began work. This project involved an experimental study: the students at this junior-senior high school would be exposed to a new clinic. A specific control group in the form of another high school was not used; instead, data from the city as a whole would be used for comparison purposes.

It was decided that the health clinic would be led by a family-planning nurse clinician, assisted by a clinic attendant and a social worker. This team would offer services five mornings a week. In addition, numerous other health professionals, including a physician, a pediatric nurse associate, a nutritionist, and a maternity nurse clinician, would work part-time in the school. After the planning stage, the clinic opened in April, 1973.

COLLECT THE DATA

From the start of its program, the clinic staff began collecting data. They kept records on all clinic visits, the increase or decrease of utilization, and the characteristics of clinic users. For example, the clinic was used by nearly two-thirds of the senior class in 1975–1976, about equally by males and females. Records were kept on all venereal disease (VD) tests, requests for contraceptive information, fertility rate, and dropout rates among pregnant females.

Sometimes it is useful to perform a pilot study which pretests an interview guide or questionnaire. If you want to interview women about the battered wife syndrome, it might be useful to prepare a guide and interview one or two persons, then revise the guide on the basis of your experience. If you develop a questionnaire to assess the nutritional needs of elderly persons living alone, try out the questions on some volunteers to determine their clarity and relevance.

In community health nursing, data collection can often occur as part of ongoing practice. However, unless the study has been carefully planned, you may collect data for months or years, only to discover that important questions have been omitted.

ANALYZE THE FINDINGS

In most epidemiologic studies, data analysis will consist of summarizing the findings, computing rates and ratios, and displaying the findings in tables and graphs. It is at this stage that the data is used to answer the original questions or test the original hypothesis. Does the data confirm or disprove the hypothesis?

Consider some of the findings from the study of the effects of a comprehensive clinic in a St. Paul high school. First, the data showed that the postpartum dropout rate declined from 45 percent to 10 percent. This finding lends some support to the hypothesis that the clinic would influence the educational achievement of pregnant teenagers by keeping them in their regular school. It can be shown in a *bar graph* (see Fig. 9-6).

Other findings analyzed by the nurse and health team members included the number of students treated for gonorrhea and the outcomes of that treatment, a count of persons receiving contraceptive services, the continuation rate of contraceptive use, and much additional information. Figure 9-7 shows how use of the clinic for prenatal care increased from 1973 to 1976. Figure 9-8 shows the drop in fertility rate per 1,000 students during that same period. Both of these findings confirm that the clinic had a strong positive effect on the health of this population.

DEVELOP CONCLUSIONS AND APPLICATIONS

Stating conclusions is an outcome of analysis and interpretation. The investigator summarizes the results and their meaning for the purpose of sharing this information with others. Many times the research will have direct practical application for improving health services, continuing or discontinuing services, and future research.

Many studies, as with the clinic project, combine research and intervention. For example, it was noted that each summer in New York

TOOLS FOR PRACTICE

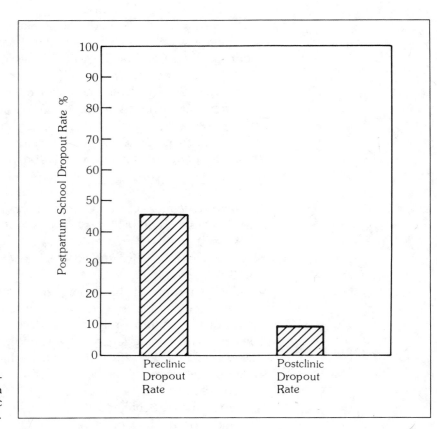

Figure 9-6. Change in postpartum dropout rate as a result of a newly established prenatal clinic in a high school.

Figure 9-7. Use of a clinic for prenatal care. Shaded areas indicate percent of students who received prenatal care. (From L. Edwards et al., An experimental comprehensive high school clinic, *Am. J. Public Health* 67(8):766, 1977. Reprinted by permission.)

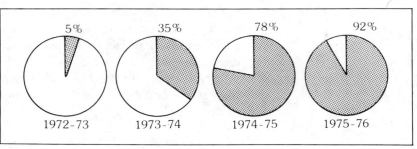

City seemed to bring on an epidemic of injured children who fell from unguarded windows. A study was conducted to determine the actual relationship of injuries to unguarded windows. As part of the study, community health nurses made follow-up visits to any home where an accident had occurred. This visit became a time for collecting data as well as educating family members in ways to prevent a recurrence of

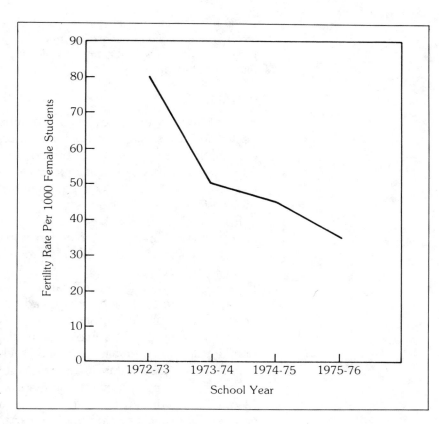

Figure 9-8. Fertility rate. (From L. Edwards et al., An experimental comprehensive high school clinic. *Am. J. Public Health* 67(8):766, 1977. Reprinted by permission.)

the accident. The New York City Health Department distributed free, easy-to-install window guards. Data collected during this project showed that a significant reduction in falls had taken place. The conclusions of the study were influential in a landmark decision by the New York City Board of Health to enact the first child accident prevention law in the United States. Passed in 1976, this law "requires owners of multiple dwellings to provide window guards where children ten years old and younger reside" [19, p. 1143].

After 4 years of operation and epidemiologic investigation, the clinic at the St. Paul junior-senior high school appeared to have proved its value. The investigators drew the following conclusions and offered recommendations for a direct application of the study [10, p. 766]:

We feel that the measurable results to date as well as the positive response of the students themselves, justify the continuation and expansion of these services within the school system. We are convinced that this mechanism provides the best hope of reducing the incidence of the "unwed mother syndrome" by interrupting the vicious cycle of out-of-wedlock pregnancy, incomplete education, alienation from friends, family, and society, and repeat pregnancy, all of which may predetermine the futures of these young parents and their offspring.

SUMMARY

Epidemiology is the study of the distribution and determinants of health and illness states in human population groups. It shares with community health nursing the common theme of the health of groups. Epidemiology can be used at three levels in community health nursing: use of existing epidemiologic data, informal investigations, and carefully designed scientific studies.

Epidemiology uses a basic model of the interaction among host, agent, and environment. Intervention may act on any of these three to prevent the spread of disease or improve health in a population. Epidemiology is based on ideas about causal relationships among these three factors. Ideas about causation have changed from the early miasma theory, contagion theory, and germ theory of disease to an emphasis on multiple causation.

Epidemiology employs two basic methods, observational and experimental. The observational method seeks to describe health-related conditions as they naturally occur. Although studies can be either retrospective or prospective, some merely describe existing conditions (descriptive studies) while others seek to explain causes (analytic studies). Epidemiologic studies of an experimental type actually intervene to expose a population of humans or animals to an illness or health condition. Observational studies can be of three types— prevalence, case-control, or cohort. In practice, all these types of studies often become combined in various ways. They also make use of quantitative concepts such as count, prevalence rate, incidence rate, mortality rate, and various types of morbidity (sickness) rates.

The investigative process of epidemiology in community health nursing includes six steps:

1. Identify the problem, which is usually some threat to the health of a population.
2. Review the literature to determine what other studies have found.
3. Carefully design the study. The investigator might decide to do an observational study or an experimental study. The methods of data collection are also identified during this step.
4. Collect the data.
5. Analyze the findings.
6. Develop conclusions and applications.

REFERENCES

1. Basco, D., Eyres, S., Glasser, J. H., and Roberts, D. E. Epidemiologic analysis in school populations as a basis for change in school-nursing practice—Report of the second phase of a longitudinal study. *Am. J. Public Health* 62(4):491, 1972.

2. Benenson, A. S. *Control of Communicable Disease in Man.* Washington, D.C.: American Public Health Association, 1975. P. 716.

3. Burnet, Sir MacFarlane. Plague. In Sir MacFarlane Burnet, *Natural History of Infectious Disease* (3rd ed.). Cambridge, England: Cambridge University Press, 1962. Pp. 323–330, 342.

4. Cameron, J., Chase, E. S., and O'Neal, S. Home birth in Salt Lake County, Utah. *Am. J. Public Health* 69(7):716, 1979.

5. Center for Disease Control. *Rubella Surveillance, Jul. 1973–Dec. 1975.* Atlanta, Ga.: Center for Disease Control, 1976. Pp. 7–11.

6. Chappell, J. A., and Taylor, M. A. H. Implications of rubella susceptibility in young adults. *Am. J. Public Health* 69(3):279, 1979.

7. Chavigny, K. Self-esteem for the alcoholic: An epidemiological approach. *Nurs. Outlook* 24(10):636, 1976.

8. Danaher, B. G., Shisslak, C. M., Thompson, C. B., and Ford, J. D. A smoking cessation program for pregnant women: An exploratory study. *Am. J. Public Health* 68(9):896, 1978.

9. Dott, A. B. Medical and social factors affecting early teenage pregnancy: A literature review and summary of the findings of the Louisiana Infant Mortality Study. *Am. J. Obstet. Gynecol.* 125:532, 1976.

10. Edwards, L. E., Steinman, M. E., and Hakanson, E. Y. An experimental comprehensive high school clinic. *Am. J. Public Health* 67(8):765, 1977.

11. Friedman, G. D. *Primer of Epidemiology.* New York: McGraw-Hill, 1974. Pp. 3, 8.

12. Lilienfeld, A. M. *Foundations of Epidemiology.* New York: Oxford University Press, 1976. Pp. 11, 218, 233.

13. Long, G., Whitman, C., Johansson, M., Williams, C., and Tuthill, R. Evaluation of a school health program directed to children with history of high absence. *Am. J. Public Health* 65(4):388, 1975.

14. MacMahon, B., and Pugh, T. *Epidemiology: Principles and Methods.* Boston: Little, Brown, 1970. P. 23.

15. Parker, B., and Schumacher, D. N. The battered wife syndrome and violence in the nuclear family of origin: A controlled pilot study. *Am. J. Public Health* 67(8):760, 1977.

16. Potter, M. E., et al. A sausage-associated outbreak of trichinosis in Illinois. *Am. J. Public Health* 66(12):1194, 1976.

17. Sanford, J., Cryer, L., Christensen, B. L., and Mattox, K. L. Patterns of reported rape in a tri-ethnic population: Houston, Texas, 1974–1975. *Am. J. Public Health* 69(5):480, 1979.

18. Selwyn, B. J. An epidemiological approach to the study of users and nonusers of child health services. *Am. J. Public Health* 68(3):231, 1978.

19. Spiegel, C. N., and Lindaman, F. C. Children can't fly: A program to prevent childhood morbidity and mortality from window falls. *Am. J. Public Health.* 67(12):1143, 1977.

20. Stahl, S. M., Laurie, T., Neill, P., and Kelley, C. Motivational intervention in community hypertension screening. *Am. J. Public Health* 67(4):345, 1977.

SELECTED READINGS

Abrahamson, J. H., et al. The contribution of a health survey to a family practice. *Scand. J. Soc. Med.* 1:33, 1973.

Anthony, N., et al. Immunization: Public health programming through law enforcement. *Am. J. Public Health* 67(8):763, 1977.

Baker, S. P. Determinants of injury and opportunities for intervention. *Am. J. Epidemiol.* 101(2):98, 1975.

Basco, D., et al. Epidemiologic analysis in school populations as a basis for change in school nursing practice—Report of the second phase of a longitudinal study. *Am. J. Public Health* 62(4):491, 1972.

Benenson, A. S. (Ed.). *Control of Communicable Diseases in Man.* Washington, D.C.: American Public Health Association, 1975.

Brown, M. M. The epidemiologic approach to the study of clinical nursing diagnoses. *Nurs. Forum* 13(4):346, 1974.

Cassel, J. C. Information for epidemiologic and health services research. *Med. Care* [Supplement] 11(2):76, 1973.

Chavigny, K. Self-esteem for the alcoholic: An epidemiologic approach. *Nurs. Outlook* 24(10):636, 1976.

Cohn, H., and Schmidt, W. M. The practice of family health care. *Am. J. Public Health* 65(4):375, 1975.

Corrigan, M., and Corcoran, L. *Epidemiology in Nursing.* Washington, D.C.: Catholic University of America Press, 1961.

Danaher, B., et al. A smoking cessation program for pregnant women: An exploratory study. *Am. J. Public Health* 68(9):896, 1978.

Donabedian, D. Computer-taught epidemiology. *Nurs. Outlook* 24 (12):749, 1976.

Drake, W. E., Jr., et al. Community action in stroke management. *Am. J. Public Health* 62(4):522, 1972.

Edwards, L., Steinman, M., and Hakanson, E. An experimental comprehensive high school clinic. *Am. J. Public Health* 67(8):765, 1977.

Fox, J. P., Hall, C. E., and Elveback, L. R. *Epidemiology: Man and Disease.* London: Macmillan, 1970.

Friedman, G. D. *Primer of Epidemiology.* New York: McGraw-Hill, 1974.

Kark, S. L. *Epidemiology and Community Medicine.* New York: Appleton-Century-Crofts, 1974.

Kirscht, J. P.   Social and psychological problems of surveys on health and illness. *Soc. Sci. Med.* 5:519, 1971.

Lauzon, R.   An epidemiological approach to health promotion. *Can. J. Public Health* 68:311, 1977.

Lilienfeld, A.   *Foundations of Epidemiology.* New York: Oxford University Press, 1976.

Long, G. V., et al.   Evaluation of a school health program directed to children with history of high absence. *Am. J. Public Health* 65(4):388, 1975.

MacMahon, B., and Pugh, T. F.   *Epidemiology: Principles and Methods.* Boston: Little, Brown, 1970.

Mauser, J. S., and Bahn, A. K.   *Epidemiology: An Introductory Text.* Philadelphia: Saunders, 1974.

Patrick, D., Bush, J., and Chen, M.   Methods for measuring levels of well-being for a health status index. *Health Sci. Res.* 8:228, 1973.

Reeder, L. G.   Social Epidemiology: An Appraisal. In E. G. Jaco (Ed.), *Patients, Physicians, and Illness: A Sourcebook in Behavioral Science and Health* (2nd ed.). New York: Free Press, 1972.

Ruybal, S. E., Bauwens, E., and Fasla, M.   Community assessment: An epidemiological approach. *Nurs. Outlook* 23(6):365, 1975.

Sackett, D. L., and Baskin, M. S.   *Methods of Health Care Evaluation.* Hamilton, Ontario: McMaster University, 1973.

Smiley, J., Eyres, S., and Roberts, D. E.   Maternal and infant health and their associated factors in an inner city population. *Am. J. Public Health* 62(4):476, 1972.

Taylor, W. C.   School children and reported hepatitis: An epidemiological note. *Am. J. Public Health* 66(8):793, 1976.

Terris, M.   Approaches to an epidemiology of health. *Am. J. Public Health* 65(10):1037, 1975.

Troop, E.   The application of epidemiological principles to community nursing. In M. Corrigan and L. Corcoran, *Epidemiology in Nursing.* Washington, D.C.: Catholic University of America Press, 1961. Pp. 244–259.

Wesson, A. F.   On the scope and methodology of research in public health practice. *Soc. Sci. Med.* 6:469, 1972.

THREE

CARE OF COMMUNITIES

TEN

THE NATURE OF FAMILIES

Imagine that you are employed as a community health nurse by an agency in Los Angeles. In a single day you might visit five families, each with different health problems. A young mother in one family seeks help in caring for her sick infant. Another family has an elderly parent recently discharged from the hospital after a stroke. The third family are Vietnamese immigrants who need instruction on the purchase and preparation of food. In the other two visits, you will check the progress of a serious burn on the arm of a ten-year-old, develop a contract for weight control with his mother, and assist a recently retired couple in adjusting to their new stage of life.

As you set out for a day of work, what kinds of things will you need to know? You will have to deal with specific health problems such as strokes, burns, and retirement. You need to know your goals, the promotion of health and self-care. You will have to rely on your knowledge of cultural differences when working with the Vietnamese family and perhaps other clients. You will need to know how to use certain tools such as problem solving and contracting. You will need to understand communication and know how to develop a helping relationship.

But do you need to know something about the nature of families? What should be known about the five families you will visit, apart from their individual members and problems? Do families, as basic units of a community, have characteristics that affect community health nursing service? The answer is an unqualified "yes." As a community health nurse, your effectiveness depends on knowing how to work with families as a unit.

CHARACTERISTICS OF FAMILIES

Let us begin with three observations. First, all families are unique. The five families you will visit have their own distinct problems and strengths. None will be exactly like any other family. As you approach the door of a large house or ring the doorbell in an apartment, you cannot assume that you know what the family inside will be like. Consequently, you will have to gather information about each particular family in order to achieve your nursing objectives.

Second, every family is like every other family. The five families you visit do have certain features that they share with all families. These universal characteristics provide an important key to understanding each family's uniqueness. Five of the most important family universals for community nursing are:

1. Every family is a small social system.
2. Every family has its own cultural values and rules.
3. Every family has structure.
4. Every family has certain basic functions.
5. Every family moves through stages in its "life cycle."

No matter how many families you might visit in the course of a year, each one will have these universal features. It will be important to know how the social system, cultural values, structure, function, and stage of development affect health care delivery. These five universals of family life provide the framework of this chapter.

Third, some families are more alike than others. Between the extremes of complete uniqueness and universal features, certain similarities among some families permit a classification of subtypes. For example, although all families have structure, the five you visit may consist of three types—three nuclear families (husband, wife, children), one nuclear dyad (husband and wife), and one multi-generation family. Knowing the range of variation within the family universals will help prepare you for the families you encounter. As we consider the universals of family life, we will also discuss those subtypes that characterize our own society; if we took a worldwide perspective, subtypes in family life would greatly proliferate, although the universals would still exist.

FAMILIES AS SOCIAL SYSTEMS

All of us fall into the trap of viewing families merely as a collection of individuals. Caused partly by our cultural value of strong individualism, this error also occurs because we encounter families through the individual members. When you sit in a living room talking with a young mother about her new infant, it is difficult to realize that all the other family members are present by way of their influence. We can see this by examining the nature of families as social systems.

INTERDEPENDENCE AMONG MEMBERS

First, all the members of a family, because they are units within a system, are interdependent. One member's actions affect the other members. For example, the community health nurse cannot expect a father's change in lifestyle to reduce his risk of coronary heart disease not to affect the rest of the family. If he cuts back on working overtime, the family's income will be reduced. If he begins to eat different foods, food preparation and eating patterns in the family will be altered. A new exercise program may upset other family routines. Furthermore, as this one member adjusts to the demands of a change in lifestyle, his ability to carry out his usual roles as husband and father may be affected.

This interdependence involves a set of internal relationships which influences the effectiveness of family functioning. There is a complex network of communication patterns among family members. It is possible to diagram the network as a family map of all the dyads, triads, and combinations of interactions that occur within families [8]. The way parents relate to each other, for instance, influences the quality of their parenting. When the lines between them are strong and nurturant, they have more to offer their children. Marital, parent-child, and sibling relationships all significantly influence family functioning (Fig. 10-1). They determine how well the family as a system handles conflict, provides a support system for its members, copes with crises, solves daily problems, and capitalizes on its own resources.

FAMILY BOUNDARIES

Second, families, as systems, set and maintain boundaries. The closeness of family relationships, which results from shared experiences and expectations, links family members together in a bond that excludes the rest of the world. Witness an example of family unity as the Pedrocelli extended family gathers for a Sunday afternoon backyard picnic. Witness, too, the distinctiveness of their family from all the others in the neighborhood. Because of the things they have in common, the Pedrocellis set and maintain boundaries that unite them and also differentiate them from others.

Families, however, are not closed systems. Their boundaries are

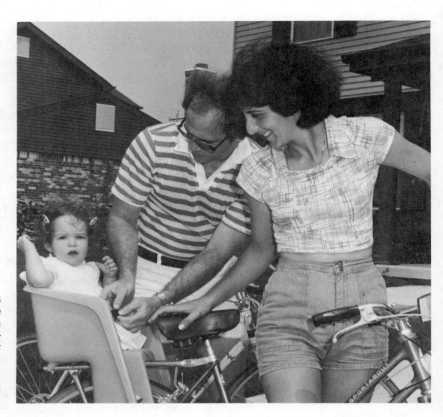

Figure 10-1. Enjoying activities together contributes to family unity and strengthens positive relationships. (From C. Schuster and S. Ashbum, *The Process of Human Development: A Holistic Approach.* Boston: Little, Brown, 1980. Photograph by Glenn Jackson.)

semipermeable, providing protection and preservation of family unity and autonomy while also allowing selective linkages with external associations. The Pedrocellis, like any family, need and have reciprocal relationships with other social systems, such as schools and work. In some instances, the outside contact is minimal and not reciprocal. Troubled families, for example, may have limited ability to reach for and utilize the resources around them; they certainly have little, if anything, to give to others in return. Their external relationships depend primarily upon the community extending itself to them. Other families, to varying degrees, establish contact with the community. They develop patterns of giving and receiving which provide them with resources in times of need. Because families are not closed systems, they also contribute to community enrichment.

ADAPTIVE BEHAVIOR

Third, families are equilibrium-seeking and adaptive systems. In accordance with their very nature, families never stay the same. They shift and change in response to internal and external forces. Internally, the family composition changes as new members are added. Roles and relationships change as members advance in age and experience, and normative expectations change as members resolve their tensions and differing points of view. Externally, families are bombarded by influences from sources such as school, work, peers, neighbors, church, and government; consequently, they are forced to accommodate to new demands. Adapting to these influences may require a family to change its behavior, goals, and even its values. Like any system, the family needs a state of quasi-equilibrium in order to function. Thus, with each new set of pressures, the family shifts and accommodates as a means of regaining balance and a normal lifestyle. There are times when a family's capacity for equilibrium-seeking and adaptation is taxed beyond its limits. At this point the system may be in danger of distintegrating; that is, family members will leave because of unresolved conflict. It is then that families may need some form of intervention, such as extended family mediation or external professional help to provide a supplemental resource for restoring family equilibrium.

GOAL-DIRECTED BEHAVIOR

Finally, families as social systems are goal-directed. Families exist for a purpose—to establish and maintain an environment that promotes the development of their members. In order to accomplish this goal, a family must perform basic functions such as providing love, security, identity, a sense of belonging, preparation for adult roles in society, and maintenance of order and control. In addition to these functions, each family member engages in tasks to maintain the family as a viable unit. We shall examine these functions and tasks in more detail shortly.

FAMILY CULTURE

SHARED VALUES AND THEIR EFFECT ON BEHAVIOR

Because every family has its own set of values and rules for operation, we can speak of family culture. Although families share many broad cultural values, they also develop unique variants. Some values will be explicitly stated: "Family matters must always stay within the family." Such values may give rise to specific operating rules: "Don't tell any of your friends how much money Daddy earns."

However, like all cultural values, many will remain at a tacit level, outside the conscious awareness of family members. These values become powerful determinants of what the family believes, feels, thinks, and does. A family that values free expression for every member engages comfortably in loud, noisy debates, while another family that values quietness, order, and control will not tolerate its members raising their voices. One family uses birth control based on beliefs about human life and parental responsibility; another family chooses not to use birth control because it holds a different set of values. How a family views education, health care, lifestyle, child rearing, sex roles, or any of the myriad other issues requiring choices, depends upon the cultural values of that family.

Family values include those beliefs transmitted by previous generations, religious influences, immediate social pressures, and the larger society. The combination of all these influences may lead a family to decide, perhaps unconsciously, that it is important to compete and succeed. Conversely, they may feel it is important to "hang loose" and never worry about tomorrow. Values become an integral part of a family's life and are very difficult to change.

PRESCRIBED ROLES

Roles, the assigned or assumed parts that members play during day-to-day family living, are bestowed and defined by the family. That is, the family determines who will play which roles and generally what each role will comprise. For instance, in one family the father role assigned to the male adult may be defined as an authoritative one that includes establishing rules, judging behavior, and administering punishment for violation of rules. In another family, the father role may be defined primarily as loving benefactor. If there is an absence of an immediate male parent, a grandfather, uncle, friend, or mother may take over the father role. Families distribute among the roles all the responsibilities and tasks necessary to conduct family living (Fig. 10-2). The responsibilities of breadwinner and homemaker, for example, with their accompanying tasks, may belong to husband and wife respectively or may be shared if both husband and wife work.

Family members often play several roles at the same time [8]. A woman, for instance, may play the role of wife to her husband, daughter to her mother living in the same home, and mother to each of her children. Even her mother role may involve wearing several different hats because it varies slightly with each child. A single parent family often combines the roles of father and mother in one person but may distribute responsibilities and tasks more widely. A grandmother or children may thus relieve the demands placed on the single parent.

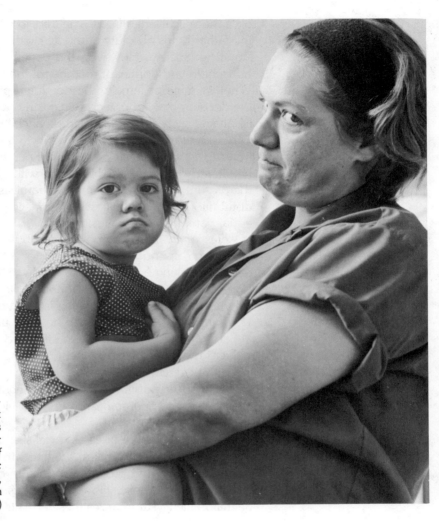

Figure 10-2. The role of disciplinarian is often difficult, but it is necessary to guide a child's socialization. (From C. Schuster and S. Ashburn, *The Process of Human Development: A Holistic Approach.* Boston: Little, Brown, 1980. Photograph by Glenn Jackson.)

Among families, there is great variation in expectations for each role and the degree of flexibility in role prescriptions. Consequently, a family may place great demands on some members while, at the same time, members may interpret their roles differently. Confusion and conflict can develop unless roles are clarified.

POWER SYSTEM

Power, the possession of control, authority, or influence over others, assumes different patterns in each family. In some families, power is concentrated primarily in one member, while in others it is distributed on a more egalitarian basis. The traditional patriarchal family, in which the father holds absolute authority over the other members, is rare in American society. However, the pattern of husband as head of the household and dominant member of the family is still frequently seen. Whether male or female, the dominant partner holds the majority of the decision-making power, particularly over the more important family affairs, such as employment, financial matters, and sexual activity. Other areas of decision making, including choices about vacations, housing, leisure activities, household purchases, and child raising, may be shared or delegated. However, with changing societal influences, the present trend among American families is toward egalitarian power distribution. Many families now practice joint decision making and equal participation by all members.

Roles often influence power distribution within the family. Along with the responsibilities attached to a role, a family may assign decision-making authority. The mother role frequently includes decision-making power regarding household management. A responsibility related to a son's role, such as lawn mowing, may empower him to decide when and how often he does the job.

Family power structure is also influenced by the amount of personal power residing in each member [7]. A mother or eldest son, for example, may exercise considerable influence over the family by virtue of personality and position rather than delegated authority. Even the child who throws temper tantrums may wield considerable power in a family.

We have viewed families as social systems. We have examined the cultural dimension of families. We know that a family is tied biologically through kinship and probably socially through choice. We know that it exists for a purpose. How, then, does one define family? Duvall's definition nicely summarizes these aspects of the family: "The family is a unity of interacting persons related by ties of marriage, birth, or adoption, whose central purpose is to create and maintain a common culture which promotes the physical, mental, emotional, and social development of each of its members" [3, p. 5].

FAMILY STRUCTURES

For many people, the term *family* evokes a picture of a husband, wife, and children living under one roof with the male as breadwinner and the female as homemaker.

This nuclear family is usually seen as the norm for everyone. Variations from this pattern have generally been treated as deviant and abnormal, even in recent studies of the family [9]. The traditional nuclear family has been sacrosanct because it is such a fundamental part of our cultural heritage, an ideal reinforced by religion, education, and other influential social institutions. Recent changes in the nuclear family have led some to predict the demise of the family itself. Yet reality insists that the nuclear model is not the only valid family form. The pressures of social conditions such as emerging new lifestyles, increasing significance of work for women, and changing sexual roles have effected changes in the American family. Approximately 12 percent of all families in the United States have a female head of household; 10 to 15 percent of couples never have children; 5 percent or more of adults will never marry; and more than 6 percent of adults live alone [4]. Although the classic family form continues to, and most likely always will, exist, there are now many variations of the nuclear model as well as emerging new patterns of family structure. Each requires recognition and acceptance by the professionals who wish to help actualize family health potential.

Families come in many shapes and sizes. We can place these varying family structures into two general categories, traditional and nontraditional.

TRADITIONAL FAMILIES

Traditional family forms are the forms most familiar to us. There is generally no question that these are families; society sanctions their legitimacy. The most obvious are husband, wife, and children living together (nuclear family), or husband and wife living together alone, either childless or with children launched (nuclear dyad). Community health nurses also work with many families that have one parent as a result of divorce, separation, or death. The nurse may visit an elderly man living alone in a high-rise apartment (single adult family) or a home where a grandmother and a divorced older daughter with her baby are living with the daughter's nuclear family (multigeneration family). Sometimes, particularly among ethnic groups, we find a group of relatives that consists of several nuclear families who live close to each other and share goods and services. Perhaps they own and run a family business together, sharing income and expenses, eat many meals together, and all have some responsibility for raising the children (kin network). Table 10-1 lists these traditional family structures.

Career patterns, particularly for women, further characterize tradi-

Table 10-1. Traditional and Nontraditional American Family Structures

Structure	Participants	Living Arrangements
Traditional		
Nuclear family	Husband Wife Children	Common household
Nuclear dyad	Husband Wife	Common household
Single parent family	One adult (separated, divorced, widowed) Children	Common household
Single adult	One adult	Living alone
Multigeneration family	Any combination of the first four traditional family structures	Common household
Kin network	Two or more reciprocal households (related by birth or marriage)	Close geographic proximity
Nontraditional		
Commune family	Two or more monogamous couples Shared children	Common household
Group marriage commune family	Several adults "married" to each other Shared children	Common household
Group network	Reciprocal nuclear households or single members	Close geographic proximity
Unmarried single parent family	One parent (never married) Children	Common household
Unmarried couple	Two adults (heterosexual, same sex, homosexual)	Common household
Unmarried couple and child family	Two adults (as above) Children	Common household

Source. Adapted from M. Sussman, Family systems in the 1970's: Analysis, policies, and programs. *Ann. Am. Acad.* 396:216, Jul., 1971.

tional family structures. Sussman distinguishes between two types of nuclear families—single career and dual career [9]. Single career families have one breadwinner, usually the husband. Both partners work in dual career families, although one partner's career, more often the wife's, may be interrupted for child raising. Nuclear dyads may also be single or dual career. Some single parent families include a working adult; others may have a single parent, such as a woman deserted by her husband and without any employable skills, who has no career. These variant structures remind us that even traditional families can assume many forms.

NONTRADITIONAL FAMILIES

Nontraditional family structures include all the newly emerging family forms; some of these forms are accepted by society and others are strongly questioned on the basis of illegitimate union. Table 10-1 lists some of the prominent nontraditional structures. One of the more well-known nontraditional family forms is composed of several unrelated, monogamous (married or committed to one person) couples living together and collectively raising their children (commune family). A variation of the commune family is the common household in which several adults are all "married" to each other; they share everything, including sex and child raising (group marriage). Occasionally a group of nuclear families, not related by birth or marriage but bound by a common set of values such as a religious system, live close to each other and share goods, services, and child-raising responsibilities (group network). Some commune and group network families select one of their members, usually a male, to be their leader, or head.

Some nontraditional families clearly form outside of marriage. One example, seen more and more in community health, is the single, unmarried parent (most often a young, unwed mother) and child (Fig. 10-3). Many adult couples form a family alliance outside of marriage or through a private ceremony not legally recognized as marriage (unmarried couple). They may range from young adults living together to an elderly couple sharing their lives outside of marriage to avoid tax penalties. Such cohabiting couples may be heterosexual, homosexual, or the same sex without a sexual relationship. In some instances, these couples have their own biologic or adopted children (unmarried couple and child family).

Varying family structures raise three important issues to consider. First, we can no longer hold to the myth that idealizes the traditional nuclear family [2]. Societal changes force us (and all who work with families) to accept many variations in family forms as valid and functional. Unless we adopt this posture and avoid judging by standards appropriate to the idealized nuclear family, we are in danger of creating even more problems for the families we attempt to serve. To hold to an ideal that parents must meet all their children's needs, for example, can lead us to conclude that parenting is defective when children have

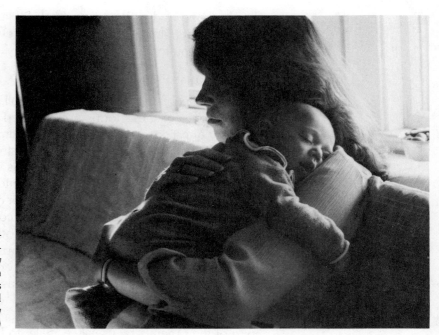

Figure 10-3. The single, unmarried parent with a child is a family form seen frequently by community health nurses. Each type of family structure has its own unique set of resources and needs. (Photograph by Jeffrey Manditch-Prottas.)

personality deficits. This expectation may be unrealistic and unattainable for dual career and, perhaps even more so, single parent families, which require supplemental resources to meet children's needs.

Second, the structure of an individual's family may change several times over a lifetime. A girl may be born into a kin network, shift to a nuclear family when her parents move away, and become part of a single parent family when her parents are divorced. As she matures, she may choose to become a single adult living alone, later part of a cohabiting couple, and still later marry and form a nuclear family. For the individual, each variant family form involves changes in roles, interaction patterns, socialization processes, and linkages with external resources [9].

Finally, each type of family structure creates different issues and problems which, in turn, influence a family's ability to perform its basic functions. Each particular structure determines the kind of support needed from nursing or other human service systems [10]. A single adult living alone, for instance, may lack companionship or a sense of being needed by other family members. A kin network family provides broad, extended family support and security but may have problems in power distribution and decision making. An unmarried couple raising a child may be parenting well but not receiving needed external support from the community in the form of recognition, approval, or assistance. Variations in structure, then, create differing family strengths and needs, an important consideration for community nurses.

FAMILY FUNCTIONS

Families in every culture throughout history have engaged in the same basic functions. From one society to the next the manner in which these tasks were performed varied. Nonetheless, families reproduced children, physically maintained their members, and provided social placement, socialization, emotional support, and social control [4]. Some societies have experimented with separation of these functions, allocating activities such as child care, socialization, or social control to a larger group. The Israeli kibbutz and Chinese commune are examples. Yet, for most peoples, the individual family unit (in its variant forms) persists, accompanied by most of the same basic functions. In American society, certain social institutions perform some aspects of traditional family functions. Schools, for example, help socialize children; professionals supervise health care; and churches influence values. Thus we see some modifications in patterns of functioning. Six functions are typical of American families today. Families provide: (1) affection, (2) security, (3) identity, (4) affiliation, (5) socialization, and (6) controls [3, 9, 11].

AFFECTION

The family functions to give members affection and emotional support (Fig. 10-4). Love brings couples together initially in our society and later produces children. In some cultures affection comes after marriage. Continued affection creates an atmosphere of nurturance and care for all family members which is necessary for health, development, and survival [1]. It is common knowledge that infants cannot survive without love. Indeed, human beings of any age require love as sustenance for growth and find it primarily in the family. Families, unlike many other social groups, are bound by affectional ties whose strength determines family happiness and closeness. Consider how the sharing of gifts on a holiday or the loving concern of a family for a sick member draws the family together. Positive sexual identity and sexual fulfillment are also influenced by a loving atmosphere. Early students of the family emphasized sexual access and procreation as basic family functions [11]. Now we recognize that families exist not only to regulate the sex drive and perpetuate the species but also to sustain life and foster human potential through a strong, affectional climate.

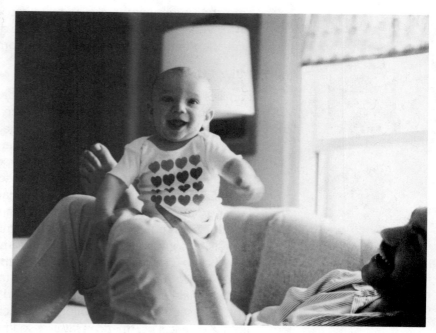

Figure 10-4. An important family function is to demonstrate affection in order to promote members' growth. A child, recognizing his father's love, responds with confidence. (Photograph by Helane Manditch-Prottas.)

SECURITY

Families meet their members' physical needs by providing food, shelter, clothing, health care, and other necessities; in so doing, they create a secure environment. Members need to know that these basics will be available and that the family is committed to providing them.

The stability of the family unit also gives members a sense of security. The family offers a safe retreat from the competition of the outside world, especially when members are accepted for themselves. They can learn, make mistakes, and grow in a secure environment. Where else does the toddler, after repeated falls, receive the encouragement to keep trying to walk; or the child, teased by a bully, regain his courage; or a parent, feeling burned out on a job, find comfort and renewal? The dependability of the family unit promotes confidence and self-assurance among its members, contributing to their mental and emotional health and equipping them with the skills necessary to cope with the outside world.

IDENTITY

The family functions to give members a sense of social and personal identity. From infancy on, the individual gains a sense of identity and worth from the family. Like a mirror, the family reflects back to its members a picture of who they are and how valuable they are to others. Positive reflections provide the individual with a sense of satisfaction and worth, such as that experienced by a girl when her family applauds her efforts in a swimming meet. Need fulfillment in the home determines satisfaction in the outside world; it particularly affects other interpersonal relationships and career choices. Roles learned within the family also give members a sense of identity. A boy growing up and learning his family's expectations for the male role soon develops a sense of the kind of person he must strive to be; often, he is expected to be strong, competitive, successful, and unemotional.

Families influence their members' social placement. That is, as a result of genetics, social class, race, economic position, and many other factors, families determine where their members will be placed in the social order. Social placement is a way of telling members who they are. For example, the members of a wealthy, influential family will be expected to follow in that family's tradition of attending Ivy League schools, mixing in upper class social circles, and selecting high status careers. A poor family, with its contrasting value system and social heritage, may influence its members to receive very little formal education and move into a trade at an early age. In fact, families influence their members' physical characteristics, intellectual abilities, educational experiences, social positions, economic levels, and religious and political affiliations. All these factors help to shape member identity.

AFFILIATION

The family functions to give members a sense of belonging throughout life. Because families provide associational bonds and group membership, they help satisfy their members' needs for belonging. We all know that we are integral, that we belong, to our families. However, the quality of a family's communication influences its closeness. If communication patterns are effective, then affiliation ties are strong and belonging needs are met. One family handles conflict over financial expenditures, for instance, by discussing differences and making compromises. A second family never resolves its financial conflicts. Instead, one member makes a selfish purchase and another member retaliates with an equally expensive personal expenditure. The healthier interactional pattern of the first family contributes to its strong sense of affiliation.

The family, unlike other social institutions, involves permanent relationships. Long after friends from school, the old neighborhood, work, or church have come and gone, we still have the family. The family provides its members with affiliation and fellowship that are unbroken by distance or time. Even when scattered across the country, family members will gather to support each other and to share in a holiday, wedding, graduation, or funeral. After separation, there is no need to reestablish ties; it is taken for granted that we belong and that we can take up where we left off. It is to the family we turn in times of happiness or need. We know we can freely share our distress and joy, call at any time, and borrow a shoulder to cry on or money to get us out of a financial bind. The durability of this affiliation remains a resource for life.

SOCIALIZATION

The family functions to socialize the young. Families transmit their culture, that is, their values, attitudes, goals, and behavior patterns, to their members. Members are socialized into a way of life that reflects and preserves that cultural heritage and, in turn, pass that heritage on to the next generation (Fig. 10-5). From infancy on, we learn to control our bowels, eat with utensils, dress ourselves, manage our emotions, and behave according to sociocultural prescriptions for our age and sex. Through this process, we learn our roles in the family. Our life-styles, the foods we prefer, our relationships with other people, our ideas about child raising, and our attitudes about religion, abortion, equal rights, or euthanasia are all strongly influenced by our families. Although experiences outside of the family also have a strong influence on roles, they are filtered through the perceptions we acquired during early socialization.

The socialization process also influences the degree of independence experienced by growing children. Some families release their maturing members by degrees, preparing them early for adult roles. Other families promote dependent roles and find release painful and difficult.

CONTROLS

The family functions to maintain social control. Families maintain order through establishment of social controls both within the family and between family members and outsiders. Members' conduct is controlled by the family's definition of acceptable and nonacceptable behaviors. From minor points such as elbows off the table to larger issues, such as standards of home cleanliness, appropriate dress, children's proper address of adults, or a teenager's curfew, the family imposes limits. Then it maintains those limits by a system of rewards for con-

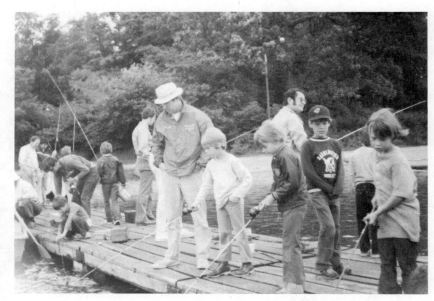

Figure 10-5. Fathers fishing with their sons reinforce the importance of a sport that many of the sons may continue to enjoy through their adult years. (From C. Schuster and S. Ashburn, *The Process of Human Development: A Holistic Approach.* Boston: Little, Brown, 1980.)

formity and punishment for violation. Children growing up in a family quickly learn what is 'right' and what is 'wrong' by family standards. Gradually family control shifts to self-control as members learn to discipline their own lives; later on, they will adopt or modify many of the same standards to use with their own children.

Division of labor is another aspect of the family's control function. Families allocate various roles, responsibilities, and tasks to their members in order to assure provision of income, household management, child care, and other essentials (Fig. 10-6).

Families also regulate the way internal and external resources are used. The family identifies internal resources, such as member abilities, financial income, or material assets, and decides how they will be utilized. For instance, a man with artistic skills may be the member to landscape the yard and a woman with mechanical aptitude the member to repair appliances. This same family may choose to drive an old car in order to spend a fair portion of its income on entertainment like eating in restaurants or going to movies. Families also determine the external resources used by their members. Some families take advantage of the many religious, health, and social services available to them in the community. They seek regular medical care, encourage their children to participate in scouting programs, become involved in

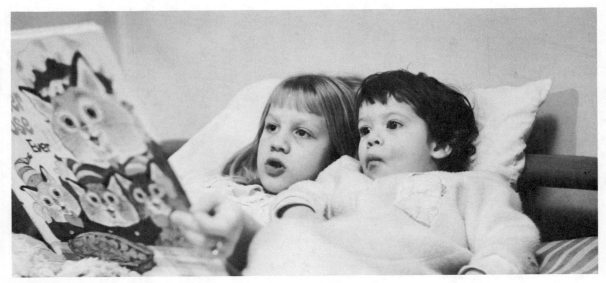

Figure 10-6. Family members all have assigned responsibilities. Older children often help with the care and training of their younger siblings. Here a young girl reads a bedtime story to her little sister. (From C. Schuster and S. Ashburn, *The Process of Human Development: A Holistic Approach*. Boston: Little, Brown, 1980. Photograph by Glenn Jackson.)

church activities, or join a bowling league. Other families, not recognizing or valuing external resources, limit their members' use of them.

Each of the six functions just described is an ongoing family responsibility, essential for the maintenance and promotion of family health [3]. Incorporated into these functions are specific tasks that a family must do to promote its growth and development. These activities are a family's developmental tasks, summarized in Table 10-2.

FAMILY LIFE CYCLE

Our examination of their nature has shown that families are social systems with cultural values, structures, and functions. A further way to understand families is to view them developmentally.

Families, while maintaining themselves as entities, change continuously. These changes occur in a sequential pattern known as the family life cycle, sometimes called the family career [1]. Families inevitably grow and develop as individuals mature and adapt to the demands of successive life changes. A family at its inception has a different composition, set of roles, and network of interpersonal relationships than at later points in time.

Consider the following example. The Jordans, a young married couple, concentrated on learning their respective roles of husband and wife and building a mutually satisfying marriage relationship. With the birth of their first child, Scott, the family composition and relationships

Table 10-2. Family Functions and Tasks

Family Functions	Associated Developmental Tasks
Affection	Establishment of climate of affection Promotion of sexuality and sexual fulfillment Addition of new members
Security	Maintenance of physical requirements Acceptance of individual members
Identity	Maintenance of motivation Self-image and role development Social placement
Affiliation	Development of communication patterns Establishment of durable bonds
Socialization	Internalization of culture (values and behavior) Guidance for internal and external relationships Release of members
Controls	Maintenance of social control Division of labor Allocation and utilization of resources

changed, and role transitions occurred. The Jordans were not only husband and wife but father, mother, and son; the family had added three new roles. Within the next four years, two daughters, Lisa and Tammy, were born. The introduction of each new member not only increased family size but significantly reorganized family living. As a result, Duvall points out, "no two children are born into exactly the same family" [3]. One by one the children entered school; Mrs. Jordan went to work for a florist; and soon Scott was leaving for college. The Jordans, like every family, were moving through the family life cycle and, in so doing, were experiencing developmental change.

DEVELOPMENTAL STAGES

Family development through the life cycle occurs in a predictable pattern of recognizable stages. Gross examination of family development shows two broad stages: *expansion* of the family as new members are added and roles and relationships are increased; and *contraction* of the family as members leave to start lives of their own. Within this framework of the expanding-contracting family are more specific stages which mark changing patterns in family growth and development. Duvall outlines eight stages in the family life cycle, which begins when a couple marries and first forms their own family, and continues through the years of having, raising, and launching children, to the empty nest, retirement, and finally death of both spouses. Figure 10-7 depicts these stages [3].

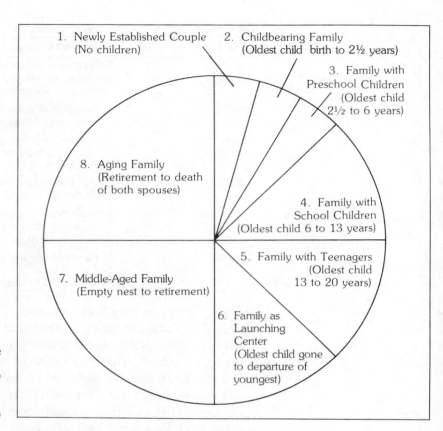

1. Newly Established Couple (No children)
2. Childbearing Family (Oldest child birth to 2½ years)
3. Family with Preschool Children (Oldest child 2½ to 6 years)
4. Family with School Children (Oldest child 6 to 13 years)
5. Family with Teenagers (Oldest child 13 to 20 years)
6. Family as Launching Center (Oldest child gone to departure of youngest)
7. Middle-Aged Family (Empty nest to retirement)
8. Aging Family (Retirement to death of both spouses)

Figure 10-7. Eight stages of the nuclear family life cycle. (Adapted from E. Duvall, *Family Development* [4th ed.]. Philadelphia: Lippincott, 1971. P. 121.)

In this model the age of the oldest child serves as a criterion for demarcation between stages. A family enters the preschool stage, for instance, when the oldest child is 2½ years of age and moves into the school stage when the oldest child is 6 years of age, even though the family may have other younger children. The size of each wedge in the circle reflects that stage's relative length. As a result of societal changes, particularly increased life span and changing roles and career patterns for women, families are having fewer children and the child-rearing period is shorter, while the median length of marriage has increased to 43.6 years [1]. As a result, couples are spending a longer portion of their lives together alone, thus expanding stages 1, 7, and 8.

To progress through the stages of the life cycle, a family must carry out its basic functions and the developmental tasks associated with those functions (see Table 10-2). Unlike individual developmental tasks, which are specific to each age level, family developmental tasks are ongoing throughout the life cycle. All families, for instance, must provide for the physical needs of their members at every stage. The manner and degree to which each function is carried out will vary, however, depending on how well members are meeting their individual developmental tasks and on the demands of each particular stage. Physical maintenance, for example, will be affected by parents' ability to accept responsibility and seek out the necessary resources to provide food, clothing, and shelter for their children. At early stages, children will usually be dependent on their parents for meeting these needs; at the school, teenage, and launching stages, however, children may increasingly contribute to home management and family income. The responsibility for these tasks shifts from parents to other family members as well.

Some functions require greater emphasis at certain stages. Socialization, for example, consumes much of a family's time during the early years of member development. These same functions and their associated developmental tasks can be further broken down into actions specific to certain stages. A family, for example, while carrying out its function of maintaining controls, sets clearly defined limits for children at the preschool stage. Do not cross the street. You may have dessert only after you finish your vegetables. Bedtime is at 8:00 P.M. During the school stage, control activities may center around allocating responsibilities and division of labor within the family. Feed the dog. Clean your room. Take out the trash. When a family reaches the teenage stage, its control function increasingly focuses on the relationships between family members and outsiders. It may regulate some activities through means such as setting a "home by midnight" limit. In other areas, such as moral conduct, controls may use family values and thus be more subtle. A family at this stage must recognize the need for young people to assume increasing responsibility for their own behavior as well as realize its own diminishing control over members. Duvall describes these activities as stage-critical family developmental tasks (see Table 10-3) [3].

NON-NUCLEAR FAMILIES

Up to this point, our discussion of the family life cycle has focused on the nuclear family. Since we encounter many nuclear families in community health, the family life cycle provides a useful means for analyzing their growth and development. However, other family structures, such as single adults living alone, single parent families, or couples who never have children, follow different life cycle patterns. They do not fit the framework just presented and require different criteria for

Table 10-3. Selected Stage-Critical Family Developmental Tasks

Stage of Family Life Cycle	Family Position	Stage-Critical Family Developmental Tasks
Married couple	Wife Husband	Establishing a mutually satisfying marriage Adjusting to pregnancy and the promise of parenthood Fitting into the kin network
Childbearing	Wife-mother Husband-father Infant daughter or son, or both	Having and adjusting to infants, and encouraging their development Establishing a satisfying home for both parents and infant(s)
Preschool-age	Wife-mother Husband-father Daughter-sister Son-brother	Adapting to the critical needs and interests of preschool children in stimulating, growth-promoting ways Coping with energy depletion and lack of privacy as parents
School-age	Wife-mother Husband-father Daughter-sister Son-brother	Fitting into the community of school-age families in constructive ways Encouraging children's educational achievement
Teenage	Wife-mother Husband-father Daughter-sister Son-brother	Balancing freedom with responsibility as teenagers mature and emancipate themselves Establishing outside interests and careers as growing parents
Launching center	Wife-mother-grandmother Husband-father-grandfather Daughter-sister-aunt Son-brother-uncle	Releasing young adults into work, military service, college, marriage, etc., with appropriate rituals and assistance Maintaining a supportive home base
Middle-aged parents	Wife-mother-grandmother Husband-father-grandfather	Rebuilding the marriage relationship Maintaining kin ties with older and younger generations
Aging family members	Widow or widower Wife-mother-grandmother Husband-father-grandfather	Coping with bereavement and living alone Closing the family home or adapting it to aging Adjusting to retirement

Source: Adapted from E. Duval, *Family Development* (4th ed.). Philadelphia: Lippincott, 1971. P. 151. Reprinted with permission.

analysis. Researchers in family theory have yet to describe non-nuclear family stages in any systematic fashion. Aldous has suggested, as one example, the following stages for families of divorced women who do not remarry [1]:

Stage 1 Establishment of the single parent family
Stage 2 Women institute or reinstitute their work-life career
Stage 3 Women with adolescents
Stage 4 Women with young adults
Stage 5 Women in the middle years
Stage 6 The retirement of women from work-life career or parental responsibilities

SUMMARY

Community health nurses' effectiveness in working with families depends on their understanding of the nature of families.

Every family is unique; its needs and strengths are different from every other family. At the same time, each family is alike because all share certain universal characteristics. Five of these universals have particular significance for community health nursing.

First, every family is a small social system. All the members within a family are interdependent; what one does affects the others and, ultimately, influences total family health. Families, as social systems, set and maintain boundaries that unite them and preserve their autonomy while also differentiating them from others. Because these boundaries are semipermeable, families can link with external resources. Families are equilibrium-seeking and adaptive systems which strive to adjust to internal and external life changes. Also, like other systems, families are goal-directed. They exist for the purpose of promoting their members' development.

Second, every family has its own culture, its own set of values and rules for operation. Family values influence member beliefs and behaviors. These same values prescribe the types of roles that each member assumes. A family's culture also determines its power distribution and decision-making patterns.

Third, every family has structure which can be categorized as either traditional or nontraditional. The most common traditional family structure is the nuclear family, consisting of husband, wife, and children living together. Other traditional structures include husband and wife living together alone, single parent families, single adult families, multi-generation families, and kin networks. Nontraditional family structures incorporate many newly emerging family forms, some recognized as legitimate by society and others not easily accepted. These variations include commune families, group marriages, group networks, a single parent family, and an unmarried couple living together.

Variant family structures remind us that the nuclear family is no longer the only viable family form; that people experience many family structures during their lifetimes; and that a family's ability to perform its basic functions is influenced by its structure.

Fourth, every family has certain basic functions. A family gives its members affection and emotional support. It promotes security through provision of an accepting, stable environment in which physical needs are maintained. A family gives members a sense of social and personal identity as well as influences their placement in the social order. It provides members with affiliation, a sense of belonging. It socializes its members by teaching basic values and attitudes that determine their behavior. Finally, the family maintains order through establishment of social controls.

Fifth, every family moves through stages in its life cycle. Families develop in two broad stages: a period of expansion when they add new members and roles, and a period of contraction when members leave. More specific developmental stages within this expanding-contracting framework can also be identified. For the nuclear family we see eight stages ranging from the newly established couple through child bearing, raising, and launching to middle and old age.

While advancing through each developmental stage in the life cycle, a family must continue to perform all of its basic functions. It must also accomplish certain tasks specific to each stage. Life cycle stages and developmental tasks will vary for families with differing structures.

REFERENCES

1. Aldous, J. *Family Careers: Developmental Change in Families.* New York: Wiley, 1978.
2. Cogswell, B. E. Variant family forms and life styles: Rejection of the traditional nuclear family. *Fam. Coord.* 24:391, 1975.
3. Duvall, E. M. *Family Development* (4th ed.). Philadelphia: Lippincott, 1971.
4. Goode, W. J. The Family as a Social Institution. In W. J. Goode, *Principles of Sociology.* New York: McGraw-Hill, 1977.
5. Hymovich, D., and Barnard, M. *Family Health Care.* New York: McGraw-Hill, 1973.
6. Pratt, L. *Family Structure and Effective Health Behavior: The Energized Family.* Boston: Houghton Mifflin, 1976.
7. Robischon, P., and Smith, J. A. Family Assessment. In A. M. Reinhardt and M. Quinn (Eds.), *Current Practice in Family-Centered Community Nursing.* St. Louis: Mosby, 1977.
8. Satir, V. *Peoplemaking.* Palo Alto: Science and Behavior Books, 1972.
9. Sussman, M. B. Family systems in the 1970's: Analysis, policies, and programs. *Ann. Am. Acad.* 396:216, 1971.
10. Sussman, M. B., and Cogswell, B. The Meaning of Variant and Experimental Marriage Styles and Family Forms. In M. Sussman (Ed.), *Non-Traditional Family Forms in the 1970's.* Minneapolis: National Council on Family Relations, 1972.
11. Zelditch, M. Family, Marriage, and Kinship. In R. E. Faris (Ed.), *Handbook of Modern Sociology.* Chicago: Rand, McNally, 1964.

SELECTED READINGS

Aldous, J. *Family Careers: Developmental Change in Families*. New York: Wiley, 1978.

Cogswell, B. E. Variant family forms and life styles: Rejection of the traditional nuclear family. *Fam. Coord.* 24:391, 1975.

Cogswell, B., and Sussman, M. Changing Family and Marriage Forms: Complications for Human Service Systems. In M. Sussman (Ed.), *Non-Traditional Family Forms in the 1970's*. Minneapolis: National Council on Family Relations, 1972.

Crawford, C. O. (Ed.). *Health and the Family: A Medical-Sociological Analysis*. New York: Macmillan, 1971.

Duvall, E. M. *Family Development* (4th ed.). Philadelphia: Lippincott, 1971.

Glasser, P. H., and Glasser, L. N. *Families in Crisis*. New York: Harper & Row, 1970.

Glick, P. C. A Demographer Looks at American Families. *J. Marriage Fam.* 37(1):15, 1975.

Goode, W. J. World revolution and family patterns. *J. Marriage Fam.* 33(11):624, 1971.

Goode, W. J. The Family as a Social Institution. In W. J. Goode, *Principles of Sociology*. New York: McGraw-Hill, 1977.

Haley, J. (Ed.). *Changing Families*. New York: Grune & Stratton, 1971.

Hill, R. B. *The Strengths of Black Families*. New York: Emerson Hall, 1971.

Hogan, P. Creativity in the Family. In *Series on Creative Psychology*. No. 2. Ardsley, N.Y.: Geigy Pharmaceuticals, 1975. Pp. 1–32.

Howard, J. *Families*. New York: Simon & Schuster, 1978.

Hymovich, D., and Barnard, M. *Family Health Care*. New York: McGraw-Hill, 1973.

Kanter, R. M. Getting it all together: Some group issues in communes. *Am. J. Orthopsychiatry* 42(4):72, 1972.

Knafl, K. A., and Grace, H. K. *Families Across the Life Cycle*. Boston: Little, Brown, 1978.

Marciano, T. D. Variant family forms in a world perspective. *Fam. Coord.* 24(4):407, 1975.

Mendes, H. A. Single-parent families: A typology of lifestyles. *Soc. Work* 24:193, 1979.

Minuchin, S. *Families and Family Therapy*. Cambridge, Mass.: Harvard University Press, 1974.

Otto, H. A. A Framework for Assessing Family Strengths. In A. Reinhardt and M. Quinn (Eds.), *Family-Centered Community Nursing: A Sociocultural Framework*. St. Louis: Mosby, 1973.

Pratt, L. *Family Structure and Effective Health Behavior: The Energized Family*. Boston: Houghton Mifflin, 1976.

Rapoport, R., and Rapoport, R. N. Men, women, and equity. *Fam. Coord.* 24(4):421, 1975.

Robischon, P., and Smith, J. A. Family Assessment. In A. Reinhardt and M. Quinn (Eds.), *Current Practice in Family-Centered Community Nursing.* St. Louis: Mosby, 1977.

Rossi, A. S. Transition to parenthood. *J. Marriage Fam.* 30:26, 1968.

Safilios-Rothschild, C. Dual linkages between the occupational and family systems: A macrosociological analysis. *Signs* 1:51, 1976.

Satir, V. *Conjoint Family Therapy.* Palo Alto, Calif.: Science and Behavior Books, 1967.

Satir, V. *Peoplemaking.* Palo Alto, Calif.: Science and Behavior Books, 1972.

Skolnick, A., and Skolnick, J. *Family in Transition: Rethinking Marriage, Sexuality, Child Rearing, and Family Organization* (2nd ed.). Boston: Little, Brown, 1977.

Skolnick, A., and Skolnick, J. *Intimacy, Family, and Society.* Boston: Little, Brown, 1974.

Sussman, M. B. Family systems in the 1970's: Analysis, policies, and programs. *Ann. Am. Acad.* 396:216 July, 1971.

Sussman, M. B. (Ed.). *Non-Traditional Family Forms in the 1970's.* Minneapolis: National Council on Family Relations, 1972.

Sussman, M. B., and Cogswell, B. The Meaning of Variant and Experimental Marriage Styles and Family Forms. In M. B. Sussman (Ed.), *Non-Traditional Family Forms in the 1970's.* Minneapolis: National Council on Family Relations, 1972.

Sussman, M. B. (Ed.). *Sourcebook on Marriage and the Family.* (4th ed.). Boston: Houghton Mifflin, 1974.

Van Dusen, R. A., and Sheldon, E. B. The changing status of American women: A life cycle perspective. *Am. Psychol.* 31:106, 1976.

Zelditch, M. Family, Marriage, and Kinship. In R. E. Faris (Ed.), *Handbook of Modern Sociology.* Chicago: Rand, McNally, 1964.

ELEVEN

FAMILY HEALTH: ASSESSMENT AND PRACTICE

Community health nursing has a long history of concern for family health. During the nineteenth century, public health nurses became aware through home visits of the significant influence that the family had on individual health. For example, many of the sick poor failed to recover because they lacked resources and support from their families. These nurses began to view client care from the more holistic perspective of family care. Nursing educators, as early as 1919, were introducing concepts of family care into curricula [2]. By 1932, the National Organization of Public Health Nursing strongly declared that *family* health was the cardinal concern of all public health nursing practice.

Although nursing continues to emphasize the family as the unit of service, a gap exists between theory and practice [3]. The problem derives in part from a health care system that fosters an individualistic orientation, often to the exclusion of the family. We have a proliferation of programs geared to individuals in specific age groups or with specific health problems. Many third party payors and reimbursement policies impose limits on the kinds of services funded, most of which are for individuals. Even public health agencies tend to organize their services around individuals. Often in response to governmental requirements, they may keep statistical records on specific disease or service categories, thus reflecting an individual rather than a family orientation. Although nurses may subscribe to the value of a family and community orientation, their experience with acute care based on the medical model often leads them to practice individualistic nursing in community health.

IMPORTANCE OF FAMILY HEALTH

NATURE OF THE FAMILY

Despite these obstacles, family nursing persists. Three major reasons underlie its continuing importance for community health. First, the family as a unit is a target for service. Much research has demonstrated that families behave as units and need to be viewed in totality for therapy to be effective [14]. The family does not simply provide the context for understanding and giving care to individuals. As we saw in Chapter Ten, it is a separate entity with definite structure, functions, and needs. The total family can be viewed as the client. In every society throughout history, the family is the most basic unit; so too in community practice [11]. It is the family, more than any other societal institution, that nurtures and shapes a society's members. Since community health practice serves population groups, we first focus on this basic societal unit, one in a series of increasingly larger communities.

EFFECT OF FAMILY HEALTH ON INDIVIDUAL HEALTH

Second, family health and individual health strongly influence each other. The health of each member affects the other members and contributes to the total family's level of health. Following her husband's stroke, for example, a woman may successfully cope with the resulting physical and emotional demands of his care but have inadequate reserves to meet effectively the needs of her children. The level at which a family functions—how well it is able to solve problems and help its members reach their potential—significantly affects the individual's level of health. A healthy family will foster individual growth and resistance to ill health and sustain its members during times of crisis. On the other hand, a family with limited capacity for problem solving and self-management is often unable to promote the potential of its members or assist them in times of need. Consider a family with an abused child. That family's level of functioning is generally very low, and the physical, emotional, and social health of each member suffers as a result.

Family health standards influence members' health practices. For instance, many individuals, even as adults, adhere to family patterns of eating, exercise, and communication. Family values influence decisions about health services such as whether or not a child receives immunizations or the mother uses birth control. Family decisions determine the kind of health care a member receives. For example, will sick members only receive care at home or will the family seek professional help? If professional advice is received, to what degree will the family carry it out? It is clear that individuals influence family health and that the family can either obstruct or facilitate individual health. The family, then, becomes an important focus for community health nursing assessment and intervention.

EFFECT OF FAMILY HEALTH ON COMMUNITY HEALTH

Third, family health affects community health. Rarely do families live in isolation from one another. Even in the most uncommunicative of neighborhoods, one family's noisy children, another family's trash-littered yard, and another's barking dog all have an impact on the surrounding families. The level at which each family functions determines whether or not it can promote a healthier community and support other families and groups rather than merely remain a liability.

Healthy families influence community health positively. Some families, for example, have temporarily housed Southeast Asian or Cuban refugees and assisted them to find employment. Others have formed community groups to encourage neighborhood safety and beautification. Many families are regularly involved in church, scouting programs, parent-teacher-student associations, or other civic activities that promote the common good.

Conversely, families with a low level of health have a negative influence on community health. Because they lack the resources to manage their own affairs, they frequently create programs and even health hazards for others. Garbage left to accumulate in a backyard, for example, attracts rats; abandoned appliances may become death traps for playing children. Regardless of socioeconomic level, a poorly functioning family becomes a drain on community resources and a threat to community health. Consider the large proportion of tax dollars and private funds that go into remedial programs for children with learning and behavior difficulties caused by problems at home, for adults with mental health problems, for the chemically dependent, and for victims of family violence, groups significantly influenced by unhealthy families. Since family health affects the health of other families, groups, and communities, nurses who assist families to develop and maintain positive health patterns and practices are also promoting community health.

CHARACTERISTICS OF HEALTHY FAMILIES

You ring the doorbell and wait. Soon someone opens the door and ushers you into the living room. You explain, in response to their quizzical expressions, that you are here to help this family sustain or raise its level of health. Of course you do not say it quite that way. Perhaps you say, "I understand you have a new baby. I'm the community nurse and I would like to assist you in any way that I can", or "I have come to see how you are getting along since your surgery." However, your job extends far beyond simply teaching infant care or postsurgical rehabilitation. This is a family, an interdependent group of people who function as a unit. That individual, the precipitating cause of the referral, is only one part of the total group upon whom you should focus. How can you sustain or raise this family's level of health? How do you determine that level?

From our discussion in Chapter Ten, we learned that families, to be healthy, must accomplish certain basic functions which they must adapt to their unique structure, environment, and needs. To develop a clearer frame of reference for understanding family health, let us consider two families in particular.

The Murphys live in a modest two-story house, clean, comfortable, and homey. There are seven of them—Jack, Bev, and their five children. Jack, now 43 years of age, has worked with the local Ford agency since high school, starting out as a mechanic and moving up to his present position of shop foreman. Bev, 41 years old, stayed home to care for the children until all were in school and then took a job as checker at a nearby supermarket. Because Bev had new responsibilities, Jack and the children took over many of the housekeeping tasks. As the Murphy children grew up, each assumed additional chores around the house as well as found jobs in the community. Two children now have paper routes, one baby-sits, one does yard work, and the oldest boy bags groceries at the market where his mother works. Each family member feels encouraged toward independence; at the same time, each member also feels supported and loved.

As a family, the Murphys do many things together. When the children were younger, they had "family night" every Friday; they played games, ate homemade goodies, and went on outings together. Church activities, baseball, and PTA functions now involve the family as a unit. Trips to their grandparents' farm in the neighboring state are delightful ways to spend the holidays or part of a summer vacation. Harmony does not always prevail with the Murphys, however. There are many disagreements over family rules, financial decisions, and other areas of family life. However, since they are accustomed to talking things over, they resolve these conflicts without difficulty. Jack and Bev together usually make the major family decisions, such as buying a car or deciding where to go on vacation. Frequently they involve the children in making decisions and encourage them to think for themselves. Around the dinner table, the Murphys often discuss current events, report on their activities, or debate various issues.

On the whole, they have had very few illnesses. There were some childhood diseases, a scattering of colds and flu, and a few broken bones over the years. Until Bev's cholecystectomy 3 years ago, none of them had undergone surgery. The family belongs to a prepaid health care plan through Jack's job and therefore is able to visit a clinic for regular checkups, immunizations, and early treatment of problems without feeling undue financial stress from health care costs. At home the Murphys eat well, and most of them are involved in some kind of exercise; even Bev, who has to watch her weight, swims regularly at the YWCA with a group of her friends from church.

The Stone family lives in the same town as the Murphys. Their sprawling rambler house in the suburbs is the center of much activity. John, 44 years old, is a professor at the community college located 4 blocks away. Because his office is so close, John often eats lunch, studies, and holds some of his classes in his home. Students also drop by frequently. Shirley, 45 years of age, became a social worker 3 years ago after going back to school. She has a heavy caseload and takes her clients' problems so much to heart that many of her evenings are spent on the phone or making extra visits. The Stones have two daughters and one son. Their 19-year-old daughter attends the community college and continues to live at home. Now the proud owner of his own car, the 17-year-old son, a junior in high school, has turned the family driveway into an auto repair shop where he and his friends spend hours tinkering with their cars. The youngest girl, a 14-year-old cheerleader in her junior high school, has a frenetic social life. The family's pets, two German shepherds and three cats, run loose and create confusion.

John has always believed that the father is the head of the house and that his responsibility is to make the rules. He expects Shirley to enforce them. Shirley, however, is disorganized and unable to discipline herself or the children; thus, assigned tasks are not done, rules are not observed, meals are almost never eaten together, and the house is never clean. John retreats to his study while Shirley spends longer hours on the job and the children go their separate ways, unconcerned about helping at home. Communication among them is infrequent. In earlier years John and Shirley were close even though Shirley always had difficulty managing the home. Since she returned to school and then to work, Shirley has been unable to keep up with the dual demands of career and homemaking. The family still expects her to do all the shopping, cooking, cleaning, and laundry. John is supportive of her professional efforts as long as they do not require him to make any adjustments in his routine and lifestyle. Shirley has a cleaning woman come once a week, but the house quickly resumes its perpetual disarray.

The Stones spend very little time together as a family, and consequently know almost nothing about each other's activities, interests, or needs. John, frustrated at not getting a promotion this year, has become more reclusive and has begun to drink heavily. Feeling inadequate about her inability to manage her life, Shirley has stepped up her work activities, drinks coffee excessively, and takes 2 or 3 Valium each day. Their son, kicked off the football squad for violating training rules, uses his car as an outlet for aggression and to attract attention. Unbeknown to her parents, the younger daughter has been smoking marijuana for the past 6 months.

Some families, like the Murphys, are healthy. Others, like the Stones, are not. Still others are somewhere in between. In fact, family health, like individual health, ranges along a continuum from wellness to illness. A family may be at one point on that continuum now and at a much different point 6 months from now. Family health refers to the health status of a given family at a given point in time. What is it that tells us the Murphys are a healthy family and the Stones are not?

A cursory view shows that the Murphys are accomplishing their basic functions. We see indications of a loving, nurturing climate (affection). The family provides consistently for its members' physical and emotional needs (security). Each member appears to be growing in independence and successfully adding new roles (identity). The family is close and utilizes effective communication patterns (affiliation). Members' behavior appears consistent with family values (socialization), and division of tasks and use of resources are flexible and adapted to changing family needs (controls).

The Stones, on the other hand, are not accomplishing these functions. At an earlier stage, they were a close, loving family but now the members have drifted apart. There is little evidence of an affectional climate. Physical and emotional needs are met only minimally, if at all, which contributes to lack of security and inadequate identity development. Communication patterns are poor; there is little sense of affiliation. Because guidance of values and behavior is almost nonexistent now, the family has little influence on members' socialization or social control. At this point in time, we see a poorly functioning family, an unhealthy family.

Analysis of a family in terms of how it meets these basic functions, however, does not give us a satisfactory picture of its health status. More definitive criteria are needed. Recent research on families, and particularly on family health behavior, gives us new data with which to assess family health. We can now describe a healthy family more explicitly.

Healthy families have six important characteristics [11, 12]:

1. There is a facilitative process of interaction among family members.
2. They enhance individual member development.
3. Their role relationships are structured effectively.
4. They actively attempt to cope with problems.
5. They have a healthy home environment and lifestyle.
6. They establish regular links with the broader community.

Let us examine these characteristics more closely.

FACILITATIVE INTERACTION AMONG MEMBERS

Healthy families communicate. Their patterns of interaction are regular, varied, and supportive. Adults communicate with adults, children with children, and adults with children. These interactions are frequent and assume many forms. Healthy families use frequent verbal communication. Like the Murphys, they discuss problems, confront each other when angry, share ideas and concerns, and write or call each other when separated. They also communicate frequently through nonverbal means, particularly those families from cultural or subcultural groups that are less verbal. There are innumerable ways—smiling encouragingly, embracing warmly, frowning disapprovingly, being available, withdrawing for privacy, doing an unsolicited favor, serving tea, giving a gift—to convey feelings and thoughts without words. The family that has learned to communicate effectively has members who are sensitive to each other. They watch for cues and verify messages in order to assure understanding. This kind of family recognizes and deals with conflicts as they arise. Its members have learned to share and to work collaboratively with each other.

Effective communication is necessary for a family to carry out its basic functions. To demonstrate affection and acceptance, to promote

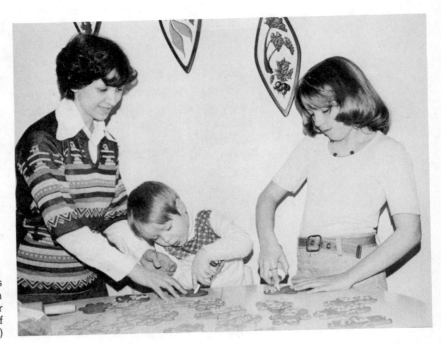

Figure 11-1. Healthy families have fun together and engage in activities that promote their members' growth. (Courtesy of the *Mt. Vernon News.*)

identity and affiliation, and to guide behavior through socialization and social controls, family members must communicate. Like the correlation between a high degree of communication and high degree of effectiveness in organizational functioning, families' facilitative communication patterns promote the health and development of their members [11] (Fig. 11-1).

ENHANCEMENT OF INDIVIDUAL DEVELOPMENT

Healthy families are responsive to their individual members' needs and provide the freedom and support necessary to promote each member's growth. "The level of health will be greater in families which support their members' personal needs and interests, assist the members' efforts to cope and function, and tolerate and encourage members' moves toward self-actualization" [11, p. 125]. If a father in a healthy family loses his job, his family will work to support his ego and help him use his energy constructively to adjust and find new work. The healthy family recognizes the growing child's need for independence, which it fosters through increasing opportunities for the child to try new things alone. This kind of family can tolerate differences of opinion or lifestyle. It is able to accept each member unconditionally and respect each one's right to be his or her own self. Within an appropriate framework of stability and structure, the healthy family encourages freedom and autonomy for its members. Patterns for promoting individual member development will vary from one family to another, depending on its cultural orientation. The way autonomy is expressed in an Italian American family will differ from its expression in a Chippewa Indian family. Yet each family can promote freedom and autonomy. The result of promoting individuality is an increase in competence, self-reliance, social skills, intellectual growth, and overall capacity for self-management among family members [11].

EFFECTIVE STRUCTURING OF RELATIONSHIPS

Healthy families structure their role relationships to meet changing family needs over time. In a stable social context, some families may establish member roles and tasks, such as breadwinner, primary decision maker, and homemaker, which are maintained as workable patterns throughout the life of the family. Families in rural areas, isolated communities, or religious and subcultural groups are more likely than others to retain role consistency because they face few, if any, external pressures or needs to change. The Amish communities in the midwest have maintained marked differentiation in family roles for more than 100 years.

However, in a technologically advanced industrial society such as ours, most families must adapt their roles to be consistent with changing family needs created by external forces. As women choose to or must enter the work force, for instance, family roles, relationships, and tasks need to change to meet the demands of the new situation [13]. Many husbands assume more homemaking responsibilities; fathers engage in child raising; children, along with the adults in their families, assume shared decision making and more equal distribution of power. The latter may be essential for the survival of a single parent family in which the children must assume adult responsibilities while the parent is working to support the family [8].

Changing life cycle stages require alterations in the structuring of relationships. The healthy family recognizes its members' changing developmental needs and adapts parenting roles, family tasks, and controls to fit each stage. Jobs around the house increase in complexity and responsibility as children are capable of handling them. Rules of conduct relax as members learn to govern their own behavior.

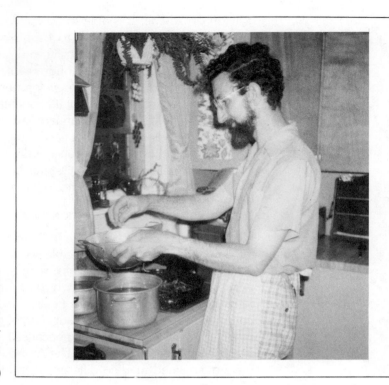

Figure 11-2. Many men today assume responsibility for home maintenance tasks, particularly in dual career or single parent families. (From C. Schuster and S. Ashburn, *The Process of Human Development: A Holistic Approach.* Boston: Little, Brown, 1980.)

ACTIVE COPING EFFORT

Healthy families actively attempt to overcome life's problems and issues. When faced with change, they assume responsibility for coping and seek energetically and creatively to meet the demands of the situation. One family dealt with the increased cost of food, for example, by raising all their own vegetables, doing home canning and freezing, cutting down on meat, substituting other protein foods, and eating at restaurants less. The result was a 25 percent decrease in their overall food expenses. Healthy families are open to innovation. Their coping ability is enhanced by receptivity to new ideas and means for solving problems (Fig. 11-2). The family that responds to gas shortages and increased gas prices by deciding to cut down on daily travel may only be adding to their difficulties. On the other hand, a family facing the same problem may solve it by exploring new ways to reach destinations. These might include increased use of public transportation, car pools, walking, bicycling, or skiing to school or work; rearranged schedules to avoid frequency of trips to regular destinations; and shopping ahead to avoid last minute trips to stores. In contrast to those who passively and fatalistically limit themselves to working with only the most obvious aids, healthy families actively seek and use a variety of resources to solve problems. They may discover these resources within the family or they may find them externally; they engage in self-care. For example, a professional couple who were faced with the expense of daytime baby-sitting arranged their schedules so that they could take turns staying home with the baby. Later, they joined a cooperative preschool which allowed their child to attend daily but required parental participation only one day a week. After having additional children, the parents, more financially able, hired live-in help. They were able to help themselves as well as accept outside help.

HEALTHY ENVIRONMENT AND LIFESTYLE

Another sign of a healthy family is a healthy home environment and lifestyle. Healthy families create safe and hygienic living conditions for their members. For instance, the healthy young family removes the potential hazards of exposed electric outlets and cleaning solvents from the reach of crawling infants. Older families recognize a greater potential for falls resulting from poor eyesight and coordination; they install good lighting and sturdy railings. These same families are concerned about cleanliness as a means of reducing infections and the spread of disease-causing organisms. Healthy families promote a healthy family lifestyle by encouraging an appropriate balance of activity and rest; they foster a nutritionally sound diet and promote regular exercise. The emotional climate of a healthy family is positive and supportive of member growth (Fig. 11-3). Such a family, like the Murphys, demonstrates caring, encourages and accepts expression of feelings, and respects divergent ideas. Members can express their individuality in the way they dress or decorate their rooms. The home environment makes family members feel welcome and accepted. As a result of all these emphases, individual members in a healthy family engage in positive personal health practices that range from regular toothbrushing all the way to coping effectively with a death in the family.

REGULAR LINKS WITH THE BROADER COMMUNITY

Healthy families maintain dynamic ties with the broader community. They participate regularly in external groups and activities, often in a leadership capacity. We may see them join in local politics, participate in a church bazaar, or promote the school's paper drive to raise money for science equipment. They use external resources suited to their family's needs (Fig. 11-4). For example, a farm family with teenagers,

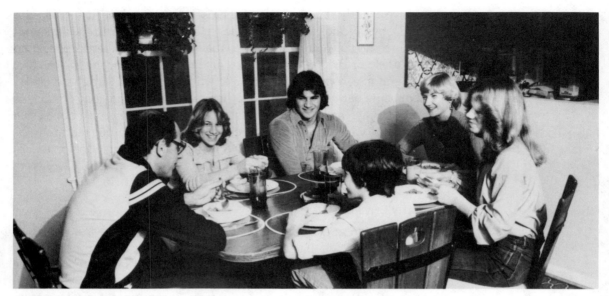

Figure 11-3. A positive, supportive emotional climate is a sign of a healthy family. (Photograph by John Neubauer for *People.* © 1979 Time, Inc.)

recognizing the importance of peer group influence on adolescents, became very active in the 4-H Club. Another family, in which the father was out of work, joined a job transition support group. The Murphys chose a health care plan that met their family's health care needs. Healthy families also know what is going on in the world around them. They show an interest in current events and attempt to understand significant social, economic, and political issues. This ever-broadening outreach gives families knowledge of external forces which might influence their lives. It exposes them to a wider range of alternatives and a variety of contacts, which increases their options for finding resources and strengthens their coping skills.

FAMILY HEALTH ASSESSMENT

A family's level of health may be elusive unless we have some means for assessment. As with the Stones and the Murphys, we may have a general idea or intuitive sense about whether or not a family is healthy. More difficult is knowing how healthy. What is that family's level of health? Assessing family health in a systematic fashion requires two tools: (1) a conceptual framework upon which to base the assessment, and (2) an instrument for measuring a family's level of functioning within that framework. The six characteristics discussed in the previous

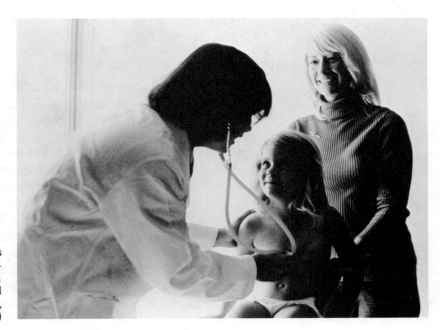

Figure 11-4. Healthy families seek out and use external resources such as regular health care. (Courtesy of the Harvard Community Health Plan, Boston.)

section provide us with a description of healthy families which serves as our framework for assessing family health. Various instruments can be used; we shall examine two in the context of five guidelines to follow when assessing family health.

GUIDELINES FOR FAMILY HEALTH ASSESSMENT

FOCUS ON THE FAMILY, NOT THE MEMBER

Family health is more than the sum of its individual members' health. If we were to rate the health of each person in a family and then combine those scores, we would still not know how healthy that family was. To assess a family's health, we must consider that family as a single entity and appraise its aggregate behavior. As we consider each criterion in the assessment process, we ask, "Is this typical of the family as a whole?" Assume that you are assessing the communication patterns of a family. You notice that there is supportive interaction between two members in the family. What about the others? Further observation shows good communication among all but one member. You may decide that, in spite of that one person, the family as a whole has good communication. When individual member behavior deviates from the aggregate picture, you will want to note these differences. They can influence total family functioning and will need to be considered in nursing care planning.

UTILIZE ASSESSMENT QUESTIONS

The activities of any investigator, if fruitful, are guided by goal-directed questions. When solving a crime, a detective has many specific questions in mind. So, too, does the physician attempting a diagnosis, the teacher trying to discern a student's knowledge level, or the mechanic repairing your car. Similarly, the nurse determining a family's level of health has specific questions in mind. It is not enough to make family visits and merely ask members how they are. If relevant data are to be gathered, relevant questions must be asked. Figure 11-5 provides a set of questions that we may use to assess a family's health. Built upon the framework of the characteristics of a healthy family, these questions guide our thinking and observations. They direct our attention to specific aspects of family behavior in order that the goal of discovering a family's level of health can be achieved. Consider the characteristic, Active Coping Effort. When visiting a family, you watch for signs of their response to change and their problem-solving ability. You ask yourself, "Does this family recognize when it needs to make a change?" or "How does it respond when a change is imposed?" Perhaps a health problem has arisen: for instance, the baby has diarrhea. Does the family assume responsibility for dealing with the problem? Do they consider a variety of ways to solve it? How do they respond to your suggestions? Do they seek out resources on their own, such as reading about causes of infant diarrhea or consulting with you, their doctor, or a clinic? How well do they use resources, once identified? Do they take a problem, try creative methods for solving it, and see it through to resolution? As you focus on these behaviors, you are asking yourself goal-directed questions aimed at finding out the family's coping skills. This investigation will be one part of your assessment of the family's total health picture.

The set of questions presented in Figure 11-5 is one useful way to appraise family health. Another, more open-ended format is used by some community health nursing agencies. This approach, displayed in Figure 11-6, proposes assessment categories as a stimulus for nursing questions. When exploring family support systems, for example, the nurse will ask, "What internal resources or strengths does this family have?" "Who, outside of the family, can they and do they turn to for help?" "What agencies, such as churches, clubs, or community services, do they use?" The open-ended style of this assessment tool allows the nurse to raise a variety of questions aimed at determining family health.

ALLOW ADEQUATE TIME FOR DATA COLLECTION

Accurate family assessment takes time. An appraisal done on the first or second visit will most likely give only a partial picture of how that family is functioning. You need time to accumulate observations, make notes, and see all the family members interacting together in order to make a thorough assessment. To appraise family communication patterns, for instance, you will want to observe the family as a group, perhaps at mealtime or during some family activity. They will need to feel comfortable in your presence in order to respond freely; it takes time and patience for such an ambience to develop.

Consider one nurse's experience. Joe Burns had talked with the Olson family twice, first in the clinic and then at home. Since Mr. Olson had not been present either time, Joe asked to see the family together and arranged an evening visit. The Olsons were receiving nursing service for health promotion. They were particularly interested in discussing discipline of their young children and contracted with Joe for six weekly visits to be held in the late afternoon when Mr. Olson was home from work. Joe's assessment began on his first contact with the Olsons. He made notes on their chart and, guided by questions similar to those in Figure 11-5, he kept a brief log. After the fourth visit, he filled in an assessment form to keep as a part of the family record. It was not until then that Joe felt he had enough data collected to make valid judgments about this family's level of health.

ASSESSMENT CAN BE QUANTITATIVE AS WELL AS QUALITATIVE

Any appraisal of family health must be qualitative. That is, we want to determine the presence or absence of essential characteristics in order to have a data base for planning nursing action. To guide our planning more specifically, we can also determine degrees of the presence or absence of these signs of health. This is a quantitative measure. We are not just asking whether a family does or does not engage in some behaviors; we are asking how often. Is this behavior fairly typical of the family, or does it occur infrequently? Figure 11-5 demonstrates one way to measure quantitatively. If we were to use this tool to assess the Murphy family's ability to enhance individuality, for example, we could score their behavior on a scale from zero to four, zero meaning never and four meaning most of the time. After several observations we would probably conclude that they responded appropriately to the

FAMILY ASSESSMENT

Family Name _____

Family Constellation

Member	Birth Date	Sex	Marital Status	Education	Occupation	Community Involvement

Financial Status _____

Using the following scale, score the family based on your professional observations and judgment:

0 = Never   3 = Frequently
1 = Seldom   4 = Most of the time
2 = Occasionally   N = Not observed

	score	date	score	date	score	date	score	date

Facilitative Interaction Among Members

   a. Is there frequent communication among all members?
   b. Do conflicts get resolved?
   c. Are relationships supportive?
   d. Is there love and caring between members?
   e. Do members work collaboratively?

Comments _____

_____

                               Totals

Enhancement of Individual Development

   a. Does family respond appropriately to members' developmental needs?
   b. Does it tolerate disagreement?
   c. Does it accept members as they are?
   d. Does it promote member autonomy?

Comments _____

_____

                               Totals

score	date	score	date	score	date	score	date

Effective Structuring of Relationships
    a. Is decision making allocated to appropriate members?
    b. Do member roles meet family needs?
    c. Is there flexible distribution of tasks?
    d. Are controls appropriate for family stage of development?

Comments _____

_____

                                              Totals

Active Coping Effort
    a. Is family aware when there is a need for change?
    b. Is it receptive to new ideas?
    c. Does it actively seek resources?
    d. Does it make good use of resources?
    e. Does it creatively solve problems?

Comments _____

_____

                                              Totals

Healthy Environment and Lifestyle
    a. Is family lifestyle health promoting?
    b. Are living conditions safe and hygienic?
    c. Is emotional climate conducive to good health?
    d. Do members practice good health measures?

Comments _____

_____

                                              Totals

Regular Links with Broader Community
    a. Is family involved regularly in the community?
    b. Does it select and use external resources?
    c. Is it aware of external affairs?
    d. Does it attempt to understand external issues?

Comments _____

_____

                                              Totals

Figure 11-5. Family assessment
               using questions.

```
┌──────────────────────────────────────────────────────────────────────────────┐
│                            FAMILY ASSESSMENT                                    │
│                                                                                 │
│  Family Name                                                                    │
│                                                                                 │
│  Family Constellation                                                           │
│                                                                                 │
│  Member names              Occupation              Educational background       │
│                                                                                 │
│                                                                                 │
│                                                                                 │
│                                                                                 │
│  Significant change in family life                                              │
│                                                                                 │
│  Coping ability of family                                                       │
│                                                                                 │
│  Energy level                                                                   │
│                                                                                 │
│  Decision-making process within the family                                      │
│                                                                                 │
│  Parenting skills                                                               │
│                                                                                 │
│  Support systems of the family                                                  │
│                                                                                 │
│  Use of health care (include plans for emergencies)                             │
│                                                                                 │
│  Financial status                                                               │
│                                                                                 │
│  Other impressions                                                              │
│                                                                                 │
│  Signature of Nurse _____ Date _____      │
└──────────────────────────────────────────────────────────────────────────────┘
```

Figure 11-6. Open-ended family assessment. (Adapted from forms used by Chisago, Mille Lacs, and Ramsey County Public Health Nursing Services in Minnesota, 1979.)

members' developmental needs (a. under Active Coping Effort) most of the time. Opposite a. on the assessment form, we would place the numeral 4 and the date of our assessment.

The value of developing a quantitative measure is to have some basis for comparison. We can assess a family's progress or regression by comparing its present score with its previous scores. Had we conducted a family health assessment 6 months ago on the Stones, for instance, and compared it with their present level of health, we would probably have discovered a drop in their scores in several areas. Many of their communication patterns, role relationships, and coping skills, in particular, would show signs of deterioration. A scored assessment gives us a vivid picture of exactly which areas need intervention. For this reason, it is useful to conduct periodic assessments. Some have suggested that assessments be conducted every 3 months [5]. In this manner, we can monitor the progress of high-risk families through the early introduction of particular preventive measures, should we see a trend or regressive behavior in some area. Periodic quantitative assessments also provide a means of evaluating the effectiveness of nursing action. We can point to documented signs of growth.

Quantitative data serve another useful purpose. We can compare one family's health status with that of another family in our caseload as a basis for priority setting and nursing care planning. The difference in the levels of health between the Stones and the Murphys tells us that the Stones need considerably more attention right now.

USE FAMILY ASSESSMENT TOOLS WITH CAUTION

While we seek to validate data, our assessment of families is still based primarily on our own professional judgment. Assessment tools can guide our observations and even quantify those judgments, but ultimately any assessment is subjective. Even though we observe that the Murphys make good use of their prepaid health plan, our decision that the use of this external resource is contributing to their health is still a subjective one. This decision is not bad. Indeed, effective health care practice depends on sound professional judgment. However, we must, at the same time, be cautious about overemphasizing the value of an assessment tool. It is not infallible. It is only a tool and should be used as a guide for planning, not as an absolute and irrevocable statement about a family's health status. This caution is particularly important when dealing with quantitative scores, which may seem to be objective.

Ordinarily, it is best to conduct assessment of a family unobtrusively. The tool is not a questionnaire to be filled out in the family's presence; its purpose is to guide your observations and judgments. Before going into a family's home, you may wish to review the questions while sitting in your car. You may find it helpful to keep the assessment tool in your briefcase for easy reference during a visit. Depending upon your relationship with a family, you may make notes during or immediately after the encounter. Like Joe, you may choose to keep a short log—an accumulation of notes—until you have enough data to complete your assessment form.

Occasionally, a family with high self-care capability may be involved in the assessment. You will want to introduce the idea carefully and use your judgment to determine when the family is ready to engage in this kind of self-examination.

FAMILY HEALTH PRACTICE

Family nursing is a kind of nursing practice in which the family is the unit of service. It is "not merely a family-oriented approach in which family concerns that affect the health of the individual are taken into account" [12]. But how does one provide health care to a collection of people? While there are some who claim such service cannot be done [7], we have increasing scientific evidence that supports its feasibility and, in fact, its necessity. It does not mean that nursing must relinquish its service to individuals. On the contrary, one of the distinctive contributions of nursing as a profession is its holistic approach to individual needs. In community health nursing, we rise to the challenge of adding a unique kind of service, one that has been neglected for too long—service to population groups that start with the family.

Several principles can clarify our understanding of family nursing and guide our practice with families.

PRINCIPLES OF FAMILY HEALTH PRACTICE

WORK WITH THE FAMILY COLLECTIVELY

To practice family nursing, we must adopt a different mind set. For the moment, we need to set aside our usual focus on individuals and remind ourselves that several people together have a collective personality, collective interests, and a collective set of needs. Viewing a group of people as one unit becomes less difficult when we examine the way we often think. We often speak, for instance, of some organization as conservative or liberal. We say that a group has taken a stand on abortion or that a business needs to become better organized. In each case, we view the group collectively, as a single entity with attributes and activities in common. So it is with families. A family has its own personality, interests, and needs.

Working with several people at the same time is not as difficult as it may initially seem. We have all experienced being part of a group that was treated as a single unit. A coach admonishes his team, "Let's practice the pivot turn one more time." A teacher says to a group of twelve-year-olds, "Now, class, I'd like you to divide into groups of four each and prepare a three page paper on how we can enjoy winter. This will be due in one week." A mother addresses her family, "This house has got to be cleaned before Grandma gets here." The church school teacher, during final Christmas play rehearsal, begs the cast to review their lines. In each instance, the group as a whole is addressed.

Group action is expected. Evaluation of the outcomes will be based on what the group does collectively.

With families, our approach is very similar. As much as possible, we want to involve all the members during nurse-client interaction. This approach reinforces the importance of each individual member's contribution to total family functioning. We want to encourage everyone's participation in the work that we and the family jointly agree to do. Like the coach, we want to help them work together as a team for their collective benefit.

Consider how we might work with the Stone family collectively. An initial contact by phone call or home visit could be used to determine whether they were interested in family nursing. If not, individual members might want service, and a family focus could be introduced at a later point in time. Assuming the Stones want family care, we would ask to meet with the entire family to discuss what the service had to offer and what they would hope to gain from it. We would explain that each person must be involved and committed to the agreed-upon goals; that, like a team of oarsmen, the family would have to pull together to accomplish the purpose of the visits. To help the Stone family improve its health status, we might jointly decide to work first on family communication patterns. A session of brainstorming could uncover many causes of poor communication. More brainstorming might suggest solutions and plans for action. On each visit we would view the Stones as a group. We would expect group responses and actions. Evaluation of outcomes would be based on what the family did collectively.

START WHERE THE FAMILY IS

When working with families, we begin at their present, not their ideal, level of functioning [7]. Although the nurse may recognize that the Stones need to develop more facilitative interaction, the family may not wish to, or be ready for, work on their communication patterns. To discover where a family is, we act in two ways. First, we conduct a family assessment to ascertain their needs and level of health. Concurrently, we determine their collective interests, concerns, and priorities.

The Kegler family illustrates this principle. Marcia Kegler brought her baby to the well-child clinic once but failed to keep further appointments. Concerned that the family might be having other difficulties, the community health nurse made a home visit. The mobile home was cluttered and dirty; the baby was crying in his playpen. Marcia seemed disinterested in the nurse's visit. She listened politely but had little to say, only repeating that everything was okay and that the baby was doing fine. He was just fussy now because he was teething, she explained. As they talked, Marcia's husband Bob, a delivery van driver, stopped by to pick up a sports magazine to read on his lunch hour. The three of them discussed the problems of inflation and how expensive it was to raise a child. The nurse reminded them that the clinic was free, and that they could at least get good health care without extra cost. They agreed without enthusiasm. After Bob left, the nurse spent the remainder of the visit discussing infant care with Marcia, particularly emphasizing regular checkups and immunizations.

The next visit also focused on the baby, but the nurse had an uncomfortable feeling that this family was not really interested in her help. After consulting her supervisor, the nurse did what she wished she had done in the first place. She asked to talk with Marcia and Bob together and explained frankly why she had first come to their home and what she could offer in the way of counseling, teaching, support, and referral to other community resources. She then asked them what, if anything, would they like. What were their concerns? The Keglers were more than responsive. There followed a listing of financial difficulties so long that sometimes they had felt like giving up. Yet the Keglers believed they would eventually overcome their problems if they just had "someone to lean on," as they put it. Their greatest concern at this point in time was for friends. They were new in the city, and both their families lived some distance away on farms. The neighbors were friendly but not close enough to confide in.

Now the nurse could start where this family was. In addition to providing needed support herself by focusing on the parents instead of the baby, the nurse also introduced them to a young couples' group which met at the community center. She had learned that, although their baby's health should be a concern, the Keglers' present social needs were greater and required her attention first.

FIT NURSING INTERVENTION TO THE FAMILY'S STAGE OF DEVELOPMENT

Although every family engages in the same basic functions, the tasks to accomplish these functions vary with each stage of the family's development. A young family, for instance, will appropriately meet its members' affiliation needs by establishing mutually satisfying relationships and meaningful communication patterns. As the family enters later stages, these bonds change with the release of some members into new families and the loss of others through death. Awareness of the family's developmental stage enables the nurse to assess the appropriateness of the family's level of functioning and to tailor intervention accordingly.

A nurse's work with the Roberts family exemplifies this principle. The Roberts, a couple in their midsixties, had recently moved to a retirement complex. They had received nursing visits following Mrs. Roberts' stroke 3 years previously but requested service now because Mr. Roberts was feeling "poorly" all the time. He thought that perhaps his diet and lack of activity might be the causes and hoped the nurse would have some helpful suggestions. The couple had eagerly awaited Mr. Roberts' retirement from teaching, planning to be lazy, travel, visit all their children, and do all those things they never had time to do when they were young. Now neither of them seemed to have any energy or capacity to enjoy their new life. The move from their home of 28 years had been difficult; they were still trying to find space in the tiny apartment for their cherished books and mementos, many of which had had to be discarded.

The nurse recognized that this family was experiencing a situational crisis (leaving their home of 28 years) and a developmental crisis (entering retirement and the aging stage). Many of the Roberts' expectations for this new life stage were unrealistic; they had not adequately prepared themselves for the adjustments that the loss of their home and retirement would demand. Through discussion, the nurse was able to help the Roberts understand their situation and feelings. They decided on a series of nursing visits focused on adapting to retirement and aging as well as agreed that the Roberts needed a support group of other persons who were experiencing some of the same difficulties. Such a group was currently meeting in the retirement center; they joined it. Because this nurse was able to help the Roberts through the crisis in a supportive and nonjudgmental manner, she found them receptive later to discussing preparation for the inevitable loss and bereavement that would occur when one of them died. She was suiting her nursing intervention to this family's stage of development.

RECOGNIZE THE VALIDITY OF FAMILY STRUCTURAL VARIATIONS

Many families seen by community health nurses are nontraditional in structure, particularly single parent families and unmarried couples. Other families are organized around nontraditional patterns; for example, both parents may have careers or a husband may care for children at home while his wife financially supports the family. There are reasons for these variant structures and organizational patterns. They result from social change—change in employment practices, welfare programs, economic conditions, sex roles, status of women and minorities, birth control, divorce, war, and many other areas. Such variations in family structure and organization lead to revised patterns of family functioning. Member roles and tasks often differ dramatically from our expectations, as in a family with a single parent who works full time while raising children, or a dual career marriage in which both partners have undifferentiated roles. Community health nurses, many of whom are accustomed to traditional family patterns, may find such variations difficult to understand or accept unless they recognize their validity.

There are two important aspects to consider in this principle. First, what is normal for one family is not necessarily normal for another. Each family is unique in its combination of structure, composition, roles, and behaviors. As long as a family carries out its functions effectively and demonstrates the characteristics of a healthy family, we must agree that its form, no matter how variant, is valid.

Second, families are constantly changing. Marriage transforms two people into a married couple without children. Adding children changes this family's structure; divorce again alters structure and roles. Remarriage with the addition of children from another family changes the family again. Children grow up and leave the home while the parents, together or singly, are left to adjust to yet another family structure. And so it goes. Throughout the life cycle, a family seldom stays the same for very long. Each of these changes forces a family to adapt to its circumstances. Consider the young woman with a baby whose husband deserts her. She has no choice but to assume a single parent role. Each change also creates varying degrees of stress and demands considerable adaptation energy on the family's part. Many family changes are predictable; they are part of normal life cycle growth. Some are not. The nurse's responsibility is to help families cope with the changes while remaining nonjudgmental and acceptant of the variant forms encountered.

Homosexual unions are difficult for some nurses to deal with. Not always recognized as a valid family form for religious or other reasons, the nurse may feel uncomfortable relating to homosexual families. Yet the nurse's responsibility remains the same. Like any family, homosexual couples need to carry out basic functions and develop characteristics that promote their collective health. The nurse can view these, and all families, as unique groups, each with its own set of needs, whose interests can best be served through unbiased care.

EMPHASIZE FAMILY STRENGTHS

Too often, without meaning to derogate, we focus our attention on family weaknesses, referring to them as needs or problems. It seems to suit our role as helper to look for things that need help. This negative emphasis can be devastating to a family and demolish any hopes of a truly therapeutic relationship: no one likes to be criticized, people with a lowered self-image (comprising a large share of the community health nurse's case load) least of all. Instead, families need their strengths reinforced.

Emphasizing a family's strengths makes that group of people feel better about themselves. It fosters a positive self-image and promotes self-confidence. It energizes the family to cope more effectively with life. This is not to say that we ignore problems. On the contrary, our assessment should explore all aspects of family functioning to determine both strengths and weaknesses. We need a total picture to achieve adequate perspective in nursing care planning, and we work on problems when the family is ready and chooses to. Yet, even as you become aware of a family's various behaviors, emphasize the positive ones. Emphasizing strengths says, in effect, "proof that you are important to me is that I see many good things about you."

Family strengths, according to Hill, are "those traits which facilitate the ability of the family to meet the needs of its members and the demands made upon it by systems outside the family unit" [4]. Not all traits that appear positive are necessarily strengths, however. Before the nurse selects a trait to emphasize, it is important first to examine it closely and ask whether or not that behavior is actually facilitating family functioning. A strong work orientation may be a strength when balanced with play and relaxation. But a family obsessed by work is experiencing this trait as a weakness. Hott suggests that the differentiating factor between whether a trait is a strength or a weakness is the amount of free choice, as opposed to compulsive drive, exercised [5].

Some traits we may consider possible strengths to emphasize are basic family functions, family developmental tasks, and characteristics of family health. For instance, we might wish to commend a family that meets its members' physical, emotional, and spiritual needs, shows respect for various members' points of view, or fosters self-discipline in its children [10].

We see a vivid illustration of this principle in the family nursing care of the Stevensons. The community health nurse made an initial home visit after referral by an outpatient physician who was concerned about possible child abuse. Alice Stevenson had brought her baby to the emergency room for treatment of a head laceration. He had fallen off the table while she was changing him, she claimed. Bruises on his arms made the physician suspicious, but Alice explained those as caused by his older brother's rough play. The nurse opened the visit by stating she was simply following up on the emergency room treatment and wanted to see how they were progressing. She made no mention of child abuse. She observed the mother and children closely, looking for small things to compliment Alice on while learning all she could about the family background. Because the nurse appeared approving rather than suspicious or judgmental, Alice agreed to further visits.

During a later session Alice admitted to the nurse that she had dropped the baby on purpose. She could not get him to stop crying, no matter what she did; she just could not endure it any longer. There had been other times when she had physically abused him, too. She had not wanted this baby at all; her husband had gotten her pregnant and then left her shortly before the baby was born. Like many abusive parents, Alice had unrealistic expectations for her children's behavior as well as very inadequate self-esteem [6]. Realizing that Alice would be particularly vulnerable to any criticism, the nurse concentrated on her strengths. She complimented her on how well she managed her home and dressed the children, on maintaining her job, and on reading stories to the three-year-old boy. It took many visits before Alice trusted the nurse, but in time they were able to discuss her feelings frankly and work toward improving this family's health. Emphasizing strengths had provided a bridge for the Stevensons into a helping relationship.

SUMMARY

The family as the unit of service has received increasing emphasis in nursing over the years. Today family nursing has an important place in nursing practice, particularly in community health nursing. Its significance results from recognition that the family itself must be a target of service, that family health and individual health strongly influence each other, and that family health affects community health.

Healthy families demonstrate six important characteristics:

1. There is a facilitative process of interaction among family members.
2. They enhance individual member development.
3. Their role relationships are structured effectively.
4. They actively attempt to cope with problems.

5. They have a healthy home environment and lifestyle.
6. They establish regular links with the broader community.

To assess a family's health systematically, the nurse needs a conceptual framework upon which to base the assessment and an instrument for measuring the family's level of functioning within that framework. The six characteristics of a healthy family provide a framework that community health nurses can use. We discussed two instruments, an assessment tool using questions and an open-ended assessment form, which can facilitate specific assessment of family health.

During assessment, the nurse focuses on the family rather than the individual member, utilizes relevant assessment questions, allows adequate time for data collection, considers collection of quantitative as well as qualitative data, and uses the assessment instruments with caution.

Community health nurses enhance their practice with families by observing five principles:

1. Work with the family collectively.
2. Start where the family is.
3. Fit nursing intervention to the family's stage of development.
4. Recognize the validity of family structural variations.
5. Emphasize family strengths.

REFERENCES

1. Duvall, E. M. *Family Development* (4th ed.). Philadelphia: Lippincott, 1971.
2. Ford, L. C. The Development of Family Nursing. In D. Hymovich and M. Barnard, *Family Health Care.* New York: McGraw-Hill, 1973.
3. Freeman, R. B. *Community Health Nursing Practice.* Philadelphia: Saunders, 1970.
4. Hill, R. B. *The Strengths of Black Families.* New York: Emerson Hall, 1971.
5. Hott, J. R. Mobilizing Family Strengths in Health Maintenance and Coping with Illness. In A. Reinhardt and M. Quinn, *Current Practice in Family-Centered Community Nursing.* St. Louis: Mosby, 1977.
6. Kempe, C. H., and Helfer, R. E. (Eds.). *Helping the Battered Child and His Family.* Philadelphia: Lippincott, 1972.
7. Kinlein, M. L. Point of view on the front: Nursing and family and community health. *Fam. Community Health* 1:57, 1978.
8. Mendes, Helen A. Single-parent families: A typology of life-styles. *Soc. Work* 24:193, 1979.

9. National Organization for Public Health Nursing. *Principles and Practice of Public Health Nursing Including Cost Analysis.* New York: Macmillan, 1932.

10. Otto, H. A. A Framework for Assessing Family Strengths. In A. M. Reinhardt and M. Quinn (Eds.), *Family-Centered Community Nursing: A Socio-cultural Framework.* St. Louis: Mosby, 1973.

11. Pratt, L. *Family Structure and Effective Health Behavior: The Energized Family.* Boston: Houghton Mifflin, 1976.

12. Robischon, P., and Smith, J. A. Family Assessment. In A. M. Reinhardt and M. Quinn (Eds.), *Current Practice in Family-Centered Community Nursing.* St. Louis: Mosby, 1977.

13. Safilios-Rothschild, C. Dual linkages between the occupational and family systems: A macrosociological analysis. *Signs* 1:51, 1976.

14. Satir, V. *Conjoint Family Therapy.* Palo Alto, Calif.: Science and Behavior Books, 1972.

SELECTED READINGS

Archer, S. E. Family: A Model of an Open System. In S. E. Archer and R. Fleshman (Eds.), *Community Health Nursing: Patterns and Practice.* North Scituate, Mass.: Duxbury Press, 1975. Pp. 30–37.

Crawford, C. O. (Ed.). *Health and the Family: A Medical-Sociological Analysis.* New York: Macmillan, 1971.

Darrill, J., and Hyde, J. Working with high-risk families: Family advocacy and the parent education program. *Children Today* 4:23, 1975.

Ford, L. C. The Development of Family Nursing. In D. Hymovich and M. Barnard, *Family Health Care.* New York: McGraw-Hill, 1973.

Gelles, R. J. Demythologizing child abuse. *Fam. Coordinator* 25(2):135, 1976.

Glasser, P. H., and Glasser, L. N. *Families in Crisis.* New York: Harper & Row, 1970.

Hill, R. B. *The Strengths of Black Families.* New York: Emerson Hall, 1971.

Hogan, P. Creativity in the Family. *Series on Creative Psychology, No. 2.* Ardsley, N.Y.: Geigy Pharmaceuticals. Pp. 1—32.

Hott, J. R. Mobilizing Family Strengths in Health Maintenance and Coping with Illness. In A. Reinhardt and M. Quinn (Eds.), *Current Practice in Family-Centered Community Nursing.* St. Louis: Mosby, 1977.

Hymovich, D., and Barnard, M. *Family Health Care.* New York: McGraw-Hill, 1973.

Kempe, C. H., and Helfer, R. E. (Eds.). *Helping the Battered Child and His Family.* Philadelphia: Lippincott, 1972.

Knafl, K. A., and Grace, H. K. *Families Across the Life Cycle.* Boston: Little, Brown, 1978.

Lockhart, C. A. Family Assessment of Coping Ability. In S. E. Archer and R. Fleshman (Eds.), *Community Health Nursing: Patterns and Practice.* North Scituate, Mass: Duxbury Press, 1975. Pp. 333–336.

Mendes, H. A. Single-parent families: A typology of life-styles. *Soc. Work* 24:193, 1979.

Minuchin, S. *Families and Family Therapy.* Cambridge, Mass.: Harvard University Press, 1974.

Murphy, N. Training professionals to support and increase the competence of young parents. *J. Nurs. Educ.* 17(7):41, 1978.

Murray, R., and Zentner, J. *Nursing Assessment and Health Promotion through the Life Span.* Englewood Cliffs, N.J.: Prentice-Hall, 1975.

Otto, H. A. A Framework for Assessing Family Strengths. In A. Reinhardt and M. Quinn (Eds.), *Family-Centered Community Nursing: A Sociocultural Framework.* St. Louis: Mosby, 1973.

Pratt, L. *Family Structure and Effective Health Behavior: The Energized Family.* Boston: Houghton Mifflin, 1976.

Robischon, P., and Smith, J. Family Assessment. In A. Reinhardt and M. Quinn (Eds.), *Current Practice in Family-Centered Community Nursing.* St. Louis: Mosby, 1977.

Rossi, A. S. Transition to parenthood. *J. Marriage Fam.* 30(2):26, 1968.

Satir, V. *Conjoint Family Therapy.* Palo Alto, Calif.: Science and Behavior Books, 1967.

Satir, V. *Peoplemaking.* Palo Alto, Calif.: Science and Behavior Books, 1972.

Skolnick, A., and Skolnick, J. *Family in Transition: Rethinking Marriage, Sexuality, Child Rearing, and Family Organization* (2nd ed.). Boston: Little, Brown, 1977.

Smiley, O. R. The famiily-centered approach—A challenge to public health nurses. *Int. Nurs. Rev.* 20(2):49, 1973.

Sobol, E. G., and Robischon, P. *Family Nursing: A Study Guide* (2nd ed.). St. Louis: Mosby, 1975.

Steward, R. F. The Family that Fails to Thrive. In D. Hymovich and M. Barnard (Eds.), *Family Health Care.* New York: McGraw-Hill, 1973.

Sweeney, B. Family-centered care in public health nursing. *Nurs. Forum* 9:169, 1970.

Tapia, J. A. The nursing process in family health. *Nurs. Outlook* 20(4):267, 1972.

Watts, R. J. Dimensions of sexual health. *Am. J. Nurs.* 79(9):1568, 1979.

TWELVE

WORKING WITH GROUPS

Groups are an important focus of community health nursing service. We meet the collective needs of many elements of the community population through work with groups. Each collection of people—a parenting group, a mastectomy club, a group of Southeast Asian refugees learning a new culture, a school health committee, or a group of discharged mental patients—has different needs. Some groups function for the purpose of problem solving; others for sharing, support, learning, or therapy. Whatever the reason and whether the nurse acts as leader or member, the use of basic knowledge about groups will enable the nurse to facilitate group process and outcomes.

All of us have had experience with groups. Our first group encounter is with the family, which is known as a primary group because it is one of several basic, informal social groups to which we belong during our lifetime [15]. As we grow, our primary groups extend to include our childhood peer group, associations with our neighbors, friendship groups, and other social affiliations. Informal and generally social in nature, primary groups function with spontaneous and unstructured communication.

In addition to primary groups, we also experience secondary, or formal, group relationships [12]. These groups usually exist for a specific purpose and include professional associations, therapeutic groups, work-related relationships, educational gatherings, and community affiliations. Examples are a student council, an exercise group, a patients' rights committee, and an assertiveness training class. These groups emphasize completing a job and accomplishing specific goals.

Although we spend much of our adult lives participating in formal and informal groups, how well do we understand such groups and how they function? With an increasing number of the community health nurse's activities taking place in groups—client groups, community groups, work groups, and others—the nurse's need for group skills becomes ever more important. This chapter examines groups and ways in which we can work more effectively with them.

The framework for our discussion involves the major processes in which a community health nurse will be involved while working with groups:

1. *Preparing for group work* occurs before the group begins, but may continue after the group forms. Preparation involves knowing the nature of groups, types of groups, and their functions and needs.
2. *Starting a group* involves specific activities to help the group begin work.
3. *Building group cohesiveness* is essential during the early growth of a group.
4. *Working with a group* involves recognizing its developmental phases, assuming appropriate leader and member roles, and solving various sorts of problems that arise.
5. *Terminating a group* begins early in the group's life and requires specific interventions.
6. *Evaluating a group* occurs in two dimensions: we examine group process as well as the outcomes of the group's work.

PREPARING FOR GROUP WORK

A group is two or more persons engaged in repeated, face-to-face communication, who identify with each other and are interdependent. This definition suggests several characteristics found in groups. A group is always a collection of people but never so large that members cannot maintain direct communication with one another [6]. Because their collective social interaction influences the way they think, members assume similar values and norms and establish a sense of belonging to each other. Konopka refers to this characteristic as the development of "bonds," the links that connect individuals and create a group from a mass of loosely related people [7]. Furthermore, the members of a group are interdependent; that is, they need and help each other. As Konopka points out, human beings need to belong to groups. "Group life . . . gives the individual security and nourishment so that he can fulfill his greatest promise while helping others to fulfill theirs too" [7, p. 22]. At the same time, the group molds its members' behavior and attitudes, thus developing its own personality, or "syntality" [16].

Let us look at some examples of how these group characteristics influence the health of clients. Steve discovered that he had epilepsy when he was 15 years of age. The fact was difficult to accept, particularly because he had just been elected captain of his swim team. He was told that epilepsy meant an end to his future in swimming. After a seizure at work, his boss fired him. A period of several months of bitterness and frustration followed, and then he was invited to attend an epilepsy club recently formed in his high school. This group knew what it was like to be epileptic. Many of them had undergone similar experiences to Steve's and could truly empathize with him. The sense of belonging that developed for Steve soon erased his feelings of loneliness and gave him a new sense of hope. The attitudes and behavior of the group gradually shaped his own feelings to the point where he could accept his diagnosis and start developing constructive plans for his life.

A group of elderly persons started a bridge club in their retirement building. Although conversation covered many topics, several members initially were reluctant to discuss the future. "I have no future," one said. "I'm just biding my time until I die." Group comradery and influence gradually changed this attitude to fit the group norm of having a good time together and looking forward to living a long time.

Not all groups influence people positively. Take the case of Tommy, 13 years of age, who has gone from petty theft to armed robbery as a result of gang pressure. Or consider Nancy, once a promising student, now a hard drug user. Her friends made fun of anyone who did well in school and, instead, promoted drug taking as a condition for group membership.

Groups are powerful. While groups meet basic individual needs for belonging, security, safety, and the oppotunity to help others, they also shape their members' thinking and behavior through internal processes of acceptance and rejection (Fig. 12-1). We have seen that they can be either a constructive or destructive force in people's lives. Our concern in community health is to facilitate their constructive use for client health.

TYPES OF GROUPS

Community health nurses work with many different kinds of groups. Since each group forms for some purpose, we shall categorize them according to their primary goal. There are five types of groups with which community health nurses work: learning groups, support groups, socialization groups, task accomplishment groups, and psychotherapy groups.

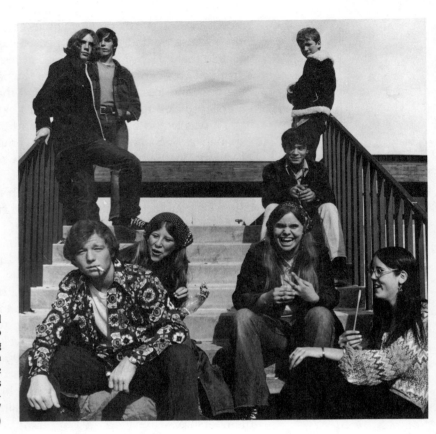

Figure 12-1. Adolescents feel strong pressure to conform to their group's standards. Acting tough and laughing at each other's jokes are some of the ways this group influences its members' behavior. (Photograph by Rondal Partridge/BBM.)

LEARNING GROUPS

The primary goal of a learning group is to have its members gain understanding in order to effect behavior change in some specified area of need. Perhaps like many community health nurses, you have led a prenatal group. The parents-to-be have many practices to learn, such as exercises, diet, breathing techniques, and what to do during labor and delivery. For each topic, you make certain that the needed information is covered and, when appropriate, demonstrate its application. You expect the parents-to-be to practice their new skills regularly at home and ask them to display their understanding by demonstrating what they have learned to the group. You have met the goals of this learning group when the members have assimilated knowledge to the point that it changes their behavior (Fig. 12-2).

A class can be a learning group, but the two are not usually the same. No doubt you have sat in many classes where, other than a brief

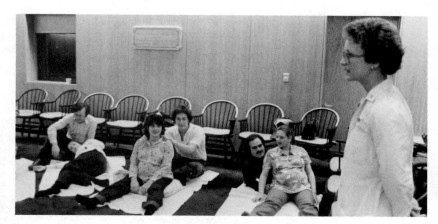

Figure 12-2. This childbirth education class enables couples to practice techniques that will facilitate the birth experience. (Courtesy of Beth Israel Hospital, Boston. Photograph by Michael Lutch.)

conversation or two with a neighbor, you have had little interaction with the other class members. That class is not a true group. The members of a group have repeated, face-to-face communication. They identify with each other and are interdependent. These characteristics typify a learning group, whose function is to utilize the benefits of group identity and interaction to accomplish learning and behavior change. Classes and learning groups share a common advantage of transmitting information more efficiently to a number of people than a one-to-one basis allows. However, learning groups, in contrast to most classes, use group commitment and reinforcement to produce desired behavior changes. They may actually practice natural childbirth, control hypertension, or maintain a postcoronary diet and exercise program. Individuals in these groups not only learn what to do and how to do it (the limit of most classes), but also have the advantage of group influence to promote and stabilize their practices at a healthier level.

The composition of a learning group varies with each situation and depends upon the group's goals. When a group goal is to teach assertiveness to females, for example, the membership would most likely be limited to women. A group goal aimed at preparing people for retirement would probably include members at midlife or approaching retirement. The composition of many learning groups, such as those concerned with weight loss, leadership training, or learning how to manage diabetes, is determined by its members' shared interest in the topic. The chief common denominator of most learning groups, however, is that the members are people who desire to gain information about some subject and better themselves as a result.

The nurse may start some learning groups; others, particularly self-help groups such as Weight Watchers or Alanon groups, will not require this kind of initiative. The nurse's role, therefore, will vary depending upon whether she initiates and leads the group, participates as a member, or participates as an outside consultant. Nevertheless, the nurse's role in any learning group includes providing some degree of structure and focus to the group's activities. The nurse also utilizes the basic teaching-learning principles described in Chapter Seven to encourage client interest in, and application of, the information presented.

SUPPORT GROUPS

The primary goal of an emotional support group is to maintain healthy behaviors and prevent maladaptive coping patterns among its members [8]. In community health we encounter many people who already have good health practices but who need help during times of stress. The support of other people enables them to adapt and preserve their healthy behaviors. Support groups meet this need. A woman alone found adjustment to the ordeal of a mastectomy painfully difficult. Feelings of loss, disfigurement, changed body image, and fear of the cancer returning, in addition to her physical weakness and discomfort, were almost more than she could handle. A single woman, she was convinced that no man would ever want to touch her. She was invited to join a mastectomy club and, through this group, found the comfort and courage that she needed to face her situation. The other members had also had mastectomies. They shared a common experience and could empathize with her feelings. The support and acceptance of the group gave her the strength to put her life back together again.

Support groups, also called therapeutic groups [9], are composed primarily of emotionally healthy (not needing psychiatric help) people caught in some change or crisis. A laryngectomy club or a divorce support group, for example, contains people involved in situational crises who need therapeutic reinforcement. A developmental crisis, such as entering parenthood, may prompt others to form a parenting group for the purpose of reassurance and reinforcement of personal resources. The need for support during adaptation to job change prompted one church to form its Job Transition Support Group for members and others in the community. So great was the need and so successful the group that, in 1980, the group celebrated its third anniversary. Groups such as this often have secondary learning goals. For instance, one week the Job Transition Support Group heard a lecture on the interview process, but its primary goal remained emotional

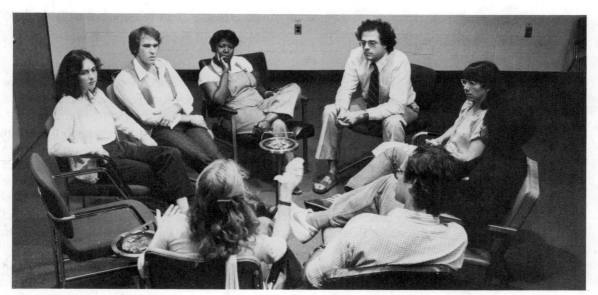

Figure 12-3. Members of this support group listen and share their feelings with one another.

support. The support group provides members with comfort and courage to face the difficulties of their present situation. It seeks to maintain and utilize their existing strengths; it helps them cope successfully and regain their equilibrium (Fig. 12-3).

Support groups sometimes serve an advocacy role as well. They can plead the cause of their members whose physical and emotional health, job security, or social status may be threatened because of their current problem. Alcoholics Anonymous, while primarily a support group, represents a strong social force working in favor of its members' rehabilitation and constructive participation in the community. The Gray Panthers, a senior citizens' lobby group, promotes the causes of the elderly while providing them with a group with which they can identify and from which they can derive sustenance. A support group for epileptics rallied around a member who had been fired from her job when her boss discovered her diagnosis. The nurse leader of the group, accompanied by two of the group members, met with the boss, explained epilepsy, and convinced him that the woman's condition was under control. She kept her job.

Nurses working with support groups aim to facilitate group interactions, but their most important role is to model acceptance and caring. Demonstrating a warm, understanding attitude with, for example, a stop smoking group or a group of individuals grieving the loss of a spouse encourages members to assume these same caring feelings and to create a supportive climate. This approach energizes individuals to resume responsible, healthy behaviors.

SOCIALIZATION GROUPS

Occasionally we encounter clients from another culture or subculture who must learn new social roles in order to achieve a positive level of health. Their old patterns of behavior are inappropriate, nonfunctional, sometimes detrimental, or at least a source of uneasiness in the larger society. Some Native Americans, accustomed to living on a remote reservation, have difficulty adjusting to urban living. Southeast Asian refugees, flocking to American cities in increasing numbers, experience even greater culture shock. Contrasting patterns of eating, living, raising children, and health practices, as well as language barriers and value differences, all call for adaptation in order for these clients to function in the new culture. Even American veterans who have served in the armed forces overseas experience some degree of culture shock upon returning to the United States. They must adjust to new values, clothing styles, social relationships, and political and economic changes. Some individuals in our society have lived in a confined subculture, such as a mental hospital, a prison, or a school for the deaf, and upon discharge must learn new ways of behaving. All of these individuals can benefit from a socialization group.

The primary goal of a socialization group is to help its members learn new social roles. A socialization group must not be confused with a purely social group. Nurses will want to be aware of social groups and their functions. For example, lonely, isolated individuals may benefit greatly from joining a bridge club, bowling league, or bird-watching group. Such groups offer friends, enjoyable activities, and support. The elderly, for instance, may need information about an activities group in their area and encouragement, even assistance, to participate. However, this chapter is concerned with groups in which the community health nurse works. Socialization groups bring together people who are adapting to a new culture or subculture. They offer the nurse an opportunity to capitalize on the benefits of group influence to help these people learn new social skills that will promote their physical and emotional health.

The nurse's role in a socialization group is first to demonstrate caring and acceptance of the group's members, to respect their present values and behaviors. The nurse also provides structure and focus to the group process. For example, with discharged mental patients or a refugee enculturation group, the nurse can encourage members to share their experiences and help them learn new ways of coping with this culture. The mental patients may discuss how to interview for a job, how to meet people, or how to behave at parties. Topics such as shopping in a supermarket, how to ride a bus, or what to expect when you go to a health clinic would be a few of those discussed in the refugee group. The nurse uses group support to give these people courage to give up their familiar practices and group influence to help them learn new roles.

PSYCHOTHERAPY GROUPS

Psychotherapy groups are formed for people who need treatment of an emotional disturbance. Many clients in community health have emotional problems ranging from minor neuroses to severe maladjustments. Psychotherapy groups can serve the needs of families in which child abuse or parent abuse occurs, married couples in conflict, chemically dependent persons, and those with suicidal impulses. These individuals may be referred by a family member, neighbor, professional worker, or agency. They may also refer themselves. Some receive group therapy following individual counseling; others are able to gain all the help they need from a psychotherapy group alone.

The primary goal of psychotherapy groups is to provide members insight into themselves and to help them change their behavior [8]. The group focuses on how its members relate to themselves and to each other; it becomes a "social microcosm" [8, p. 10]. That is, the group serves as a minisociety, allowing members to display their negative feelings and behaviors in an accepting and corrective milieu. An occasional group member may not be ready or willing to participate in self-change and may need to be counseled in some other setting.

Some nurses in community health have advanced training and experience in group psychotherapy and serve as therapists for these groups. More often, the community health nurse is a cotherapist working with a psychiatrist, psychologist, or psychiatric social worker. For example, a nurse and psychiatric social worker co-led a psychotherapy group for delinquent adolescent girls. Among other behaviors, they focused on the girls' tendency to "run away," to avoid anything perceived as unpleasant. The nurse's role included demonstrating acceptance and caring, encouraging the girls to share their feelings, helping them to understand the reasons behind their feelings and behavior, and providing structure and focus to the group process.

TASK-ORIENTED GROUPS

A final category of groups with which community health nurses work includes all those groups whose primary goal is to accomplish some predetermined task. In community health there are many complex problems to solve, decisions to make, and tasks to accomplish that require a collaborative effort. Nursing staff in a public health agency disagree over the proper method for supervising home health aides. A day care center needs new health and safety policies. Community residents are concerned about a rising incidence of vandalism in their area and want to develop some constructive program to keep children and teenagers busy. The local elementary school wants help in planning a health fair. Mothers attending the well-child clinic would like to make the waiting room more pleasant and interesting. Each of these tasks will need a group of people contributing their unique perspectives and skills and working together to address the issue. Community health nurses play a significant part in this process.

Membership in task-oriented groups varies but generally encompasses clients, community residents, and health-related professionals. Client task-oriented groups often form spontaneously out of a desire to improve the current situation. With minimal assistance from their community health nurse, several elderly clients, feeling lonely and useless, established a foster grandparents program. Volunteering their services through local churches and clubs, these retirees soon had more requests than they could handle. As foster grandparents, they met real needs of children in the community and also contributed to their own enjoyment and satisfaction. The community health nurse may work with a group of clients whose goal is to accomplish some task but whose collaboration also serves other health-related functions. One such group was the well-child clinic mothers who wanted to redecorate the waiting room. The nurse helped them plan and implement a fund-raising rummage sale and worked as a group member during the redecoration. Group cohesiveness developed as a result of the many hours spent together, and the nurse was able to form an ongoing mothers' support group with these women.

Community residents frequently initiate task-oriented groups in which community health nurses participate. A school nurse was asked to lead the elementary school task force to plan its health fair. Two community health nurses served on a local community council's planning committee to develop a hypertension screening program. In contrast, the nurse may initiate a task-oriented group involving community

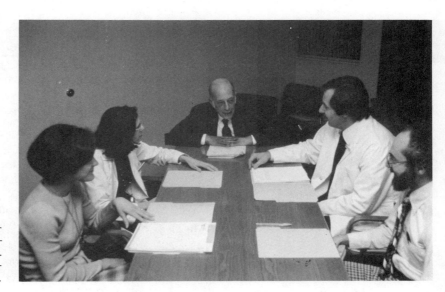

Figure 12-4. This group of professionals is meeting to accomplish a health planning task. (Courtesy of the Harvard Community Health Plan, Boston).

residents. A community health nurse influenced some concerned Native Americans to form a committee to raise the health consciousness of the people on their reserve. She met with the committee weekly for 3 months and accompanied its chairman when he presented their recommendations to the tribal council. She assisted the woman who started the weekly health column, one element of the committee's health consciousness-raising plan, for the tribal newspaper. In another instance, a community health nurse initiated a task-oriented group in order to develop a friendly visitor program for elderly shut-ins.

Professional task-oriented groups are a frequent part of community health nursing practice (Fig. 12-4). They might include an agency team meeting, a state nursing association subcommittee, a state health planning commission, or an environmental safety task force. In these groups, the nurse, whether leader or member, works with other health-related professionals to accomplish specific tasks. For example, a community health nurse in St. Paul chaired a subcommittee of the Metropolitan Health Board to study ways and means of facilitating greater collaboration between health care agencies. In addition to consumer members, the committee included health care administrators from public and private agencies, nurses, physicians, and health planners.

The nurse's role in task-oriented groups varies depending upon whether the nurse is the leader or a member of the group. This chapter

Table 12-1. Types of Groups in Community Health

Type of Group	Primary Goal	Membership	Nurse's Role
Learning	Develop and apply knowledge	People desiring information and improvement in their lives	Provide structure and focus for group process
Support	Maintain healthy behavior and prevent maladaptive coping	Emotionally healthy people needing support during change or crisis	Present role model of acceptance and caring Facilitate group interaction
Socialization	Learn new social roles	People adapting to a new culture or sub-culture	Offer acceptance and caring Provide structure and focus for group process
Psychotherapy	Gain insight into self and change behavior	People needing treatment of an emotional disturbance	Offer acceptance and caring Encourage sharing of feelings Help members understand the reasons behind their feelings and behavior Provide structure and focus for group process
Task-oriented	Accomplish task	People assigned to or volunteering to complete a job	Facilitate progress toward goal achievement

will examine group leader and member roles in more detail later. In either case, however, the nurse works to facilitate group progress toward goal achievement.

Table 12-1 summarizes the five types of groups with which community health nurses work by listing each type's primary purpose, membership, and nurse's role.

ESSENTIAL GROUP NEEDS

Group needs differ from individual needs. We are all familiar with various definitions of individual needs, such as those outlined in Maslow's *Hierarchy of Needs* or Erikson's *Eight Ages of Man*. These needs include belonging, recognition, generativity, and self-actualization. For individuals to achieve a maximum level of functioning, their basic needs must be met. A group, as an entity, has a different set of needs that must be satisfied and maintained in order to allow optimal group functioning. Gouldner and Gouldner describe four essential group needs [3].

SHARED GOALS

First, a group needs an agreed-upon goal and a shared understanding about the means for its achievement. No group can function for long if its members have different ideas about what it is trying to accomplish.

A learning group on family planning, for instance, can make little progress if some members define it as a sex education class, others join to help influence people against abortion, and some use it as a social outlet. The group must be solidly behind the stated goals if members are to work together and accomplish desired results.

CONSISTENT NORMS

Second, the group needs consistency in its norms. That is, there must be some continuity and stability in the internal rules and policies, spoken and unspoken, that govern the group's actions [8]. Every group has to establish ground rules for operating. These rules govern areas such as membership eligibility, attendance requirements, whether or not new members can join after the group is in progress, what kind of participation is expected of each member, and what is expected of the leader. If rules and policies are ignored or frequently broken, the structure of the group is weakened, members do not feel secure, and the group eventually is unable to function.

MOTIVATION

Third, a group needs members motivated to do their various jobs. Many variables influence motivation; among them are leader power and charisma, degree of member commitment to group goals and group success, how well individual needs are being met, group cohesiveness, and members' sense of belonging. Group goals can be accomplished only through collaborative effort: unless members do their share of the work, the job does not get done. Nor can the group function if members are lazy or morale is low. Each member has a unique role to play and, as for any system, the group's viability depends on the proper functioning of all its parts.

COMMUNICATION

Fourth, every group needs stable communication channels among the members. No group can function without a dependable system for giving and receiving information. The effectiveness of a divorce support group depends on members' ability to share their feelings of anger, rejection, or loneliness freely and to receive accepting, understanding responses in return. The work of a committee to study safety hazards in a summer camp cannot be done without an active exchange of ideas. Were it not for demonstrated acceptance and caring, and constant two-way communication to help members gain insight into their feelings and behavior, a psychotherapy group would have minimal success. In order to function, all groups require viable lines of communication.

GROUP FUNCTIONS

Every group serves two types of functions: a task-related function and a group maintenance function [12]. The task function focuses on completing the job while the maintenance function deals with how members are interacting. The former is goal-related and instrumental; the latter member-related and interpersonal.

Consider how a student council operates. Part of the group's focus will be on the task dimension. Members will explore ideas, make plans, decide on jobs to be done, keep discussion on target, and make certain that members have done their delegated tasks. The other part of the group's concentration is on the maintenance dimension, which includes responsibilities such as keeping up group morale, making certain that individual members' needs are met, encouraging and praising member accomplishments, and mediating conflicts.

A well-functioning group emphasizes both task and maintenance concerns [4]. You may have experienced membership in a group that focused so heavily on tasks the interpersonal dimension was neglected. This situation happens most often in task-oriented groups, such as committees, where the job to be done becomes so important that it is accomplished at the expense of members' feelings. Internal dissatisfaction develops, resulting in poor attendance, disruptive behavior, or withdrawal. Everyone expects and needs to get something from group membership; if they do not, they will either drop out or possibly disrupt the group in some way. On the other hand, a group that concentrates too heavily on the interpersonal dimension may have happy members but not accomplish its goals. An appropriate balance between task and maintenance functions is needed.

STARTING A GROUP

When any group is about to be formed, certain questions must be answered. Who should the members be? What is the best size for this group? What are the group's needs, and what should its goals be? Where should it meet, and what type of physical arrangements would most enhance its purpose? How can members be oriented to facilitate effective group development and group process? We shall consider the answers to each of these questions separately.

SELECTING MEMBERS

We determine who a group's members will be by considering several factors. We need to know the group's general purpose. If it is task-oriented, its members should be people who have expertise or skills pertinent to accomplishing the task. If its purpose is support, the members will be people who are experiencing change or crisis and need emotional reinforcement. In other words, the members should have something in common that relates to the group's primary goal.

Members should also exhibit similarities relative to the group's specific goals. Sometimes age- or sex-specific membership is necessary. For example, a support group for men in midlife crisis would limit its membership to middle-aged men. A preschool mothers' group aiming to understand early childhood growth and development and learn appropriate mothering responses would limit its membership to young mothers. In other groups, the members may be very dissimilar in age, sex, or social role, but have some other common denominator. A weight loss group, for instance, might be composed of members with a variety of ages and sexes since obesity is their shared concern. The epileptic support group mentioned earlier included young people from grade school through high school. Their variant ages and sexes gave a broader range of perspectives to group discussion and further enhanced the group's value. Their common denominator was epilepsy.

Members should choose to be part of the group. Any group member who does not participate willingly is not likely to benefit from, or contribute positively to, the group. If, for example, a client is coerced into a psychotherapy group or a professional is drafted reluctantly to serve on a health committee, we may see nonparticipation, conflict, or disruption in group process.

One should also select members on the basis of their commitment to the group's success. People who are genuinely interested in the group's goals and motivated to work for their accomplishment will gain more from the group experience and make a greater contribution to its process and outcomes. We see strong evidence of this contribution particularly in self-help groups, such as Alcoholics Anonymous, where group loyalty and commitment accomplish significant results.

Finally, leaders are helped by selecting members with whom they enjoy working and are more likely to be effective. Some leaders enjoy working with challenging groups, such as drug addicts, while groups with a strong commitment to change may be more satisfying for others. As Loomis points out, "therapists should be encouraged to become familiar with their own personal characteristics and preferences in the selection of clients" [8, p. 52]. This factor clearly affects a group's success.

DETERMINING GROUP SIZE

Not long ago a community health nurse and seven other professionals formed a task force to study service delivery problems and make recommendations to a county board. The group met for several months and formed a good working relationship. However, its final product, a set of recommendations, met with resistance from county agencies not represented on the original task force. They insisted on expanding the task force and restudying the problems. Now composed of 22 members, the group met frequently but made almost no progress. Most of the leader's energy was spent resolving conflicts and attempting to pacify a few vocal members who dominated the discussion with lengthy diatribes defending their agencies' territoriality. Many members could not or chose not to participate. Attendance began to drop. As the deadline drew near, the leader, in desperation, appointed a subcommittee of five members to draft a proposal to which the larger group could respond. The draft, with minor changes, was approved, and the task force limped to its final conclusion with participation from about half of the original group.

Why was the first task force so successful and the second not? Because group size affects performance. The larger the group, the longer it takes to reach decisions, especially if consensus is required. In addition, the subgroups which almost always develop within larger groups can polarize interests, create conflicts, and impede group progress.

Group size also influences satisfaction. We have known for many years that as a group expands, the individual member's satisfaction declines [15]. The larger the group, the less likely is the opportunity for all members to participate. In a large group, a few people usually do most of the talking while the rest are either intimidated, bored, or dissatisfied to the point of choosing not to participate.

Large groups do exist; examples are professional nursing groups, parent-teacher-student associations, student bodies, and older adults clubs. In order to meet specific group needs, however, we must divide groups into smaller ones of workable size. Loomis emphasizes, "It is not good clinical practice to remain with too large a group simply because there are not enough funds available to start a second group.

Client needs and group task should be the primary consideration in determining group size'' [8, p. 61].

Determining the number of members in a group varies depending upon the situation and the group goals. To allow an appropriate mix of members and enough people to promote good interaction, a group should have at least five or six members. Ten to twelve members is considered the maximum size before subgroups start to form. The optimal size for any talk-oriented group that aims at problem solving, support, learning, insight, or behavior change is six to ten members [8]. The choice of seven members is often preferred for providing the best balance of variety of ideas with opportunity for all members to participate.

SETTING GROUP GOALS

We set goals and objectives on the basis of needs. A community health nurse, working with an interpreter, started a socialization group for deaf high school students. These young people attended a state residential school for the deaf and would soon be graduating. They were concerned about functioning in a hearing world, about getting jobs, developing a social life, applying to colleges, and planning careers. They had needs. On the basis of these needs, the group established its goals and objectives.

Every group must identify its needs before setting goals. Needs assessment involves collecting and interpreting data, and reaching a diagnosis about needed changes. A detailed discussion of needs assessment and goal setting is provided in Chapter Five. In order to set goals and objectives with a nursing leadership training group, for instance, we ask the members what they think they need, and we probably evaluate their leadership knowledge and skills. On the basis of this data, we determine this group's specific needs, needs such as how to make decisions, how to plan, and how to delegate. Then the goals and objectives can be established.

Setting goals is a group activity involving all members. Unless members participate in this process, it is possible that their expectations for the group will differ from others. Members and leader together need to agree on the group's major goals and its specific objectives, the activities that will ensure the desired outcomes. It is often helpful to negotiate a group contract in which the nurse/leader and members mutually agree on their expectations for the group and the manner in which the outcomes will be achieved. Negotiating a fee for service with some groups is an important element in the contract and contributes to group commitment [8].

MAKING PHYSICAL ARRANGEMENTS

Where, how, and when a group meets significantly influences its productivity. The meeting place must be conveniently located, perhaps near a bus line, in order to be accessible to members. It must also have appropriate facilities, such as wheel chair access or parking space, to accommodate members' needs.

Space is another consideration. Some groups, such as an exercise group or a first-aid demonstration class, need a larger meeting area in order to accomplish their goals. Other groups function best in a more intimate setting which is conducive to sharing and expression of feelings; for them, a smaller room works best.

Seating arrangements can influence group process. If chairs are set in classroom style, there is a tendency for members to direct their comments only to the leader. Many task-oriented groups, such as committees, work around long tables. It is difficult for members along the sides of the tables to have eye contact with others along the same side. As a result, communication is inhibited and group cohesiveness is slower to develop. To facilitate communication in all directions, a circular seating pattern in which every member can see every other member is most useful.

A comfortable atmosphere, compatible with group goals, is important. A group dealing with feelings may find softer chairs or even sitting on the floor relaxing, informal, and conducive to free expression, while a "think" group may need firmer seating. Background noise, a room that echoes, distracting posters, or distasteful decorations may often detract from group productivity.

Finally, the time when a group meets is also important. Dates and times should fit members' schedules so that all can attend, and length and frequency of meetings should enhance group goals. A support group, for instance, may find it most helpful to meet weekly to receive frequent reinforcement. Other groups, such as some learning or task groups, may need more time between sessions to practice new skills or research a problem.

ORIENTING GROUP MEMBERS

Three points need emphasis to ensure smooth functioning as a group starts. First, be certain that all the members agree on the group's goals.

Members should agree as early as possible in the life of the group to erase misconceptions and to help solidify the group behind its purpose.

Second, new group members need to know how the group will function; they must begin to establish its structure and rules for operating. Structure refers to the way a group defines and regulates its members' behavior in terms of roles, communication patterns, and power relationships within the group [12]. It must be clear from the beginning of any group who, if anyone, is leader and what that person is expected to do. Expectations for the members should be clearly spelled out, and special roles, such as a time keeper in a discussion group or a referee for debates, should be assigned. More specific leader and member roles will emerge during the life of the group; we will discuss these later. Communication patterns evolve as group members work together, but awareness from the start of how members communicate is important. The interaction networks tend to be most effective in groups whose members are all free to communicate with each other as well as with the nurse/leader [15].

Power structure in informal groups often fluctuates depending upon which members have the most influence, while formal groups, such as an agency's nursing organization, generally have a stable, clear-cut structure of power, influence, and authority. In any group, however, decisions can be made to designate who has power to do what. For example, the leader of a learning group may have absolute power over all decisions, or the group may choose a completely democratic format with decision-making power distributed among the members. Rules governing group action also need to be established early. The group must decide on matters such as attendance, physical arrangements, and whether smoking will be permitted.

Third, members need to hold the same expectations for the group's outcomes. The anticipated final product of the group can be restated and discussed to make certain that everyone understands and agrees that this is the outcome they want. Part of this discussion should include how the group will evaluate its final product. How will they know when their goals have been met? Some groups will find it easier to evaluate than others. A stop-smoking group or a weight loss group, for instance, will have clear standards for measuring their success. An assertiveness training group for women may decide that its outcome is the ability of every member to assert herself appropriately in public and will evaluate this outcome by having each member describe one such experience. A divorce support group may have more difficulty agreeing on outcomes but perhaps will choose to measure them in terms of each member's satisfaction, feelings of comfort, or self-confidence.

BUILDING GROUP COHESIVENESS

Group cohesiveness is the sum of all the forces that influence members to stay in a group. These forces include whether (1) a member's needs can be met in the group, (2) group goals are consistent with member needs, (3) members expect the group to benefit them, and (4) members actually perceive that the group is benefitting them [8]. These are positive forces that attract members toward the group. In some instances, negative outside pressures may also promote group cohesiveness.

Cohesive groups display certain characteristics which begin early in the group's development and increase over time. There is an attraction of members to the group and a sense of pride in membership, which intensifies as the group becomes more successful. Pride is usually accompanied by an emotional commitment of the members to the group and manifests itself in increasing loyalty and high morale. The members feel good about one another and their group identification. They are loyal to each other and to the group's goals and values and, in some instances, may talk, dress, or act in similar ways. They work well together and enjoy spending time together, even outside of the regular group meetings.

During the life of every group there are times of internal problems and external threats. Group cohesiveness helps a group to weather these times. When the members of a parenting group disagreed among themselves over ways to discipline children, their closeness and unity as a group helped them over this period of conflict and prevented the group from disintegrating. The members of a chemical dependency group discovered that their funding source had been cut off and that there would be no more money for medications or consultation. Because of the members' commitment to remaining together, they sought and found new resources and continued working on their goals.

Group cohesiveness is as important to the group as the nurse-patient relationship is to individual therapy [18]. Research demonstrates that there is a positive correlation between group cohesiveness and positive group therapy outcomes [8]. Thus it becomes essential to foster group cohesiveness in the groups with which we work.

We build cohesiveness in a group by making certain that its four basic needs are met. First, there must be agreement among all members on the group's goals and the means by which these goals will be achieved. No group will be cohesive if members disagree on or misunderstand the goals. To avoid misunderstanding, members need to know exactly what the goals mean, have a clear (preferably written) statement of them, agree on the methods and actions to use in implementing them, and have a sense of hope that they are attainable. Second, group norms, the standards for acceptable behavior in the group, must be continuous and stable to help the group function. These norms are developed through discussion between leader and members as to what is expected and acceptable behavior. Formal groups tend to define norms at the start. Norms often develop more gradually in informal groups. Third, there must be group motivation. Clarity and feasibility of goals can help members feel that working for the group is worthwhile. The leader can be a strong motivator by giving individual members recognition and positive reinforcement and by promoting the member's sense of belonging and participation. Fourth, communication channels within the group must remain viable. It is often up to the leader to monitor communication networks and make certain that they function effectively. Members, too, can help to facilitate a good exchange of information and feelings, but the group may need an outside process observer to make objective recommendations for improving its communication patterns.

Several factors can block group cohesiveness from developing or remaining [8]. Open membership, particularly with an unlimited number of sessions, sometimes makes it difficult for a group to stabilize its norms. Some groups, such as Alcoholics Anonymous or Weight Watchers, overcome this difficulty by having established goals and norms for the group which essentially do not change as new members join. In a less formal group with open membership, such as an "ostomy" club, the nurse/leader can help the founding members to develop a charter or written statement describing the group's general purpose and policies. Then, as new members enter and old ones leave, there can be some flexibility within this structure to allow specific goals and norms to reflect the changing membership's needs. That is, both goals and norms would have to be renegotiated depending upon the rate of member turnover. When members move in and out of a group very rapidly, it is almost impossible to establish cohesiveness. In general, the more stable the membership, the more likely is the achievement of group cohesiveness.

Other blocks to group cohesiveness include members who do not conform to norms or agree with goals, the formation of competitive subgroups, or a leader-centered group. Deviant members can sometimes be persuaded to change their behavior or perhaps to leave the group. Strong group agreement on goals and norms prevents competition and allows the formation of positive subgroups which enhance cohesiveness. One can also minimize splintering by keeping the subgroups task-specific and time-limited. Responsible group leadership focuses on uniting the group behind its goals and maximizing its potential to meet client needs.

Some groups need cohesiveness more than others. Without a close working relationship, a support group, for example, will probably not be able to function while a learning group may be able to accomplish its goals; however, the learning group's full potential cannot be realized without group cohesiveness.

WORKING WITH THE GROUP

Let us say you have prepared for a group by gaining an understanding of the types of groups and their needs. Then you actually started a group and worked to build cohesiveness; the group appears to be moving along well. Between this initial period of establishing a group and the final period of terminating it, you will be working with an ongoing group. This work requires an understanding of the phases of group development, the different roles that leader and members can play, and the ways problems can be resolved.

PHASES OF GROUP DEVELOPMENT

Groups, like individuals, go through predictable growth phases. It is easiest to observe these phases in groups whose membership is constant; it is more difficult to distinguish the phases in groups whose membership or goals frequently change. The phases are dependence, counterdependence, and interdependence [1, 4].

DEPENDENCE

During this first phase members depend on the leader for guidance and direction. They are still sorting out why they are there and what their roles will be; they do not question the leader's authority. It is during this phase that members are most concerned with inclusion in the group [13]. It is a time of personal contact and encounter. Members want to be part of the group but still feel some conflict in giving up their personal identity. Dependence has been called the "childhood" stage of group development [4].

COUNTERDEPENDENCE

As members become more comfortable in their roles, they also become more assertive. Conflict and power struggles develop, and acceptance of the leader's authority diminishes. The major issue in the counterdependent phase is control. Who has power and authority? Who will influence and control? Who will be controlled? It is an "adolescent" stage of group development.

INTERDEPENDENCE

Finally, group members learn to work out their relationships. They make decisions together, engage in open communication, manage conflict successfully, and experience satisfaction in the entire group's accomplishments. During this phase, the issues revolve around communicating and meeting individual needs to express and receive affection. Subgroups, and even pairing of members occur to handle intimacy needs. Interdependence is a "mature" phase of group development which may take weeks, months, or even years for a group to reach, depending upon the stability of the membership. Some groups never achieve interdependence.

While monitoring a group's development, we will notice that as each new issue arises the group will again progress through the developmental phases with regard to that issue. "A particular developmental stage . . . is never fully completed for all time; rather, as circumstances change, the same developmental [stage] may crop up again and again" [12, p. 184]. For example, a nursing team in a community health agency has been working on solving case problems. During the past 5 months the team members have worked through their dependence on the team leader and their conflicts over different ways to manage family problems; now they are communicating well and assuring everyone the opportunity to express ideas. They are experiencing the interdependent phase on this issue. Recently the team was told that they would have to redistribute members' geographic work boundaries. Feeling insecure and uncertain about how to accomplish this task, members initially looked to the team leader for suggestions (dependent phase). Soon they recognized advantages and disadvantages of various proposals for redefining work boundaries, ignored the leader, and began arguing among themselves over how to decide. Power struggles signal that they are currently in the counterdependent phase on this issue.

Knowing the phases of group development helps us recognize where a group is and what to expect from the members. Groups must be allowed to progress through each phase at their own pace; this progress can be greatly enhanced by an understanding and facilitative leader.

LEADER ROLE

The group leader has a specific responsibility: to help the group achieve its goals. Sometimes a formal, designated leader assumes this role; at other times, an informal leader emerges to help focus the group's energy on its business. The nurse may be either a formal leader, an informal leader, or only a member. All the members, including the leader, must be committed to working together to accomplish the group's goals. Leadership style influences this task. Whether the leader should assume an autocratic (leader-centered, persuasive) style, a democratic (member-centered, problem-solving) style, or a laissez-faire (noncentered) style depends upon the group's needs. Each style has advantages as well as disadvantages, although the democratic style works best in most situations. Leadership styles are presented in more detail in Chapter Fifteen. During the group process, the leader exercises some unique functions and employs certain techniques.

FUNCTIONS

Leader functions include a variety of activities designed to strengthen the group's ability to achieve its purpose. Important ones are [12]:

Obtain and receive information.
Help diagnose group goals, obstacles, and consequences of decisions.
Facilitate communication.
Help integrate varying perspectives and alternate possibilities for action.
Test and evaluate proposals and decisions.

TECHNIQUES

To carry out these functions, the leader needs skill in the use of certain techniques or leader interventions [12].

SUPPORT

Support means to create an encouraging climate that reinforces positive behaviors and makes members feel secure and accepted. A leader could use this technique by telling the group, "You have made real progress today. Several people shared feelings as well as ideas, and you have all listened attentively and accepted these comments without judging them."

CONFRONTATION

Confrontation is a technique that counters negative behavior through constructive feedback. We may direct it toward an individual member or the group as a whole. It consists of making direct, honest, reflective statements about how behaviors appear to us. People do not always want to hear these statements, but they may be necessary to facilitate group progress. It is helpful to combine support with confrontation.

ADVICE AND SUGGESTION

Advice and suggestion is another technique to use when leader expertise or perspective is needed. Be careful to use it only when members are unable to solve problems for themselves.

SUMMARIZING

Summarizing means providing the group with a concise, descriptive review. We may wish to summarize the group's actions to date, its progress in relationship to goals, its unresolved issues, and other areas of functioning. The value of this technique is to refocus group attention for future planning.

CLARIFICATION

Clarification is used to prevent confusion or distortion of ideas. A leader could use this technique by saying, "From the comments I've heard, it seems to me that the group would like to switch to Tuesdays. Is that correct?"

QUESTIONING

Probing and questioning is a useful technique for gaining information and greater understanding. By asking questions we can help members explore ideas in greater depth.

REFLECTION

Reflection can be used to mirror back people's ideas, feelings, or behaviors. To reflect ideas, we repeat, paraphrase, or highlight comments in order to facilitate communication. For example, when a member says, "I don't agree," a reflective response is, "You don't agree?"; thereby the person receives an opportunity to further discuss the idea. Reflecting feelings means restating to the group or member the feelings we think are being conveyed. If a learning group complains, "We've never had to do anything like this before," the leader may reflect back, "You seem to be a little frightened of doing this." To reflect behavior we simply describe the behavior we see, thus allowing the group to clarify the meaning. We can say to the group, "I notice that you've become silent since I made that last suggestion."

INTERPRETATION AND ANALYSIS

Interpretation and analysis is a technique that seeks to uncover the underlying meaning of group comments and behaviors. In using this technique, we summarize our observations of the group and then offer an analysis of their behavior's deeper meaning or reason. The leader might say, "I notice that several of you who are usually active have not participated in the past two sessions. I wonder if the decisions about this issue seem to be a foregone conclusion, and you feel it's useless to say anything?"

LISTENING

Listening attentively shows the group that the leader is interested in them and what they have to say. It also provides a positive model for group members to use with each other. Attentive listening helps sharpen the focus of the conversation by allowing specific responses to the comments being made.

MEMBER ROLES

A new mothers' group has been meeting weekly now for a month and a half. As their leader, you notice that each person's behavior is unique in some way. Susan, for instance, asks many questions and also tends to agree with whoever is speaking. Diane, on the other hand, is full of ideas and frequently offers suggestions or proposes some new plan of action. Then there is Maureen. Her friendly, warm responses seem to make the others feel better in contrast to Fran's constant complaining. Verona has been especially helpful to you by keeping the group on track, helping to smooth out differences, and encouraging others to participate in the discussion. Each of the five women has assumed different group member roles.

Every group needs its members to perform specific roles. Member roles serve one of two basic functions necessary for a viable group—task or maintenance functions. Some roles are task-related: they help the group do its work. Diane, for instance, is an initiator of ideas, and Susan is both an information seeker and follower. Verona orients the group to its goals (keeps it on track). These are task roles. Other roles are maintenance-related: they deal with group members' participation.

Maureen encourages members by showing acceptance and support while Verona serves as gatekeeper, keeping communication channels open and facilitating member involvement. Both women play maintenance roles.

The most common task and maintenance roles are listed below [10, pp. 28–30]:

TASK ROLES

Initiator   *Proposes tasks, goals, or actions; defines group problems; suggests a procedure*

Information seeker   *Asks for factual clarification; requests facts pertinent to the discussion*

Opinion seeker   *Asks for a clarification of the values pertinent to the topic under discussion; questions values involved in alternative suggestions*

Informer   *Offers facts; gives expression of feelings; gives an opinion*

Clarifier   *Interprets ideas or suggestions; defines terms; clarifies issues before the group; clears up confusion*

Summarizer   *Pulls together related ideas; restates suggestions; offers a decision or conclusion of the group to consider*

Reality tester   *Makes a critical analysis of an idea; tests an idea against some data to see if the idea would work*

Orienter   *Defines the position of the group with respect to its goals; points to departures from agreed-upon directions or goals; raises questions about the direction which the group discussion is taking*

Follower   *Goes along with movement of group; passively accepts ideas of others; serves as audience in group discussion and decision*

MAINTENANCE ROLES

Harmonizer   *Attempts to reconcile disagreements; reduces tension; gets people to explore differences*

Gatekeeper   *Helps to keep communications channels open; facilitates the participation of others; suggests procedures that permit sharing remarks*

Consensus taker   *Asks to see if the group is nearing a decision; sends up a trial balloon to test a possible solution*

Encourager   *Is friendly, warm, and responsive to others; indicates by facial expression or remark the acceptance of others' contributions*

Compromiser   *Offers a compromise which yields status when his own idea is involved in a conflict; modifies in the interest of group cohesion or growth*

Standard setter   *Expresses standards for the group to attempt to achieve; applies standards in evaluating the quality of a group process*

All of the roles just listed are needed for a group to function effectively [4]. Some members will play several overlapping roles while others will play only one or two. You can determine the roles your group's members are playing by having an outside observer evaluate your group or by using one of various member participation checklists [2, 5, 11]. Should a vital role, such as gatekeeper, be missing from your group, you and the group may wish to ask someone to assume this role.

Some roles are dysfunctional; they hinder the group from reaching its goals. Fran's constant complaining is an example of a dysfunctional role which inhibits communication and demoralizes the group. Other behaviors, such as being aggressive, blocking, dominating, distracting, or seeking recognition or sympathy, are also dysfunctional. These roles cannot be ignored. The group must identify and deal with them. During the group meeting the leader may redirect the focus back to the topic if someone disrupts by saying, for example, "I'd like to hear other people's ideas too." When disruptive behavior is persistent, a technique such as reflection or interpretation and analysis may be a constructive way to deal with it. Confrontation should be used with discretion, particularly in front of the group, since it may be too threatening and counterproductive.

SOLVING GROUP PROBLEMS

Many difficulties arise during the life of a group. We have dealt with a few such as how to start the group, avoid blocks to group cohesiveness, and deal with dysfunctional behavior. Three group problems in particular are worthy of further discussion. They are interpersonal conflict, dominance, and nonparticipation.

RESOLVING CONFLICTS

Conflict, by itself, is neither good nor bad. It is a form of tension frequently found in groups which may be used constructively by broadening the group's outlook and sharpening its problem-solving skills, or destructively by dissolving group cohesiveness.

Conflict arises when one or more members take sides against others in the group. There is sharp disagreement, arguing, tension, and impatience. Conflict may occur because one or more members are seeking special status or making a power play, because some members have vested interests in or loyalty to another conflicting organization, or because members have overinvested in the group's productivity [2].

Managing conflict means taking neither the extreme of flight (avoidance) or of fight (head-on confrontation), but rather a realistic attitude aimed at maximum gain for all those concerned. It is called a Win/Win approach [4, 17].

Lose/Lose   you lose/I lose
Win/Lose   you win/I lose
Lose/Win   you lose/I win
Win/Win   you win/I win

In using the Win/Win approach, we encourage people to work together to benefit all parties. We examine all the issues at stake and maximize the opportunity for everyone to satisfy at least some of their desires. Win/Win refocuses energy into problem solving instead of competition.

There are four steps we can take to resolve conflicts. First, acknowledge that there is a conflict and reach agreement on its definition in the group. People may not be arguing different points, after all. Second, identify possible areas of agreement. There are nearly always some points that are not mutually exclusive. Third, determine the changes each party in the dispute must make to resolve the problem satisfactorily. Fourth, keep the focus of the conflict on issues rather than people. Personal attack will stalemate any attempt at resolution and may even strengthen the conflict [15].

DEALING WITH EXCESSIVE PARTICIPATION OR NONPARTICIPATION

Most groups need a relative equality of member participation for group work to be effective. To allow a full diversity of views, to foster cohesiveness through members' self-expression, and to make best use of the group's time, each member should have a fair share of the group's attention. Either nonparticipation or excessive participation will disrupt the group.

Excessive participation of members in the form of monopolizing conversation can produce feelings of anger and frustration for the leader and the group. Dominant members may be trying to cover up anxiety or seeking attention, recognition, and approval. However, their compulsive talking and apparent insensitivity to their effect on the group only create dislike and disrespect. Other members feel cheated out of their share of the group's time. The group cannot benefit from a complete range of member contributions.

The leader copes with a dominant member by first trying supportive interruption. "Your point is well-taken but, in the interest of time, we need to allow others to express their views." If the member is not responsive to this approach, try another technique, such as reflection: "You seem to be doing most of the talking today." You might offer an interpretation: "I wonder if you are talking so much because you feel a little anxious about something, perhaps about how the group sees you?" Even confrontation may be necessary. It is also possible that the group is permitting the dominant member to monopolize as a way of avoiding its own responsibility. In that case, confrontation of the group may be needed.

A member may refuse to participate as a result of apathy, lack of commitment to the group's goals, anger, fear of ridicule, timidity, or poor self-image. When other members do not know why this person is quiet, they begin to feel uncomfortable (Is this person judging us, ridiculing us, or not liking us?) and resentful (It is unfair of members not to carry their share of the group's work). The silence of several members may indicate an angry reaction to a few who are dominating or discomfort in the presence of conflict. When the entire group is silent or apathetic, they may be responding to the leader's style or the current task, which may seem unimportant or too difficult.

Nonparticipation must be diagnosed before the leader can intervene. Diagnosis can be made by offering a reflective or interpretive statement such as, "I've noticed that there is very little participation in the group today. Are people uncomfortable with this topic or perhaps with the way I'm leading the group?" or "Susan, you haven't said much in the last few sessions. Is the rest of the group not giving you a chance?" From member responses and discussion, the leader learns the reasons behind the nonparticipation and then can take appropriate action. Nonintervention is sometimes best if it appears that too much group time and energy will be spent on the problem or if nonparticipation is infrequent. Occasional silence, particularly in one individual, may only be temporary. As the group becomes increasingly supportive and accepting, such individuals may gradually feel secure enough to start participating on their own.

TERMINATING THE GROUP

Termination is an extremely important phase in the life of a group [8]. Like any ending, including death, termination involves a mixed set of feelings which the group must face, explore, and resolve. Members must cope with feelings of loss and grief at leaving people to whom they have become attached. They must deal with a sense of success or failure depending on whether their goals were met. They must recognize that they will no longer experience the group's support and other benefits. Termination is important because it is a time in the group's life when members have an opportunity to analyze the meaning of the group experience, which they can build on when planning for the future. Successful termination creates a sense of completion and a positive attitude toward future group experiences.

Termination is an issue that must be dealt with in every group. Most health care groups mark a beginning to their work and an ending when that work is complete. For these groups, the entire group will terminate. Other groups have an open-ended membership; thus the group (e.g., an ongoing support group) remains while members come and go. In these instances, the individual member terminates. Leaders, too, sometimes leave a group, perhaps for health reasons or a job change. Whether it is the entire group or an individual who is terminating, all the group members are affected. Positive leader intervention can make the difference in whether or not a group terminates successfully.

PREPARING FOR TERMINATION

Ideally, we establish criteria for termination at the onset of the group. If the criteria are built into individual and group goals, clients know that, upon completion of their goals, it will be time to terminate. A failure on the part of many leaders, however, is not to explain these criteria fully to clients. The subject of termination is even avoided by some leaders, which suggests they may be denying its reality because they do not want to face the pain of separation. Part of the leader's responsibility, as early as possible in the life of the group, is to clarify with the group the exact conditions and date for termination.

Termination may be defined in terms of time (number of sessions or specific target date), behavior (when specific behavior changes have occurred), or circumstances (moving, job change, health). For example, a parenting group may choose to meet for 12 sessions and then terminate. If additional needs are identified at the end of that period, the group can renegotiate for more time. The members of a psychotherapy group will most likely decide that termination is appropriate when they see the desired changes in their behavior. Circumstances, such as moving or job change, are usually known far enough in advance to allow the group time to prepare adequately for termination.

WORKING THROUGH TERMINATION

When facing termination, group members may experience a mixture of feelings, such as sadness, anger, joy, or fear. They may deny the possibility of termination altogether. Members' behavior gives the leader clues about their reactions to termination. For instance, members who were formerly open in sharing feelings may become defensive and superficial. Others may appear angry and upset for no apparent reason. People may start to make plans for getting together beyond the termination date. Some may withdraw, come late, or act as if the group were no longer important to them. None of these are healthy responses and require intervention.

Leader intervention during the termination process includes the following. First, help the group to identify and acknowledge that termination is occurring. Members must accept its reality. Second, assist group members to find appropriate alternatives for meeting the needs that the group has met. Fear of having to function without the group drives some members to return to old, unhealthy behaviors such as smoking or overeating after having not smoked or gone off their diets for months. Instead, encourage members to assess what the group has been providing for them and identify other ways to meet these needs outside of the group. For instance, one woman who was leaving an assertiveness training group decided to meet weekly with a friend for continued reinforcement of her new behaviors. The leader should allow enough time before termination for members to accomplish this task. Third, give group members an opportunity to express and deal with their feelings, which need to be worked through until the group senses that its business is finished. Finally, you can facilitate termination by having the group evaluate its progress. "Here is where we were when we started. Look how far we have come" is a message which helps people leave with a sense of accomplishment and a positive outlook on the future.

EVALUATING GROUP EFFECTIVENESS

Group evaluation includes two important areas, process measurement and outcomes measurement. The first examines ongoing group interaction, and the second looks at the group's final product.

PROCESS EVALUATION

It is important for groups to conduct periodic self-examinations. Leaders and members both need to hear reactions to their performances.

Are they conducting their roles effectively? Are they making progress toward their goals? This information is vital to making improvements in the way members work together.

Process evaluation can be done in several ways. One useful method is to have an outside observer sit in on the group, watch for specific behaviors, and then give reactions to the group. The observer can use one of several guides available for this purpose [2, 11]. Another method is to have a group member act as an impartial observer during a session in which the member only observes and refrains from participating. The group itself may diagnose its health by periodically or even regularly using some form of checklist or questionnaire, followed by discussion [2, 4, 5]. The kinds of behaviors to observe will vary with each group; generally, however, a group needs to examine all of the roles listed earlier and ask questions pertaining to areas such as communication skills and patterns, responses to leadership style, group climate, stage of group development, and progress on group objectives. Sweeney has developed a useful set of criteria which appraises the strength and effectiveness of groups in terms of their physical, interpersonal, intrapersonal, and community dimensions [14].

MEASURING GROUP OUTCOMES

To determine the effectiveness of any group, we must measure its outcomes. Did the group accomplish its objectives? Are the group members different now than they were when the group started? Clear goals and specific objectives are the keys to unlocking the answers to these questions. Goals spell out the overall purpose of the group; objectives narrow goals down into specific behaviors that we can measure. For example, the group's goal may be to learn the techniques of natural childbirth. Objectives should describe separate behaviors, such as specific breathing techniques or exercises, that demonstrate the accomplishment of the goal. Thus we look to objectives that describe outcome behaviors as our criteria for measuring the group's performance. If members can and do demonstrate ability in the breathing techniques and the exercises (or any other behaviors outlined in the objectives), then we can say that the group goal has been accomplished.

Some groups' goals are more difficult to evaluate than others, but all can be measured to some degree. A group of women with mastectomies may have a goal of learning to accept their own bodies. They can identify specific behaviors that will tell them when they have met this goal. The behaviors may include looking in the mirror without wincing, admitting to having undergone a mastectomy to another person outside the group, or wearing form-fitting clothing and not feeling overly self-conscious.

The group should participate equally with the leader in the evaluation process. Group members' own observations, insights, and feedback are essential to collecting the necessary data for evaluating the objectives. If specific behavior changes, such as staying on a special diet or exercising daily at home, are part of the objectives, then further supporting data can be solicited from family members or friends.

SUMMARY

Groups are an important part of community health nursing service. A group is two or more persons who engage in repeated, face-to-face communication, identify with each other, and are interdependent.

In preparing to work with groups, the community health nurse must understand different types of groups, their essential needs, and their primary functions. There are five major types of groups encountered by community health nurses:

1. Learning groups are those in which the primary goal is to gain an understanding in order to change behavior in some specified area.
2. Support groups aim to provide emotional reassurance and maintain healthy behaviors.
3. Socialization groups help members to learn new social roles and skills.
4. Psychotherapy groups are formed for people who need treatment of an emotional disturbance.
5. Task-oriented groups include all the groups whose primary goal is to accomplish some predetermined task.

Individuals have needs; so do groups. The groups with which community health nurses work need clear, shared goals and an agreement about how to reach those goals. They need consistent group norms and individuals motivated to participate in the group. Finally, every group needs stable communication channels among the members. Groups have two primary types of functions—task-related functions and group maintenance functions.

Starting a group involves determining the criteria for membership and then selecting people who are committed to the goals of the group. It is important to determine the optimal size of the group, set clear group goals, make physical arrangements for the group, and orient the members.

Every group varies in terms of the degree of cohesiveness experienced by members. The community health nurse can build a cohesive group by assuring that its four basic needs are met and avoiding certain barriers such as open membership. Building group cohesiveness must be an ongoing process in any group.

Working with a group is enhanced by recognizing the phases of group development: dependence, counterdependence, and inter-dependence. The group leader has specific functions and ways to carry out those functions. Every group also needs its members to carry out specific roles such as initiator, information seeker, informer, and clarifier. Many difficulties arise during the life of a group. In particular, the community health nurse must be alert to resolving conflicts, dealing with those who monopolize the group, and handling the nonparticipant member.

Every group must deal with the issue of termination, the last phase in the life of a group. It is important to prepare members for termination early in the life of a group and to work through the feelings generated by termination.

Group evaluation involves assessing the ongoing group interaction as well as the final outcome. Periodic self-evaluations are useful strategies for evaluating the process of group experience. Measuring the outcomes determines to what extent the group's goals were achieved. The entire evaluation process should involve both the leader and group members.

REFERENCES

1. Bennis, W. G., and Shepard, H. A. A theory of group development. *Hum. Relations* 9:415, 1956.
2. Bradford, L., Stock, D., and Horwitz, M. How to Diagnose Group Problems. In S. Stone, et al. (Eds.), *Management for Nurses.* St. Louis: Mosby, 1976.
3. Gouldner, A., and Gouldner, H. P. *Modern Sociology.* New York: Harcourt, Brace & World, 1963. P. 104.
4. Guthrie, E., and Miller, S. *Making Change: A Guide to Effectiveness in Groups.* Minneapolis: Interpersonal Communication Programs, 1978.
5. Hill, W. F. *Learning Through Discussion: Guide for Leaders and Members of Discussion Groups.* Beverly Hills, Calif.: Sage, 1962. Appendix.
6. Homans, G. C. *The Human Group.* New York: Harcourt, Brace & World, 1950. P. 1.
7. Konopka, G. *Group Work in the Institution.* New York: Whiteside, 1954.
8. Loomis, M. E. *Group Process for Nurses.* St. Louis: Mosby, 1979.
9. Marram, G. D. *The Group Approach in Nursing Practice* (2nd ed.). St. Louis: Mosby, 1978.

10. Mill, C. R., and Porter, L. C. What to Observe in a Group. In C. Mill and L. Porter (Eds.), *Reading Book.* Washington, D.C.: National Training Laboratories Institute for Applied Behavioral Science, 1976. Pp. 28–30.

11. Pfeiffer, J., and Jones, J. E. (Eds.). *A Handbook of Structural Experiences for Human Relations Training,* Vol. 1 (Revised). La Jolla, Calif.: University Associates, 1974.

12. Sampson, E., and Marthas, M. *Group Process for the Health Professions.* Somerset, N.J.: Wiley, 1977.

13. Schutz, D. *The Interpersonal Underworld.* Palo Alto, Calif.: Science and Behavior Books, 1966. P. 168.

14. Sweeney, B. Learning groups: Survival level, growth level. *J. Nurs. Educ.* 14:20, 1975.

15. Tubbs, S. L., and Moss, S. The Small Group: Therapeutic Communication. In S. Tubbs and S. Moss, *Human Communication: An Interpersonal Perspective.* New York: Random House, 1974.

16. Uris, A. *Techniques of Leadership.* New York: McGraw-Hill, 1964. P. 58.

17. Veninga, R. The management of conflict. *J. Nurs. Adm.* 3:13, 1973.

18. Yalom, I. D. *The Theory and Practice of Group Psychotherapy.* New York: Basic Books, 1975. P. 45.

SELECTED READINGS

Anderson, J., et al. Group theory integrated: A model for baccalaureate nursing programs. *J. Nurs. Educ.* 16(9):16, 1977.

Benne, K. D. The Current State of Planned Changing in Persons, Groups, Communities and Societies. In W. G. Bennis, et al. (Eds.), *The Planning of Change* (3rd ed.). New York: Holt, Rinehart & Winston, 1976.

Bennis, W. G., and Shepard, H. A. A theory of group development. *Hum. Relations* 9:415, 1956.

Berne, E. *The Structure and Dynamics of Organizations and Groups.* New York: Lippincott, 1963.

Bormann, E. G., and Bormann, N. C. *Effective Small Group Communication* (2nd ed.). Minneapolis: Burgess, 1976.

Bradford, L., Stock, D., and Horwitz, M. How to Diagnose Group Problems. In S. Stone, et al. (Eds.), *Management for Nurses.* St. Louis: Mosby, 1976.

Burnside, I. M. *Working with the Elderly: Group Processes and Techniques.* North Scituate, Mass.: Duxbury Press, 1978.

Cartwright, D., and Zander, A. (Eds.). *Group Dynamics: Research and Theory* (3rd ed.). New York: Harper & Row, 1968.

Cathart, R. S., and Samovar, L. A. (Eds.). Small Group Communication: A Reader (2nd ed.). Dubuque, Iowa: Brown, 1974.

Chopra, A. Motivation in task-oriented groups. *J. Nurs. Adm.* 3(1):15, 1973.

Dyer, W. G. Working with Groups. In A. Reinhardt and M. Quinn (Eds.), *Family-Centered Community Nursing: A Socio-cultural Framework.* St. Louis: Mosby, 1973.

Ebersole, P. P. Group Work with the Aged: A Survey of the Literature. In I. M. Burnside (Ed.), *Nursing and the Aged.* New York: McGraw-Hill, 1976.

Guthrie, E., and Miller, S. *Making Change: A Guide to Effectiveness in Groups.* Minneapolis: Interpersonal Communication Programs, 1978.

Henkel, B. O. Solving Health Problems Through Small Group Action. In B. Henkel, *Community Health* (2nd ed.). Boston: Allyn and Bacon, 1970. Pp. 338–347.

Hill, W. F. *Learning Through Discussion: Guide for Leaders and Members of Discussion Groups.* Beverly Hills, Calif.: Sage, 1962.

Larson, M., and Williams, R. How to become a better group leader? Learn to recognize the strange things that happen to some people in groups. *Nursing '78* 8(8):65, 1978.

Lieberman, M., Yalom, I., and Miles, M. *Encounter Groups: First Facts.* New York: Basic Books, 1972.

Loomis, M. E. *Group Process for Nurses.* St. Louis: Mosby, 1979.

Marram, G. D. *The Group Approach in Nursing Practice* (2nd ed.). St. Louis: Mosby, 1978.

Mill, C. R., and Porter, L. C. What to Observe in a Group. In C. Mill and L. Porter (Eds.), *Reading Book.* Washington, D.C.: National Training Laboratories Institute for Applied Behavioral Science, 1976. Pp. 28–30.

Ohlsen, M. M. *Group Counseling* (2nd ed.). New York: Holt, Rinehart & Winston, 1977.

Pfeiffer, J. W., and Jones, J. E. (Eds.). *A Handbook for Structured Experiences for Human Relations Training,* Vol. 1 (Revised). La Jolla, Calif.: University Associates, 1974.

Sampson, E., and Marthas, M. *Group Process for the Health Professions.* Somerset, N.J.: Wiley, 1977.

Shaw, Marvin E. *Group Dynamics: The Psychology of Small Group Behavior.* New York: McGraw-Hill, 1971.

Sweeney, B. Learning groups: Survival level, growth level. *J. Nurs. Educ.* 14(3):20, 1975.

Tubbs, S. L., and Moss, S. The Small Group: Therapeutic Communication. In S. Tubbs and S. Moss, *Human Communication: An Interpersonal Perspective.* New York: Random House, 1974. Pp. 231–257.

Veninga, R. The Management of Conflict. *J. Nurs. Adm.* 3:13, 1973.

Yalom, I. D. *The Theory and Practice of Group Psychotherapy.* New York: Basic Books, 1975.

Thirteen

Organizations and Population Groups

Community health nursing offers us a dual challenge: to promote the health of individuals and, at the same time, promote the health of aggregates. We have already discussed how the care of communities involves working with two kinds of aggregates, families and groups. In this chapter we will consider two additional aggregates, organizations and populations.

Let us begin with a nurse who described her experience of broadening her focus to include these larger aggregates. She was employed by an agency we will call Wilford County Public Health Nursing Service.

CASE EXAMPLE

"I received a referral to see a family whose fifteen-year-old daughter, Mary Jo, had run away from home for the third time. She was obese (215 pounds) and flunking out of school. There were so many problems in that family—unemployment, poor diet, stress, family conflict, another daughter's recent delivery of a sick illegitimate baby, and the obesity of the mother and all three daughters—that I hardly knew where to begin, but the parents were willing to work with me. We discussed their concerns and started with their biggest worry, the running away of Mary Jo. We finally found her. She and another girl who was also flunking out of school had hitchhiked to the city to find jobs but had no luck and ended up at the YWCA. When they got home, we had some long talks, and she agreed to stay and give it another try.

Up to this point, I felt some success in working with this family, and Mary Jo in particular. Then, an offhand comment made by Mary Jo shifted my attention to a larger aggregate.

'I know a lot of other girls at school in the same boat as me,' she said. I asked her what she meant. 'Well, there's a lot of others who don't give a damn about school and feel that life is pretty worthless.' I should have followed up on that remark right away, but I didn't. Then a girl committed suicide in that same school, one of *my* schools. I felt terrible. If some kind of effort had been made to reach those kids who were hurting emotionally, maybe that girl would be alive today. I had spent a lot of time with Mary Jo and her family, but it wasn't too late to work with other girls. We started to look at the needs of the whole population of adolescent girls. Then we went into both of my schools and started working with their organizations. We did something about those other students and, would you believe, we now have 35 girls coming to our Teen Topics meetings after classes on Tuesdays in one school and Thursdays in the other.''

Since nurses have traditionally worked with individuals and families, it was not surprising that this nurse focused on Mary Jo. Here was a family that needed and, in fact, asked for help. The nurse understandably gave care where a need had been clearly identified. In contrast, a whole population of girls plus two high schools appeared to be an amorphous mass of people, too indistinct to be assessed, too nebulous to treat as a whole, and too large for one nurse to serve. But was it? Belatedly, this nurse discovered that she could assess and meet the needs of larger aggregates. In this case, the aggregates included both a population group and two organizations.

An *organization* is an association of people that is organized into a formal structure around agreed-upon goals and tasks. The two high schools cited in the above example are organizations, as are the Wilford County Public Health Nursing Service, Sunset Nursing Home, Bell Telephone Company, Highland Park Health Center, and the Kansas Farm Bureau. A *population* or *population group,* on the other hand, is a large, unorganized aggregate of people, based on one or more common characteristics. The adolescent girls cited in the above example constitute a population. All the elderly in the United States is another population; those elderly confined to nursing homes are still another population group. Electricians who work in the communications industry make up a population; so do all farmers in the state of Iowa.

It is easy to see that populations and organizations are almost always interrelated. If you set out to promote the health of adolescent girls (a population), you will almost certainly become involved with schools or other organizations. A program to reduce accidents among farmers (a population group) might easily involve organizations like 4-H clubs, the Kansas Farm Bureau, or a farmers' cooperative. The intersection of organizations and populations occurs in almost all community health practice. Although your primary goal might be to promote the health of

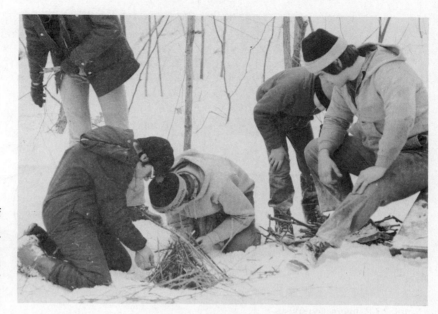

Figure 13-1. The Boy Scouts of America is a formal organization. These scouts learn winter camping and survival skills in keeping with their organization's purpose to develop character and promote affiliation. (Courtesy of the *Mt. Vernon News.*)

an organization, you will probably also become involved with assessing and serving a population. If your primary goal is to promote the health of a particular population, you will at the same time usually become involved in one or more organizations. Because organizations and populations interact, this chapter discusses them together.

ORGANIZATIONS

Every organization involves a collection of people who are working together in some fashion. They have prescribed responsibilities in order to ensure optimal functioning and achievement of the organization's purpose. Organizations are formal entities with distinct names, stated goals, and recognized role structures (Fig. 13-1).

The structure and functioning of an organization revolves around its goals. Four interacting subsystems form an organization: (1) an administrative-structural subsystem, (2) a communicative subsystem, (3) an economic/technologic subsystem, and (4) a social subsystem [7]. Like a family or group, an organization establishes authority and prescribes roles for its members (the administrative subsystem). It establishes information and decision-making patterns (the communicative subsystem). It develops a system and technology for maintaining control and accomplishing its work (the economic/technologic subsystem). It also meets member needs and promotes member motivation

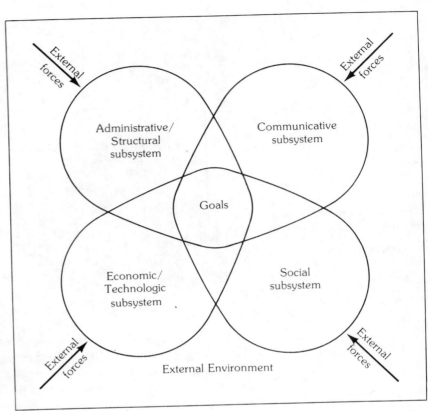

Figure 13-2. Interacting subsystems within an organization. (Adapted from P. Hersey and K. Blanchard, *Management of Organizational Behavior: Utilizing Human Resources* [3rd ed.]. Englewood Cliffs, N.J.: Prentice-Hall, 1977. P. 8.)

(the social system). As illustrated in Figure 13-2, a healthy, well-functioning organization exhibits effective, balanced interaction among its four subsystems. Each subsystem, in turn, maintains a central focus on the organization's goals.

Community health nurses may view organizational health from two perspectives. First, they may examine the health of the organization itself as a social system. Are its four major subsystems interacting effectively? Is each receiving proper emphasis in the organization? Are all subsystems contributing to accomplishment of the organization's goals? Is the organization as a whole responding appropriately to its external environment? This perspective of organizational health is generally the concern and responsibility of those in management positions. A community health nurse directing a nursing agency, for example, will need to assess and plan for the health of that organization. She may notice that staff members are not carrying out assignments effectively because job descriptions are unclear and the orientation program is inadequate. The administrative/structural subsystem needs correction. She may also recognize a need for technologic improvement in the agency's functioning, such as installation of a computer to facilitate record keeping. In addition to internal management of the organization, the nursing director will also consider the needs and pressures imposed by external forces such as budget restraints, legislative mandates, or consumer demands.

A second perspective for viewing organizational health focuses on the organization's members. Nurses working within the context of any organization must be aware that, just as family health affects individual health, the health of an organization influences the health of its members. Whether or not the nurse is responsible for the health of all the organization's members, as might be the situation at the Ford Motor assembly plant, the nurse still needs to recognize the impact of an organization's proper functioning on its members' well-being. If Highland Park Health Center has a poor communication system and a low concern for individual needs, then staff and patients, denied adequate information and feedback, may experience tension, anxiety, and decreased incentives to cooperate or participate in the center's activities. St. Clair Island Prison is another example of an unhealthy organization. Because it has a poorly functioning system for delivering health care to its inmates, like so many prisons today, prisoner health is directly affected [21]. Health screening, triage for sick call, and emergency treatment have been grossly inadequate. Dental and psychiatric needs have not been met. The organizational structure of the prison, the desire to maintain security, and budgetary constraints all combine to preserve the present inadequate system under the direction of the prison warden. A new program, managed by health professionals, could develop the needed, comprehensive preventive and primary care services.

On the other hand, a health organization such as the Kansas Farm Bureau positively influences and may actively promote its members' health. Seventy percent of the Kansas Farm Bureau headquarters' 420 employees are participating in its new wellness effort. Members may select programs in physical fitness, stress management, control of alcohol abuse, weight reduction, improvement of dietary habits, accident prevention, and stop-smoking clinics [22].

The health of an organization has a wide-ranging impact. As we have discussed, an organization's level of wellness influences its own internal functioning and affects the health of its members. Furthermore, an organization is a unit whose viability influences the larger community of which it is a part. Healthy organizations contribute significantly to community effectiveness because organizations that function well interact smoothly with the rest of the community and generate valuable products and services. In community health nursing, we are particularly concerned with organizational wellness as it affects the quality of life and health of community residents.

Nursing practice with an organization may seem foreign to some of us. Yet, more and more, nurses are moving into larger arenas, recognizing aggregate needs, and dealing with them.

POPULATION GROUPS

A population group is a large, unorganized aggregate based on one or more common demographic features. In contrast to an organization, a population group is a loose collection of people. Members share a set of defining criteria but do not share common goals or participate in a structure. That is, when we designate a special population, we identify one or more environmental or personal characteristics that the group of people have in common [23]. They might share the feature of age, as in a pediatric population or a population group of the elderly. The defining characteristic might involve language; consider the Spanish-, Italian-, French-, Native American-, or Vietnamese-speaking populations within our country. Some population groups, such as blue-collar, pink-collar, and migrant workers, are defined in terms of their common employment (Fig. 13-3). Other population groups share a common diagnosis; we may speak of the diabetic population, or the populations of stroke or automobile accident victims. We often define populations in terms of their potential vulnerability to health problems; for instance, we identify populations at risk for coronary heart diease, home accidents, or family abuse. The special population groups of unwed teenage mothers in a city, managers demonstrating stress symptoms in a specific corporation, and farm workers in the state who have experienced accidents with machinery in the past year all share a clear set of defining criteria. These criteria describe the population group.

The purpose for designating a population group arises from some special need residing in that collection of people. When a number of school children in the same school district contract measles, the nurse may study all the children of that district as a population group to determine immunization levels and institute preventive immunization programs. There may be a large group of elderly people living alone in a community who are at risk for developing physical and emotional health problems because they do not utilize available resources. A

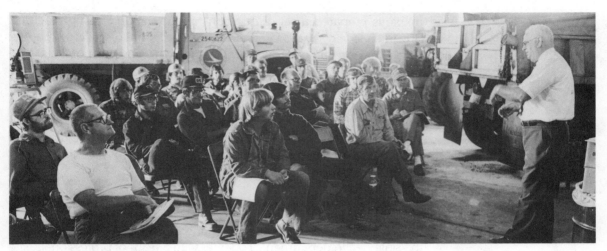

Figure 13-3. These farm workers comprise a population group. Here they meet to learn in an agricultural training session. (Courtesy of the *Mt. Vernon News.*)

significant number of employees with hypertension in an organization may attempt to function with their problem unrecognized and untreated. Community health professionals, therefore, single out population groups for the purpose of meeting health needs. The groups themselves become units for study and service.

ASSESSING ORGANIZATIONS AND POPULATIONS

Nurses can employ many different assessment strategies for studying the needs of organizations and populations. Four strategies are especially useful.

OBSERVATION

Observation can provide valid information about both these aggregates. It is often one of the best ways to begin any assessment. In the course of daily practice, nurses can watch for evidence of existing or potential problems. For example, after one nurse noticed symptoms of malnutrition in some migrant children, she broadened her observations to include the entire migrant community. Many of these hard-working people showed evidence of being undernourished. A nurse at a community college observed that several faculty members were frequently tense and fatigued. She began to pay attention to these indicators of stress when she participated in various college committees.

INTERVIEWING

Interviewing, a second assessment strategy, can offer detailed information about an organization or a population. The nurse working with migrants prepared a set of questions about diet and eating practices. She interviewed several families in their shacks and discovered they ate no protein or dairy products, but rather white bread, potatoes, and occasional vegetable scraps stolen from the fields. Their income was too meager to allow purchase of better foods. At the community college, the nurse interviewed several selected faculty members and discovered that the source of pressure was a crisis-oriented administration. Requests for department reports came at the last minute; every decline in enrollment brought announcements of possible faculty layoffs.

EPIDEMIOLOGIC SURVEY

The nurse concerned about migrant nutrition took her initial findings to the state health department. Together with a team of professionals, she helped design an epidemiologic survey, a third assessment strategy. Even in an organization such as a community college, however, it is possible to conduct an epidemiologic survey. In her role as a member of the president's council, the nurse pointed out the level of stress and tension among faculty; others agreed that the level was also high among staff members. She then suggested that an anonymous questionnaire to both faculty and staff might be useful in identifying causes and planning ways to reduce the stress. She became part of a team that planned this institutional survey.

USE OF EXISTING DATA

A fourth assessment strategy uses existing data. We can learn a great deal about a population group by examining information that has already been collected for other purposes. Census records, community demographic data, or surveys done by other community organizations can often provide needed information for assessment and health planning for population groups. Statistics on infant morbidity and mortality from automobile accidents, for example, as well as records describing infant car seat use could assist in a study to promote the safety of the infant car-riding population. Most organizations have records of activities, health of members, and statements about their goals. Many have conducted past surveys, which offer a gold mine of organizational data.

To clarify how nursing is practiced at the organization and population group levels, as compared to the individual, family, and group levels, aggregate nursing will be examined more specifically. We shall consider its practice in the context of three important foci in community health—school health, occupational health, and health of the elderly.

SCHOOL HEALTH

In community health practice, nursing service to a school-age population rightfully includes service to the school as an organization. The two are intertwined. That is, the health of the school as an organization cannot help but influence the health of school children and will directly determine whether or not an effective school health program is administered. The health of the school (an organization) and the health of school children (a population group) are simultaneous concerns of community health nursing. We shall view the two levels of concern together.

As we examine school health and the role of the school nurse, we must keep in mind that service to organizations and population groups requires a special mind set. We must shift from a focus entirely on individual school children or small groups of children to one that includes aggregates. In order to show how this shift can be made, let us consider what your role as school nurse would involve.

Imagine that you, a community health nurse, recently became school nurse for Keeler Elementary School. You have been working with families and groups in the community for almost a year, but you have not done school nursing before. Since it is summer and school has not yet started, you take time to get acquainted with the school and the nurse's role.

Mrs. Murray, the principal, is happy to talk with you. She comments that she expects the nurse to keep the children as healthy as possible and be the major consultant on health matters in the school. Because she is very busy with administrative concerns she prefers that you carve out your own role, although she wants to be kept informed of your plans. She describes the school to you. Built 40 years ago, Keeler has 353 students in grades kindergarten through sixth, with 14 teachers; its pupil-teacher ratio is 25:1. The teachers give some health instruction to their classes. Mr. Jones, a fourth grade teacher, was a medical corpsman in the army and handles first-aid problems for the school when the nurse is not there. Two PTA mother-volunteers keep the student health records in order. You can ask for more help if you need it. Mrs. Murray gives you material to read that describes school health services generally.

NURSING SERVICES

You learn that school health services incorporate three functions: health services, health education, and improvement of the school environment [17]. Health services include programs such as vision and hearing screening, psychological testing, health examinations, emergency care, and referrals. There are special correction and training services for speech, hearing, or mental health problems. Student and family counseling are important components; there is a program of communicable disease control. School health services also include health appraisal and services for school personnel.

The health education function of school health services involves planned and incidental teaching of health concepts, classes in health science and healthful living, and use of educational media, library resources, and community facilities. These activities aim to integrate health information with students' daily living experiences, to build positive attitudes toward health, and to establish sound health practices.

The third function of school health services is the promotion of healthful school living. Emphasis on a healthful physical environment includes proper selection, design, organization, operation, and maintenance of the physical plant. Consideration should be shown for areas such as adaptability to student needs, safety, visual, thermal, and acoustic factors, aesthetic values, sanitation, and safety of the school bus system. Healthful school living also emphasizes planning a daily schedule that monitors healthful classroom experiences, extra class activities, school lunches, emotional climate, program of discipline, and teaching methods. It also seeks to promote the physical, mental, and emotional health of school personnel.

HEALTH TEAM

You are impressed with all that can be done in school health and explore the subject further through reading and interviewing school personnel. It quickly becomes apparent that school health, like all health programs in the community, requires a team effort. Although the school nurse plays a central role, she collaborates with many other individuals. The school principal influences all phases of the school health program. Mrs. Murray, for example, can promote good school health through actively supporting all the school's health services, setting policies, and tapping community resources. She can reinforce positive efforts, ranging from health teaching to good housekeeping by the custodian, within the school. Because of the principal's influential

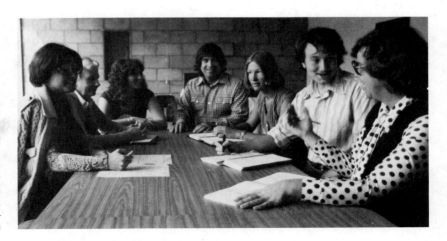

Figure 13-4. A school nurse, third from right, meets with a developmental specialist, a psychologist, a speech therapist, two teachers, and a social worker. Their combined knowledge and efforts are essential for promoting a comprehensive school health program. (Courtesy of La Esperanza Developmental Center, San Mateo, Calif.)

position, it is absolutely essential that the nurse maintain a positive working relationship with her.

Teachers, whether they are involved in regular instruction, physical education, or special education classes, play a major role in school health. Because they spend so much time with students, their observations, health teaching, and personal health habits have a profound effect on student health and the quality of school health services. Nurse and teachers must collaborate constantly.

Other health team members, such as health educators, health coordinators, psychologists, audiologists, counselors, dentists, dental hygienists, social workers, or health aides, may be present depending on the size and financial resources of the school. All team members, including students, parents, and the custodian, have a specialized role complementary to that of the school nurse. Consultation and referral between team members are crucial to implementing the school health program (Fig. 13-4).

The school physician may work full-time or part-time, or be available on a consultation basis. This role focuses largely on advising and consulting in policy and medical-legal matters. The physician often serves as liaison with the community and other health agencies and consults with those who plan and develop school health programs. The physician may also become involved in some student health appraisal and health problem intervention [19]. A good working relationship between the school nurse and school physician is important. The nurse's role, while complementary to and unique from the physician's, nonetheless may need clarifying and interpreting to maximize the effectiveness of their collaboration.

You want to learn more about the school nurse's role. You consult with your nursing supervisor who explains the difference between specialized school nursing and the generalized school nursing which you will be expected to practice.

SPECIALIZED AND GENERALIZED NURSING ROLES

School nurses operate from one of two administrative bases. In many localities, school nurses are hired through the public school system and maintain a specialized, school-based service. There is growing conviction that such nurses should work under the jurisdiction of the board of health rather than the board of education. With professional instead of educational supervision, better utilization of the nurse and greater quality of health care service would be ensured [8]. An advantage of the specialized school nurse role is that the nurse can concentrate all her time and effort on the school health program and thus develop specialized skills in school health assessment and intervention. A disadvantage is that school nurses' practice is often limited to the school setting. A specialized role may prevent the school nurse from assessing preschoolers, providing health service to families of school children, or making broader community assessments and contacts.

School nurse practitioners, nurses with advanced preparation and experience in child care and school health, assume an even more specialized and expanded role, that of identifying and managing many of the health problems of school children. They have made a significant contribution to the provision of primary health care to school children. They have an important but different function from that of school nurses who are community health nurses.

Generalized school nurses work within the framework of generalized community health nursing, serving private and sometimes public schools as part of their case loads. The advantage of a generalized school nurse role is the broader community base from which the nurse can operate. This base allows contact with preschoolers and families, strengthened knowledge of the community and its resources, and integration of in-school and out-of-school care [6]. Humes also argues, "A public health nurse working in the schools tends to have more of a working knowledge of the general health needs of the community. With this kind of background information she is better able to view student health problems in a community context" [8, p. 396]. A disadvantage of the generalized role, however, is that the nurse often has less time to meet school health needs.

Whether specialized or generalized, the primary functions of the school nurse are to prevent illness and to promote and maintain the health of the school community. A philosophy of school nursing, adopted in Minnesota, is suggested by your supervisor as a basis for your school nursing practice [16, p. 3]:

All children and their families have a right to education which guides them toward self-awareness and self-realization in meeting the needs of complex living. The focus of public health school nursing is the self-motivation of individuals and families to seek and maintain optimum health. The partnership of public health school nursing and education is essential for increasing high level wellness of students, their families, school personnel, and the community.

The community health nurse not only serves individuals, families, and groups within the context of school health, but also the school as an organization and its membership (students and staff) as population groups.

School has started, and the three days a week you spend at Keeler never seem to be enough time to finish all there is to do. You have already looked through student records to determine children with health problems and followed up on your findings. You sent five children home with notes recommending dental work; sent little Norma, a new kindergartner, to the audiologist after testing her hearing; and referred Jimmy Hansen for psychological testing. You found out that Tommy Sandberg had a convulsive disorder but did not take his medication regularly. You visited his family, explained the need for consistent treatment and medical supervision, had him start on a regular treatment program, and gave him his medication during school hours. Many individual children in your school show signs of improved health as a result of your efforts. Several families of children in the school are now part of your regular case load. The group you started with sixth graders on how to become good baby-sitters is going well. Yet there are so many children you have not assessed. Moreover, what about the teachers' needs? You know that you are not really providing service to the whole school community. You realize that you must shift your focus.

NURSING GOALS

Previously your primary goal as a school nurse had been to assess and promote the health of the preschool and school age child. Changing your focus means you now adopt a broader set of goals for school nursing which involve the school organization and population levels. At the individual, family, and group levels, you aim to:

1. Assess the health and developmental status of the preschool and school-age child.
2. Promote and maintain optimal health of students, families, and school personnel.
3. Implement an appropriate plan for the education and care of each exceptional and each handicapped child.*

At these levels, you concentrate on selected individuals, selected families, or special groups needing nursing or other professional intervention. Many of these clients will be referred to other community resources for assistance. You plan to get to know personally each member of the school faculty and staff, including the secretary and their custodian, in order to cultivate their good will, sharpen their observation skills regarding the students, and assess their own health needs. A faculty or staff member who is not well physically or emotionally may significantly influence the health of the school community.

ORGANIZATION LEVEL

At the organization level, you aim to:

1. Establish and revise school and district health policies, administration, and philosophy pertaining to school health services.
2. Develop and maintain a system of emergency care.
3. Provide for school safety and a healthful school environment.
4. Facilitate comprehensive community health care planning and resources development to include the health needs of the preschool and school-age populations and their families.*

This level requires more attention than you have given to it in the past. True, you have worked out a system with Mr. Jones to handle basic first-aid for injuries and have updated physician orders to cover emergencies. Now you make certain everyone understands what to do and where to go in the event of an emergency such as a tornado. Some school safety issues have been addressed, but now you need to examine the overall safety of the building and check with administration about safety of the school buses. You look into the effectiveness of fire drills and alternate routes for emptying the building. You oversee the handling of dangerous materials in the science laboratories.

*Adapted from Minnesota Nurses' Association, School Nurse Branch, Goals of School Nursing: An Interpretative Tool. St. Paul, Minn.: Minnesota Nurses' Association, 1974.

The school environment needs more careful assessment. You start checking the nutritional value of the school lunches and the ventilation of classrooms. You begin to analyze seating arrangements in each classroom while observing students and consult with teachers about your observations. The dingy halls of the old building soon take on a new cheerful appearance through the work of your volunteer paint crew from the PTA.

As an organization, Keeler Elementary School is functioning fairly well, you decide. The pupil-teacher ratio is slightly high by some standards, but a class of 25 students is generally considered a manageable load. To provide students with more individual attention, you suggest adding more teacher aides. Faculty on the whole get along well with each other and with Mrs. Murray. There is open communication and positive feedback. Working conditions are pleasant, and faculty requests are answered in a reasonable amount of time. There is also adequate space, equipment, personnel assistance, and support for your school health program.

To influence school health policy and resource planning, you volunteer to serve on a district committee which meets once a month. Meeting other professionals concerned about school health broadens your understanding of school and community needs and also gives you ideas on intervention strategies and how to tap community resources.

POPULATION GROUP LEVEL

At the population group level you aim to:

1. Assess the collective needs of preschool and school-age children and school personnel.
2. Identify existing and potential health problems in the school population (and in the larger community affecting it), determine those at greatest risk, develop a plan, and intervene to minimize or prevent problems.
3. Promote and maintain optimal health of the student body and the school personnel population.
4. Prevent and control communicable disease in the student population (in order to protect the well-being of students and the community).
5. Evaluate and upgrade the contribution of the school nurse role toward promoting the health of the school community.*

During a conference with your community health nursing supervisor, you review the new goals and make plans for conducting a

*Adapted from Minnesota Nurses' Association, School Nurse Branch, *Goals of School Nursing: An Interpretative Tool*. St. Paul, Minn.: Minnesota Nurses' Association, 1974.

broader assessment of the school population's health. Journal articles and discussion with other school nurses give you additional ideas. For example, one school nurse, instead of performing a routine physical examination on every child, developed a systematic method of classroom assessment. She evaluated an entire class of 25 to 30 children at one time through regular observation of their behavior and developmental status and through close consultation with teachers that alerted them about special student behaviors to observe [24]. You decide to try this method in combination with further data gathering on selected children through screening, interviews, and family visits. The yearly vision and hearing screening which you are required to give students offers another opportunity to observe them closely for signs of child abuse, malnutrition, or other physical or emotional problems that might be prevalent among this population group.

You assess preschool age children who will be starting kindergarten next year by holding a Saturday afternoon preschool fair. Invitations are sent out to all the families in the community with four-year-old children. PTA volunteers help you organize games and refreshments and conduct school tours. Registered nurse volunteers from the community assist you in cursory physical exams that include vision and hearing screening. You notify parents immediately if children need follow-up care.

While conducting this preschool assessment, you keep in mind that you want a profile of this population of four-year-olds, not just each individual child's health picture. You look for recurring problems that are common to the group, such as skin rashes, orthopedic defects, headaches, eating or respiratory difficulties, and signs of communicable diseases. Such population screening has sometimes uncovered widespread community health problems. For instance, recognition of common symptoms among Love Canal residents in New York led to a discovery that the river was contaminated with poisonous industrial wastes. In 1980, a community in Memphis, Tennessee, whose incidence of miscarriages, cancer, and infant deaths had markedly increased, discovered that nearby chemicals buried many years previously were the cause. Identifying common problems among the preschool or school-age populations enables you to take corrective action on a broader scale and thus to help many children at once as well as to take preventive action.

You begin to collect data on the needs of the school personnel population by observing and talking informally with faculty and staff.

You discover that some of the teachers seem on the verge of burning out. They do not enjoy their teaching, feel tired most of the time, take piles of work home with them every night, do not sleep well, and often feel irritable toward the children. With school administration's approval, you plan a workshop to prevent teacher burnout. Expert consultants help the teachers learn to recognize symptoms and how to avoid burnout. During the workshop the teachers develop specific plans to help them cope with their present situations and design strategies for alleviating future stress.

The three sets of goals for school nursing have helped you refocus your thinking and expand your service to include not only individual, family, and group levels of nursing intervention but school organization and school population group levels as well.

OCCUPATIONAL HEALTH

Community health nurses have a long history of involvement in occupational health. In 1895, the Vermont Marble Company hired the first industrial nurse in the United States to care for its employees and their families. It was an unusual demonstration of interest in employee welfare at that time. The nursing service, consisting almost entirely of home visiting and care of the sick, was free to employees and their families. Gradually this nursing role changed. By World War II there was a striking increase in employment of industrial public health nurses who practiced preventive medicine and health education among employees at work. In addition to emergency care and nursing of ill employees, the activities of many industrial nurses involved safety education, hygiene, nutrition, and improvement of working conditions. Yet a significantly high number of industrial accidents and sick employees kept many nurses too busy to do anything but illness care. They might see as many as 75 or more patients a day in the plant dispensary, where they provided first aid and medications [11]. More recently, employee health programs have improved as socioeconomic and political pressures have created greater safety and health standards for the work environment. These changes have caused the role of the nurse to expand and change also.

As we examine occupational health and the role of the occupational health nurse, we must remind ourselves that traditional nursing practice with individuals and groups of employees is very different from aggregate nursing. We must again broaden our perspective to include the health needs of organizations and population groups, composed now of working people rather than school children. In order to make this shift in focus, let us consider how you might practice nursing with the working community.

EMPLOYEE HEALTH PROGRAM

You have just been hired, let us imagine, as a full-time occupational health nurse for Allied Electronics, a firm which manufactures and sells electronic components and equipment. Allied's 450 employees are scattered through its sprawling 5-acre plant located on the edge of the city. At present, Allied's health program consists of several components. The health service, run by the nurse, provides emergency care for employees who are injured or become ill on the job. An on-call physician has left standing orders for the nurse to use in emergencies and sick care. Regular checking for real or potential hazards in the work environment is done through the safety division by the plant safety engineer. Allied pays for a large percentage of employee health care through its health benefits program; this fact is precisely why Allied has hired you. Health insurance premiums per employee have skyrocketed, and management is looking for alternative solutions to lower health service costs. They would like you to develop a new approach to employee health.

Occupational health programs, generally speaking, have grown tremendously since World War II. Many manufacturing plants, service organizations such as the Kansas Farm Bureau, and commercial establishments, including department stores, have instituted some kind of health program for employees. The majority of programs still concentrate on providing emergency care, but others are beginning to recognize the importance of prevention and health promotion. For example, Sperry Univac of St. Paul held an Employee Health Promotion Day, and Ball Electronics keeps employees fit with exercise breaks. The Resource Trust Company of Minneapolis pays the initial fee and half the weekly dues of any employee who attends Weight Watchers. As an added incentive, the firm reimburses the other half of the costs to employees when they meet their weight objectives [22]. Recent research has demonstrated the correlation between healthy employees and increased productivity on the job. In fact, as a result of wellness promotion, employees have shown increased self-esteem, improved job performance and job satisfaction, decreased absenteeism, and less use of company health services [9].

NURSING GOALS

A broad goal for occupational health is "the promotion and maintenance of the highest degree of physical, social, and emotional well-being of workers in all occupations" [18, p. 7]. In actual practice, this goal is only beginning to be realized in selected instances. Nevertheless, it is a worthy and, more importantly, an essential objective in the realization of an energized and productive working community.

We can address this goal more specifically through four working goals to guide occupational health nursing practice:

1. Assess the health needs of employees and intervene to promote and maintain their highest possible level of wellness.
2. Study factors in the work environment that are a real or potential hazard to employee health and take action to minimize their impact or prevent their occurrence.
3. Provide early diagnosis and prompt treatment for injury or illness on the job.
4. Provide programs for employees with disease or disability aimed at restoring and maintaining their maximum level of functioning.*

HEALTH TEAM

Even as you consider these goals, you realize that you will not be pursuing them alone. Like most community health efforts, your work will require collaboration with others. Company management and administrative personnel will be important partners with you in this venture. As Keller points out, "the philosophy and vision of these administrative persons can make or break the contribution of the nurse and the development of her full potential" [12, p. 414]. Collaboration may take time but will be worth the investment. Your goal is to gain the respect and trust of management and establish open communication lines in order that you may influence company policies regarding the nature and scope of its health program.

The company physician is another important health team member with whom the nurse collaborates. Whether a full-time, part-time, or on-call position, the physician has a strong influence on the company's health policies and programs. Development of a positive ongoing working relationship with the physician gives the nurse a powerful supporter of proposals and program efforts.

*These goals summarize a comprehensive listing of occupational health nursing competencies developed by Keller. For a complete presentation of the competencies with suggested nursing actions, see M. J. Keller in association with W. T. May, *Occupational Health Content in Baccalaureate Nursing Education*. Cincinatti: National Institute of Occupational Safety and Health, 1971.

Based in health service, usually a part of personnel services, the nurse works closely with other professional, technical, and clerical personnel, particularly those from the safety, engineering, and industrial hygiene departments. Any comprehensive assessment of employee health and safety problems, as well as any health promotion program, would require cooperation and assistance from many individuals of various departments within the organization.

Finally, the occupational health team is not complete without the workers themselves. You will want to encourage employees to identify problems and needs. They can also contribute to decision making regarding health programs. Their cooperation in implementing and evaluating programs is essential for an effective health protection and promotion effort.

As the only nurse at Allied, you will particularly need skills in effective communication, leadership, change management, and assertiveness. These tools will be crucial to effectively interpret your role and promote your ideas. Your goal is to establish positive working relationships with the other health team members, on whom your success depends.

NURSING SERVICES

Nurses involved in occupational health have a unique opportunity to help shape the health profile of the working population. The degree of that influence depends on how the nurse defines her role. Also, the nurse must be able to overcome the many obstacles incurred in the occupational setting, including restrictive company policy, misunderstanding of the nurse's role, and lack of time for innovative program development. The nurse's role in occupational health, therefore, still varies considerably. It ranges from only providing emergency care for injuries or illness on the job to establishing comprehensive programs covering health promotion, accident and disease prevention, and innovative care for disease and disability.

MEETING EMPLOYEE NEEDS

Occupational health nursing applies the philosophy and skills of nursing and community health to protecting and promoting the health of people in the context of their employment [1, 12]. In other words, the occupational health nurse relies on in-depth nursing preparation as well as strong community health background to provide her with the tools and perspectives necessary in meeting the challenges of occupational health. Many nurses in occupational health acquire additional physical assessment skills as well.

Specifically, some of your typical nursing activities in the new job will include history taking, partial physical examinations, ordering of tests, and emergency care. You will refer many employees for further treatment and follow-up care. Keeping health records will be an expected part of your job, but it can be largely delegated to clerical help. You will participate in conducting health education and health counseling sessions for groups as well as for individual employees. Health assessment, screening, and monitoring are also important aspects of your role.

In order to keep a proper perspective on your goals and also to begin developing a more innovative approach to meeting the employees' health needs (the reason you were hired), you do some strategic planning. You review your four main goals, develop specific objectives for each one, and schedule times when the activities to meet those objectives will be done.

Meeting most of the individual and group needs of employees can be accomplished by scheduling health service hours, classes, and counseling sessions. You plan time to visit departments, observe, and interview selected personnel as part of your health assessment process.

You know there is a relationship between the health of the employees (a population group) and the health of Allied Electronics (an organization). Consequently, you keep a running log of observations on how the company functions and what its effects are on the employees. For example, you notice that some departments seem to place greater stress upon their workers than other departments. Among these workers there is a higher incidence of hypertension, headaches, gastrointestinal disturbances, and other somatic complaints. You collect data on the working conditions in those departments. Is there high production pressure? Are there any opportunities to relieve stress on the job? Do workers receive any positive feedback about their work? Could the symptoms be caused or aggravated by some environmental factor such as chemicals, gasses, or noise? (See Fig. 13-5.)

ASSESSMENT STRATEGIES

To assess the health needs of the total employee population and selected smaller population groups within the company, you use several approaches. First, you enlist the assistance of the company com-

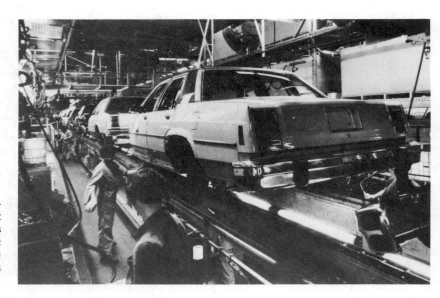

Figure 13-5. The work environment can contribute to or detract from employees' health. Effects of hazards, noise, and toxic chemicals are examples of the nurse's concerns for the workers in this Ford auto assembly plant.

puter services, compile the results of individual health histories and physical examinations, and analyze the findings. A picture emerges of dominant health problems among the employees and of the workers at greatest risk for other problems.

It appears that hypertension, overweight, excessive smoking, and inadequate exercise are the major problems common to Allied's employee population. You can attack these problems on several fronts. You start a regular program of blood pressure monitoring. The employee health education program can be upgraded with new videotapes and literature to make workers more health conscious and show them how to improve their health. Specifically, they learn how to lose weight, manage stress, stop smoking, and maintain an exercise program. More important than information, however, is motivation. You convince management that company inducements, such as Resource Trust Company's payment for Weight Watchers' costs, are important in stimulating employee participation. You tell them about the Speedcall Corporation of Hayward, California which pays its workers a $7 weekly bonus if they do not smoke on the job. After 2 years on this program, 20 out of 24 smokers had quit smoking on the job [14]. Ball Electronics gives workers time for exercise breaks [22]. A number of Milwaukee, Wisconsin companies, some of them splitting the cost between employer and employee, have enrolled employees in the Milwaukee YMCA fitness programs. Allied's management agrees to give time for exercise breaks, a weekly bonus to employees who stop smoking on the job, and a quarterly bonus to those whose blood pressure readings are within normal limits.

Another approach that you use to assess the health needs of the employee population is to conduct an environmental survey of health hazards. Using data from the safety division's regular spot checking, you collaborate with the division on systematic observations of working conditions and interviews of workers. In addition, you post suggestion boxes and gain management's approval to give any employee half a day off with pay for suggesting a safety or health improvement that is implemented into the health program. You gain further ideas from other companies' measures. For example, Scherer Brothers Lumber Company in Minneapolis has removed their cigarette machines and stocked other vending machines with nutritionally beneficial foods, such as granola bars, yogurt, iced tea, and fruit drinks. The company provides fresh fruit instead of sweet rolls to its employees without charge. It has reduced its noise levels, provided a HMO medical insurance option to encourage illness prevention, and initiated a committee of employees to plan wellness activities [15].

To assess employee population health further, you participate in a committee composed of the company physician and other personnel to analyze accidents, injuries, and illnesses. The findings reveal a high percentage of injuries and absenteeism. One possible solution is to offer incentive pay similar to the programs instituted by other companies. Parsons Pine Products, Inc., an Ashland, Oregon, manufacturing plant, had a high rate of accidents and absenteeism. Management offered incentive pay to encourage employee wellness. For each month that workers were not absent or late they received 8 hours of extra pay. In addition, if they had no injury accidents during the quarter, they received 2 more hours of pay per month. As a result, absenteeism was reduced by 30 percent, accident rates dropped from 86 percent above average to almost zero, and the company's medical insurance costs dropped [13]. Scherer Brothers also uses "wellness pay." For each month that employees are not absent from work because of illness, they receive 2 hours of extra pay [15].

Another problem uncovered in your analysis is a rising incidence of back injuries among Allied's production workers. You learn that Ball Electronics Corporation has a similar problem and consider their approach. Ball has instituted a voluntary exercise program. Once or twice a day, assembly line workers engage in 5-minute limbering and strengthening exercises near their work stations. They are also invited to use the company exercise room, attend optional exercise classes which are offered at break times (lasting five extra minutes for employees on company time) and after work, and join the company running club. The program has already resulted in improved production efficiency and job satisfaction but has not been in effect long enough to measure direct impact on back injuries [15]. In the meantime you offer literature on backache prevention and present two classes, one at noon and the other after work, on ways to strengthen back muscles and prevent injuries.

Each set of data gathered through the various assessment approaches gives you material to guide your planning and development of health programs. An important dimension in this process is accurate record keeping. Exact figures on incidence and prevalence of health problems in the company give you ammunition to justify your programs and data with which to compare the results when you evaluate program outcomes.

Occupational health nursing demands a great deal from the nurse. Individual needs in the work place will always compete for the nurse's time and attention with aggregate needs, often to the detriment of the latter. To maintain a proper focus on aggregate needs requires discipline and commitment, commitment which is based on the realization that meeting the health needs of an organization and its employee population will also greatly benefit the individuals in that organization. Cost and production incentives increasingly cause greater receptivity among employers to methods that enhance employee wellness. The time is ripe for health promotion of the working community.

HEALTH OF THE ELDERLY

The elderly constitute one of the largest population groups in our country. Hundreds of different organizations, ranging from the Gray Panthers, a national advocacy group, to a local church in a small town, provide services to the elderly. We want to discuss this population in order to illustrate four fundamental requirements for effective nursing of any population. Whether you work with schools and school-age children, business and industry, spinal injury victims, the deaf, the blind, the elderly, or any other population, these four requirements are essential:

1. View the population from the broad perspective of community health which promotes wellness.
2. Know the characteristics of the population.

3. Set aside those stereotypes based on misconceptions of the population.
4. Know the health needs of the population as a basis for nursing intervention.

Let us consider each of these requirements in the context of our elderly population.

COMMUNITY HEALTH PERSPECTIVE

In general, we can divide nursing service to the elderly into two approaches. One approach emphasizes the science of geriatrics; the other, the science of gerontology. Although these fields overlap, they tend to differ in at least one significant way. Geriatrics is the study of diseases of old age, while gerontology studies the broader phenomena of aging itself [2]. Geriatric nursing in the past has been oriented primarily toward care of the sick aged. Gerontologic nursing, a broader practice, concentrates on preventing illness and promoting the health and maximum functioning of older adults [5]. While both are important dimensions of nursing practice, a community health perspective emphasizes the gerontologic approach.

Community health nurses work with many elderly people. In one instance, the nurse may promote and maintain the health of a vigorous 80-year-old man who lives alone in his home. As another example, the nurse may give postsurgical care at home to a 69-year-old woman, teach her husband how to care for her, and help them contact needed community resources for shopping, meals, housekeeping, and transportation services. Perhaps the focus is on teaching nutrition and a healthy lifestyle to a family, including the 73-year-old grandmother who lives with them. Yet again, the nurse may lead a support group for senior citizens who have recently lost their spouses through death.

A large portion of the community health nurse's work with the elderly is at the individual, family, and group levels. However, the community health perspective also leads to working with large aggregates of the elderly. Many organizations—adult day-care centers, retirement communities, nursing homes, senior citizens centers, long-term care facilities, and old age assistance programs, to name a few—exist to serve senior citizens. In addition, there are many population groups composed of elderly persons. Consider the following: residents of a senior citizens' high-rise apartment building, retired business and professional women, elderly residents in a community at risk for glaucoma, the elderly poor, and skid row alcoholics. Organizations existing to serve senior citizens and population groups composed of the elderly are important partners in nursing intervention. We need to focus our attention on these wider levels of practice.

CHARACTERISTICS OF THE ELDERLY POPULATION

Never before in the history of our society has the population of elderly people been so large. Moreover, it is increasing in size. Twenty-two million people in the United States, 11 percent of the country's population, are over 65 years of age, and by 2020 that amount is expected to rise to 20 percent. Women outnumber men in the older population because they live an average of 7 years longer. In fact, "women outlive men every place in the world where women no longer perform backbreaking physical labor and where adequate sanitation and a reduced maternal mortality are present" [3, p. 5]. In the United States, there are 3 million more women than men, a proportion of approximately 143 women for every 100 men.

People are also living longer. In 1900 the average life expectancy in the United States was 47 years, and only 4 percent of the population were over 65 years of age. Now, as a result of improved health care, reduction in infant mortality, and new medical discoveries, the average life expectancy has increased to 71 years (67 for men, 74 for women). For those who reach age 65, the life expectancy becomes even higher by an average of 15 additional years; men can expect to live an average of 13 years, and women an average of 17 years, longer. The average life expectancies for blacks (63.8), Hispanics (mid-50s), and American Indians (47), however, are considerably lower.

Within the elderly population, the number of people living into "older" old age has increased. Almost half of the elderly are over 73 years of age, more than 1 million are 85 or more years of age, and nearly 110,000 claim to be over 100 years of age. The 75 years and over age group is the most rapidly growing segment of the entire United States population.

Other facts about the elderly are also useful for community health nurses to know. Most elderly men are married and thus have some companionship. Two-thirds of elderly women are widows. Most senior citizens live in the central part of cities (about 60 percent) or in rural areas (5 percent on farms, 35 percent in small towns). Some speculate that in 15 or 20 years this demographic picture will change and more elderly will be living in the suburbs. Nearly 25 percent of older Americans are poor, many of them living in profound poverty, unable to afford clothing, recreation, transportation, or other assets that younger people consider necessary for mental health, social status, avoidance of isolation, and personal growth.

MISCONCEPTIONS ABOUT THE ELDERLY

All of us have had personal experiences with individuals from many populations. We have watched school children play in the street; we have elderly neighbors; we have seen a blind man walking down the street. In our professional training, we encounter many sick elderly. These past experiences with individuals often become the data upon which we base our assumptions about populations. When we generalize our knowledge about a few older persons to the entire elderly population, we are operating with a stereotype. Many people, including health professionals, have such misconceptions about the elderly. These misconceptions often arise from negative personal experiences. Practitioner bias can interfere with effective practice and prevent the kind of service aging persons need or deserve. The following are some of the more common misconceptions [3, 20].

It is not true that *most old people live in institutions.* Ninety-five percent of the eldery live independently in the community. Seventy percent live in families, and 25 percent live alone or with nonrelatives. Only the remaining 5 percent live in institutions consisting of nursing homes, long-term care facilities, homes for the aged, and mental institutions.

It is not true that *chronologic age determines "oldness."* One 75-year-old man may be actively involved in community organizations, drive his own car, and play golf. He may still have some dark hair and very few wrinkles. Another 75-year-old person may be stooped, wrinkled, slow, and confined to an apartment. Most old people are quite distinct from one another, and they age at widely disparate rates. Physical, social, and mental health parameters, life experiences, as well as genetic traits all combine to make aging an individualized process.

It is not true that *most old people are senile.* Senility, while not an actual medical term, is widely cited by health professionals and laymen alike to denote deteriorating mental faculties associated with old age. Such stereotypical labelling often provides an easy escape for practitioners impatient with the older person's complaints. It interferes with proper diagnosis and treatment. Certainly arteriosclerosis and senile brain disease may cause mental disorders among the elderly. But many so-called senile cases, compounded by anxiety, loss, grief, or psychosomatic problems, are treatable and sometimes preventable.

It is not true that *all old people are content and serene.* The tranquil picture of grandma sitting in her rocker with her hands folded in her lap is misleading. It is true that many older people have learned to accept rather than fight the hardships and vicissitudes of life. Yet, for most people, old age brings increasing problems—physical, emotional, social, and financial—to harass and worry them.

It is not true that *old people cannot be productive or active.* More than 3 million Americans over 65 years of age work full- or part-time, and many others, not counted in labor statistics, work but do not report their earnings because of Social Security restrictions [3]. Healthy old people do not disengage; rather, they are active and involved. Butler and Lewis emphasize that activity instead of disengagement produces the best psychological climate for the elderly [3].

It is not true that *most older people have diminished intellectual capacity.* Studies show that intelligence, learning ability, and other intellectual skills do not decline with age [3]. Intelligence is more directly affected by health; poor health and near death cause a drop in intellectual functioning [10]. Speed of reaction tends to decrease with age, but basic intelligence does not. In fact, some abilities, such as judgment, accuracy, and general knowledge, may increase with age. Most older people are largely capable of making their own decisions; they want and need the freedom to make choices and to be as independent as their limitations will allow.

Misconceptions about their intelligence often leads to the treatment of older people as children. Practitioners who infantilize their approaches to and programs for the elderly may create self-fulfilling prophecies: old age may indeed resemble a second childhood if the elderly are stripped of their rights and dignity.

It is not true that *all old people are resistant to change.* In a study of nursing home residents, Carp concluded that rigidity is not intrinsic to aging but rather tends to result from difficult social or physical situations. When these pressures are lifted, the rigidity disappears [4]. The elderly have spent a lifetime adapting to change, with varying measures of success. The ability to change does not depend on age but rather on personality traits acquired throughout life [3]. An older person's apparent resistance to change may be a factor of his established personality. Then again, his conservatism may be caused by socioeconomic pressures. Financial concern, for example, may cause an older property owner to vote against a school levy that would increase his taxes.

HEALTH NEEDS OF THE ELDERLY

The fourth requirement for working with any population is to know their health needs. How can we help the elderly achieve their highest possible level of wellness? There are two answers to this question: (1) by knowing the characteristics of healthy aging, and (2) by knowing the health needs of the elderly as a basis for health planning.

Consider an older person who is aging at a high level of wellness.

CHARACTERISTICS OF THE HEALTHY AGED

Minerva Blackstone, affectionately called Minnie by her friends, is a lively 87-year-old woman who enjoys life. Every day, except in bad weather, she walks the half mile distance to the house of her grand-daughter, Karen, for a visit. There she works on the quilt, stretched on a frame, that she is making for Karen. Twice a week Minnie takes the city bus to the senior citizens' center to join her friends in an exercise class. Although her eyesight has failed somewhat, Minnie enjoys reading in the evening and crocheting while she watches TV. Mysteries and comedies are her favorite kinds of stories. She is not content, however, unless she has kept up on the latest political developments. She always has opinions on current events and expresses them with vigorous shakes of her curly white head at her monthly group meeting on women and politics. She has a good appetite and generally sleeps well. Minor arthritis does not hamper her activities, nor does the hypertension which she controls by taking her medication with conscientious regularity. Minnie is enjoying healthy, successful old age.

What is healthy old age? As we said earlier, the vast majority (95 percent) of the elderly, like Minnie Blackstone, are living outside of institutions and maintaining relative independence, even those with chronic diseases and other disabilities. They are able to function. The ability to function is a key indicator of health and wellness and is an important factor in understanding healthy aging. Good health in the elderly means maintaining the maximum degree of physical, mental, and social vigor of which one is capable. It means being able to adapt, to continue to handle stress, and to be active and involved. In short, healthy aging means being able to function with, and despite, disabilities, with no more than ordinary help from others [20].

Wellness among the elderly population varies considerably. It is influenced by many factors such as personality traits, life experiences, current physical health, and current societal supports. Some elderly people, like Minnie Blackstone, demonstrate maximum adaptability, resourcefulness, optimism, and activity. Others, often those from whom we tend to draw our stereotypes, have disengaged and present a picture of dependence and resignation. Most of the elderly population is somewhere in between these two extremes. Although the level of wellness varies among the elderly, that level can be raised. Our challenge in community health nursing is to maximize the wellness potential of the elderly. We must analyze and capitalize on their strengths, not focus only on their problems. As Butler and Lewis so poignantly describe it, our goal is to enable older people to thrive, not merely survive [3].

HEALTH PLANNING

How can nurses help the elderly achieve their highest possible level of wellness? The answer to this question lies in understanding healthy old age and in knowing the elderly's needs. At all stages of life, people have the same basic needs. We know that the elderly, like any age group, have physiologic, safety, love and belonging, esteem, and self-actualization needs. As we assess the health of the elderly population, however, some needs in particular demand extra attention.

Among these is the need for good nutrition. People who have maintained sound food habits throughout life need not change in old age. However, many have not established such habits. Older people need to maintain their optimal weight by eating a generally low fat, moderate carbohydrate, and high protein diet. They should avoid habitual use of laxatives, adding instead more fiber and bulk to their diet. Loss of teeth will cause some to need foods that are easier to chew. Eating should be a pleasurable experience, preferably taking place in the company of other people.

Older people continue to need exercise (Fig. 13-6). Even a daily walk can keep muscles in good tone, enhance circulation, and promote mental health. They need economic security. Worry over finances is often one of the most debilitating factors in old age. Putting older people in touch with appropriate community resources can do much to relieve this source of stress. They need independence. As much as possible, the elderly need to make their own decisions and manage their own lives. Independence helps to meet another need, that of self-respect and dignity. The elderly need to have their ideas and suggestions heard and acted upon, and to be addressed by their preferred names in a respectful tone of voice.

Older people need companionship, particularly when they live

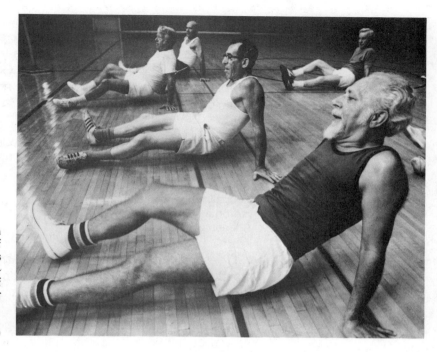

Figure 13-6. Community health nurses must learn the needs of each population group, such as elderly persons' need for physical fitness. Here a group of senior citizens exercise in their community center gymnasium. (Photograph by David Franklin. © 1979 Time, Inc.)

alone. The company of other people offers an avenue for expression and response and adds meaning to life. So, too, does meaningful activity, another very important need of the elderly. Some kind of active role in community life is essential for mental health and satisfaction. It can range from involvement in hobbies, such as gardening or crafts, to volunteer work or even full-time employment.

Our assessment of the needs of the older population must also include evaluation of the organizations serving the elderly. Are these organizations singly and collectively meeting the health needs of the elderly? Do they encourage their clients' independent functioning? Do they treat senior citizens with respect and preserve their dignity? Do they recognize the elderly's need for companionship, social status, and economic security? When appropriate, do they promote meaningful activities? Bingo and shuffleboard alone are not enough; they must be balanced with opportunities for creative outlets, continued learning, and community service.

CRITERIA FOR EFFECTIVE SERVICE

A community service delivery system for the elderly (all the organizations that collectively serve this population) should meet four major criteria. First, it should be comprehensive. Many communities provide some services, such as limited health screening or selected activities, but do not offer a full range of services that would more adequately meet the needs of their senior citizens. Gaps and duplication in programs most often result from poor or nonexistent community-wide planning. A comprehensive set of services should provide the following:

Health care services (prevention, early diagnosis and treatment, rehabilitation)
Health education (including preparation for retirement)
Recreation and activity programs
Adult day-care programs
Specialized transportation services
In-home services
Adequate financial support

A second criterion for a community service delivery system for the elderly is coordination. Often older persons go from one agency to the next; after visiting one place for food stamps, they may go to another for answers to Medicaid questions, another for congregate dining, and still another for health screening. Such a potpourri of services reflects a system organized for the convenience of providers rather than consumers. It encourages non-use. Instead, there should be coordinated, community-wide assessment and planning. Communities must consider alternatives such as multiservice agencies which can meet many needs in one location, more convenient and perhaps specialized transportation services, and more in-home services.

A third criterion is accessibility. Too often, services for the elderly are not conveniently located or are prohibitive in cost. Some communities are considering multiservice community centers which would bring programs and services for the elderly closer to home. Federal, state, and private funding sources can be tapped to ease the burden on the already economically pressured elderly population.

Finally, an effective community service delivery system for older people provides a coordinated information and referral system. Most communities need a better information network. A directory of all resources and services for the elderly with the name and telephone number of a contact person for each listing is available in some communities and should be developed in those without one. A simplified information and referral system—a system that includes one number to call to find out what resources and services are available and how to get them—is particularly helpful to older people.

SUMMARY

Community health nursing practice involves promoting the health of organizations and populations. An organization is an association of people that is organized into a formal structure around agreed-upon goals and tasks. A population is a large, unorganized aggregate of people, based on one or more common characteristics. These two levels of community health practice are interrelated. Almost any work with an organization involves one or more population groups. Working with a population group will involve numerous organizations.

Organizations achieve their goals through the functioning of four interacting subsystems: administrative/structural, communicative, economic/technologic, and social. A healthy organization is one in which there is balanced interaction among these subsystems. They all contribute effectively toward the accomplishment of the organization's goals. The health of an organization, its level of wellness, affects the health of its members. It also has an impact on the wider community.

The selection of some criteria for designating a population group depends on the goals of nursing practice. Because health problems vary with age, nurses often use age as a defining criteria for populations such as the elderly or children. Population groups are also defined in terms of their potential vulnerability to health risks. We can assess both populations and organizations by means of observation, interviews, epidemiologic surveys, and use of existing data.

This chapter examined the dynamics of organizations and populations in the context of nursing practice to schools, workers, and the elderly. In order to promote the health of the school population as well as the school as an organization, community health focuses on specific health services, health education, and the school environment. In both school and occupational health, the nurse always works with a team of professionals to accomplish health care goals. Occupational health nursing applies the philosophy and skills of nursing and community health to protecting and promoting the health of people in the context of their employment. Whether working with school populations, workers, or the elderly, the community health nurse goes beyond the needs of individuals to focus on the needs of organizations and the population as a whole. This approach requires the nurse to view the population from the perspective of wellness, to know the characteristics of the population, to set aside stereotypes and misconceptions of the population, and to know the specific health needs on which to base nursing intervention. Although these three populations are important, community health nursing seeks to promote the level of wellness among many other population groups as well.

REFERENCES

1. Brown, M. L. *Occupational Health Nursing.* New York: Springer, 1956.
2. Burnside, I. M. (Ed.). *Nursing and the Aged.* New York: McGraw-Hill, 1976.
3. Butler, R. N., and Lewis, M. I. *Aging and Mental Health: Positive Psychosocial Approaches* (2nd ed.). St. Louis: Mosby, 1977.
4. Carp, F. M. *A Future for the Aged: Victoria Plaza and its Residents.* Austin: University of Texas Press, 1966.
5. Davis, B. A. Gerontological nursing comes of age. *J. Gerontol. Nurs.* 1:6, 1975.
6. Freeman, R. *Community Health Nursing Practice.* Philadelphia: Saunders, 1970. P. 307.
7. Hersey, P., and Blanchard, K. *Management of Organizational Behavior: Utilizing Human Resources* (3rd ed.). Englewood Cliffs, N.J.: Prentice-Hall, 1977.
8. Humes, C. W., Jr. Who should administer school nursing services? *Am. J. Public Health* 65(4):394, 1975.
9. Jaffe, R. M. Science and wellness: The new medicine. Presented at the 105th Annual Meeting of the American Public Health Association, Washington, D.C., November 3, 1977.
10. Jarvik, L. F., Eisdorfer, C., and Blum, J. E. (Eds.). *Intellectual Functioning in Adults.* New York: Springer Verlag, 1975.
11. Kalisch, P. A., and Kalisch, B. J. *The Advance of American Nursing.* Boston: Little, Brown, 1978.
12. Keller, M. J. Health Needs and Nursing Care of the Labor Force. In M. J. Fromer, *Community Health Care and the Nursing Process.* St. Louis: Mosby, 1979.
13. *Minnesota Council on Health Newsletter.* Minneapolis: Minnesota Council on Health, Sept. 1978.
14. *Minnesota Council on Health Newsletter.* Minneapolis: Minnesota Council on Health, Jan. 1979.
15. *Minnesota Council on Health Newsletter.* Minneapolis: Minnesota Council on Health, Oct. 1979.
16. Minnesota Nurses' Association, Special Committee, School Nurse Branch. *Goals of School Nursing: An Interpretive Tool.* St. Paul, Minn.: Minnesota Nurses' Association, 1974.
17. Nemir, A., and Schaller, W. *The School Health Program* (4th ed.). Philadelphia: Saunders, 1975.
18. Report of the Committee on School Physicians of the American School Health Association. *J. Sch. Health* 37:395, 1967.
19. Tinkham, C. W. The Catherine R. Dempsey memorial lecture. Occu-

pational health nursing in the 1980's. *Occup. Health Nurs.* 25:7–13, 1977.

20. U.S. Department of Health, Education and Welfare, Public Health Service. *Working with Older People: A Guide to Practice.* Arlington, Va.: Division of Health Care Services, 1969. Vol. 1.

21. Weisbuch, J. B. Public health professionals and prison health care needs. *Am. J. Public Health* 67:720, 1977.

22. *Wellness Gazette.* Minneapolis: Minnesota Council on Health, Jan. 1980.

23. Williams, C. A. Community health nursing—What is it? *Nurs. Outlook* 25:250, 1977.

24. Withrow, Cora. The school nurse takes a look at her charges. *Nursing '79.* Pp. 48–51, Jan. 1979.

SELECTED READINGS

Burnside, I. M. (Ed.). *Nursing and the Aged.* New York: McGraw-Hill, 1976.

Brown, M. L. *Occupational Health Nursing.* New York: Springer, 1956.

Butler, R. N., and Lewis, M. I. *Aging and Mental Health: Positive Psychosocial Approaches* (2nd ed.). St Louis: Mosby, 1977.

Freeman, R. *Community Health Nursing Practice.* Philadelphia: Saunders, 1970.

Hanlon, J. J. *Public Health: Administration and Practice* (6th ed.). St. Louis: Mosby, 1977.

Hawkins, N. G. Is there a school nurse role? *Am. J. Nurs.* 71:744, 1971.

Hersey, P., and Blanchard, K. *Management of Organizational Behavior: Utilizing Human Resources* (3rd ed.). Englewood Cliffs, N.J.: Prentice-Hall, 1977.

Holt, S. J., and Robinson, T. M. The school nurse's family assessment tool. *Am. J. Nurs.* 79(5):950, 1979.

Humes, C. W., Jr. Who should administer school nursing services? *Am. J. Public Health* 65(4):394, 1975.

Kane, R. L., and Kane, R. A. Long-term care: Can our society meet the needs of its elderly? *Annu. Rev. Public Health* 1:227, 1980.

Keller, M. J. Health Needs and Nursing Care of the Labor Force. In M. J. Fromer, *Community Health Care and the Nursing Process.* St. Louis: Mosby, 1979.

Long, G., et al. Evaluation of a school health program directed to children with history of high absence—A focus for nursing intervention. *Am. J. Public Health* 65:388, 1975.

MacDonough, G. P. School Nursing. In M. J. Fromer, *Community Health Care and the Nursing Process.* St. Louis: Mosby, 1979.

Managan, D., et al. Older adults: A community survey of health needs. *Nurs. Res.* 23:426, 1974.

Minnesota Nurses' Association, Special Committee, School Nurse Branch.

Goals of School Nursing: An Interpretive Tool. St. Paul, Minn.: Minnesota Nurses' Association, 1974.

Nemir, A., and Schaller, W. *The School Health Program* (4th ed.). Philadelphia: Saunders, 1975.

Patti, R. J., and Resnick, H. Changing the agency from within. *Soc. Work* 17(4):48, 1972.

Richter, E., and Kretzmer, D. Prevention through pre-review in occupational health and safety. *Am. J. Public Health* 70(2):157, 1980.

Serafini, P. Nursing assessment in industry. *Am. J. Public Health* 66(8):755, 1976.

Stefl, B. M. Prevention Measures and Safety Factors for the Aged. In I. M. Burnside (Ed.), *Nursing and the Aged.* New York: McGraw-Hill, 1976.

Stone, V. Nursing of Older People. In E. Busse and E. Pfeiffer (Eds.), *Behavior and Adaptation in Late Life* (2nd ed.). Boston: Little, Brown, 1977.

Tinkham, C. W. The Catherine R. Dempsey Memorial Lecture. Occupational health nursing in the 1980's. *Occup. Health Nurs.* 25:7, 1977.

de Tornyay, R. Public health nursing: The nurse's role in community-based practice. *Annu. Rev. Public Health* 1:83, 1980.

U.S. Department of Health, Education, and Welfare, Public Health Service. *Working with Older People: A Guide to Practice*, Vol. 1. Arlington, Va.: Division of Health Care Services, 1969.

Weisbuch, J. B. Public health professionals and prison health care needs. *Am. J. Public Health* 67:720, 1977.

Withrow, C. The school nurse takes a look at her charges. *Nursing '79* 9(1):48, 1979.

Williams, C. A. Community health nursing—What is it? *Nurs. Outlook* 25:250, 1977.

Wold, S. *School Nursing: A Framework For Practice.* St. Louis: Mosby, 1981.

Zald, M. N. Organizations as polities: An analysis of community organization agencies. *Soc. Work* 11(4):56, 1966.

Zaltman, G., Duncan, R., and Holbek, J. *Innovations and Organizations.* New York: Wiley, 1973.

Fourteen

The Community: Assessment and Planning

A central theme of this book has been community health nursing's involvement in promoting the health of aggregates of people. This idea has been emphasized because, in both subtle and direct ways, our culture works against it. The value of individualism is one of the greatest barriers to carrying out the mission of community health nursing.

INDIVIDUALISM AND COMMUNITY HEALTH

Every society has a small number of core values that give meaning to life. In the United States, for example, we value success and material rewards. Such values provide motivation for millions of people. They uphold the work ethic; they become the measures by which we elevate successful and wealthy people to the status of popular heroes. The very existence of our society and its way of life depends on a deep commitment to such values. We learn them early in life and come to take them for granted as "the way things ought to be." One value that most Americans hold as God-given, a value that profoundly influences the entire practice of nursing, is individualism.

Nearly every social observer who has written about American society has identified this value. A cornerstone of our civilization, this basic premise underlies most of our institutions. "Protect the rights of the individual." "Equal justice for all under the law." "Life, liberty, and the pursuit of happiness for all individuals." More than 40 years ago, the sociologist Robert Lynd described this value: "Individualism, 'the survival of the fittest,' is the law of nature and the secret of America's greatness; and restrictions on individual freedom are un-American and kill initiative" [4, p. 60].

We reward individual effort in the school and in the workplace. Our criminal justice system punishes individual crimes far more harshly than corporate crimes. A woman who steals $5 in a southern state serves several years in prison; a large oil company that steals millions by overcharging customers pays a relatively small fine or suffers no punishment at all. Health care in our society is dominated by a commitment to the treatment of individuals. The vast majority of our research, personnel, and health care institutions engage in the care of individual illness rather than promote community health.

How does this value of individualism affect community health nursing? All nurses are first educated and trained in the individualistic perspective of clinical nursing. The individual patient is the focus of nursing service. Moreover, this early education is supported by powerful cultural premises; together, they create a mind-set which we bring into community health nursing. Unless we become aware of this mindset and consciously set it aside, our clients will remain individuals instead of families, groups, organizations, populations, and communities [6, 9].

This mind-set is influenced by three pervasive myths, all touched on in earlier chapters.

THE LOCATION MYTH

Community health nursing is only clinical nursing outside the hospital setting. This myth silently influences us to think of our task as simply nursing *in* the community. Community health nursing, from this perspective, seems to have the merit of reducing hospital costs. It is easy to think that patients do not have to spend so much time in the hospital; we can treat them and care for them in their homes. Instead, community health nursing is practice *to* and *with* the community. It may include the hospital.

THE SKILLS MYTH

Community health nursing employs only the skills of clinical nursing when working with community clients. This myth leads many nurses to assume their clinical skills are completely adequate for community nursing. It can lead us to overlook a large and sophisticated body of knowledge required for effective community health nursing. When unquestioningly accepted, this myth causes nurses to discount key concepts such as health, culture, family dynamics, and group process, or an essential epidemiologic approach.

THE CLIENT MYTH

Community health nursing involves working with communities, but the individual in a family context is the primary client. This myth prevents us from taking a wide perspective, one that sees the health of families, groups, organizations, populations, and communities as central to community health nursing practice.

In order to escape the constricting influence of this final myth, it is useful to think of six different levels of nursing practice. One level focuses on individuals; the other five involve aggregates. On a typical day, a community health nurse might well work at all six levels. In a city such as Atlanta, Georgia, you might leave an agency to visit an unmarried adolescent in the last trimester of her pregnancy. As you offer service to this individual, you will also assess her family as a group and seek to promote the health of that family. You might invite this young woman to a group of expectant mothers with whom you will meet that evening. Before noon, let us say that you stop by The Family Tree on Selby Avenue to meet with the staff for a discussion of this organization's goals. In the early afternoon you meet with other staff at your agency to discuss assessing the population of unmarried, pregnant adolescents in the city of Atlanta. Before you finish your day's work, you might stop by the city council hearing room to participate in a hearing on a local ordinance regarding abortion. Or you might visit the Georgia state legislature for a committee hearing on the use of state funds for abortion by women on welfare. These last two activities involve nursing practice at the community level.

Table 14-1 summarizes some of the major differences among the various levels of nursing practice. We have already examined the family as client, the characteristics of a healthy family, and ways to provide nursing service to families. We also examined the nature of groups, what causes groups to function effectively, and how community health nurses can work with groups. In the last chapter, we discussed organizations and populations. Now we will shift our attention to a larger aggregate, the community.

Although community health nurses work at all six levels of practice, working with communities is of primary importance for several reasons. First, the community includes all the other levels of practice. An attempt to determine the major influences on a family or organization,

Table 14-1. Levels of Nursing Practice

Client	Example	Characteristics	Health Assessment	Nursing Involvement
Individual Level				
Individual	Mr. Jones Tommy Jones	One person with various needs	Individual health assessment	A dyad; interaction with the individual
Aggregate Level				
Family	The Jones family: 7 members	A small group based on kin ties; specific roles	Family health assessment	Family visits; interaction with members as a group
Group	A parenting group An Alanon club	2 or more people; face-to-face communication; interdependency	Assessment of group effectiveness in fulfilling its functions	Group participation; having a role in meetings
Organization	Ford Motor assembly plant	A formal organization with identified goals; structured	Assessment of functional effectiveness, e.g., membership turnover	Formal role as occupational nurse or consultant
Population	Preschool children All diabetics in one state	A large, unorganized aggregate based on some demographic feature	Survey of health needs and vital statistics	Researching the population; planning and setting up services
Community	St. Paul, Minnesota Macalester neighborhood	An aggregate of people in a specific location; organized in a social system	Survey of community characteristics, such as vital statistics and competence	Membership in organizations such as health planning council

for example, leads directly to community assessment. Second, the health of individuals, families, groups, organizations, and populations is directly affected by the community. When the city of Los Angeles failed to take aggressive action to stop air pollution, this failure affected the health of millions of individuals and families. Similarly, when a community improves its water supply, this action affects the health of families, groups, and all the other levels. Third, working with communities is important because it is at this level that most health service delivery occurs. Health information is developed by community agencies, as are the services required by families and groups.

The community health nurse, then, must deal with the community as client. Understanding the community is a prerequisite for effective service at every level of nursing practice.

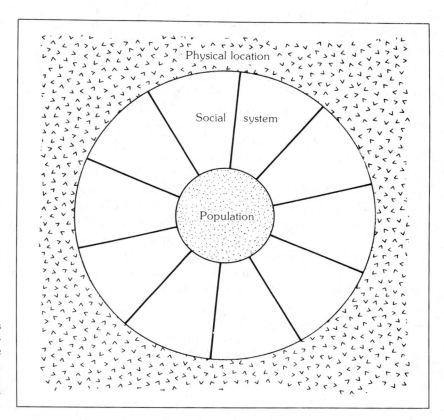

Figure 14-1. A community has (1) a physical location, represented here by the square boundary; (2) a population, shown here by the central circle; and (3) a social system, divided here into subsystems.

THE COMMUNITY AS CLIENT

Community is a term that we use in many different ways. Some people talk about the "community of professional nurses," those nurses who are trained and work in the field. On a small college campus in the south, students and faculty talk about the "college community." You probably think of your home town or city as a "community." On occasion, the President of the United States will refer to the "American community." In England and France, people talk about the "European Economic Community," and spokespeople for the United Nations refer to the "world community."

In Chapter One, we defined a community as having three features: (1) a location, (2) a population, and (3) a social system [4]. This three-dimensional view, represented in Figure 14-1, especially suits our idea of a local community. The size of a local community can vary by expanding or constricting the geographic boundary. The community of

Seattle, for example, may refer to the city as defined by all the people within the city limits. But we also speak of "greater Seattle," a community composed of the city, its suburbs, and many other small towns located near Seattle. A community health nurse might want to restrict the size of the community within Seattle to the Wallingford district. If you worked in the Washington State Health Department in Olympia, you would probably think of your community as the entire state. However, all these communities still share the three common denominators of a single location, population, and social system.

Think of these three dimensions of every community as a rough map you can follow whether you are working in a rural town of 250 people or in the city of Chicago. This concept of community is a useful tool for assessing needs or planning for service delivery, whether your particular community is a refugee camp in Cambodia or the state of New Hampshire. As we consider each dimension, we will pay particular attention to the questions you will want to ask to assess the health of a community.

LOCATION

Every community carries out its daily existence in a specific geographic location. The health of a community is affected by this location, by the location of health services, the geographic features, climate, plants, animals, and the human-made environment. The community health nurse will want to become aware of all these location variables and their implications for community health.

The location of a community places it in an environment which offers resources and also poses threats. The healthy community is one that makes wise use of its resources and is prepared to meet threats and dangers. In assessing the health of any community, it is necessary to collect information not only about these location variables, but also about how the community relates to them. Do groups cooperate to identify threats? Do health agencies cooperate to prepare for an emergency such as flood or earthquake? Does the community communicate information about resources and dangers to its members?

To guide you in assessing the health of any community is a Community Profile Inventory (Tables 14-2 to 14-4). It is divided into three parts—location, population, and social system—in order to conform to our definition of a community. Although not exhaustive, it suggests the implications for community health of each variable, provides a set of community assessment questions, and some information sources. Let

Table 14-2. Community Profile Inventory: Location Perspective

Location Variables	Community Health Implications	Community Assessment Questions	Information Sources
Boundary of community	Basis for measuring incidence of wellness and illness Basis for determining spread of disease	Where is community located? What is its boundary? Is it a part of a larger community? What smaller communities does it include?	Atlas State maps County maps City maps Telephone book City directory Public library
Location of health services	Use of health services depends on availability and accessibility	Where are major health institutions located? What necessary health institutions are outside the community? Where?	Telephone book Chamber of Commerce State health department County or local health departments Maps Public library
Geographic features	Injury, death, and destruction from floods, earthquakes, volcanoes Recreation opportunities at lakes, seashore, mountains	What major land forms are in or near the community? What geographic features pose possible threat? What geographic features offer opportunities for healthy activities?	Atlas Chamber of Commerce Maps State health department Public library
Climate	Extremes of heat and cold affect health and illness Extremes of temperature and precipitation may tax community's coping ability	What is average temperature and precipitation? What are extremes? What climatic features affect health and illness? Is community prepared to cope with emergencies?	Weather atlas Chamber of Commerce State health department Maps Local government Weather Bureau Public library
Flora and fauna	Poisonous plants and disease-carrying animals can affect community health Plants and animals offer resources as well as dangers	What plants and animals pose a possible threat to health?	State health department Poison control center Police department Emergency rooms Encyclopedia Public library
Human-made environment	All human influences on environment—housing, dams, farming, type of industry, chemical waste, air pollution, etc.—can influence levels of community wellness	What are major industries? How has air, land, and water been affected by humans? What is quality of housing? Do highways allow access to health institutions?	Chamber of Commerce Local government City directory State health department University research reports Public library

Table 14-3. Community Profile Inventory: Population Perspective

Population Variables	Community Health Implications	Community Assessment Questions	Information Sources
Size	The number of people influences number and size of health delivery institutions Size affects homogeneity of the population and its needs	What is the population of the community? Is it an urban, suburban, or rural community?	State health department Census data Maps City or town officials Chamber of Commerce
Density	Increased density may increase stress High and low density often affect the availability of health services	What is the density of the population per square mile?	Census data State health department
Composition	Composition of the population often determines the types of health needs	What is the age composition of the community? What is the sex composition of the community? What is the marital status of community members? What occupations are represented and in what percentages?	Census data State health department Chamber of Commerce U.S. Department of Labor Statistics
Rate of growth or decline	Rapidly growing communities may place excess demands on health services Marked decline in population may signal a poorly functioning community	How has population size changed over the past 2 decades? What are the health implications of this change?	Census data State health department
Cultural differences	Health needs vary among subcultural and ethnic populations Utilization of health services vary with culture Health practices and extent of knowledge affected by culture	What is the ethnic breakdown of the population? What racial groups are represented? What subcultural populations exist in the community? Do any of the subcultural groups have unique health needs and practices? Are different ethnic and cultural groups included in health planning?	Census data State health department Social and cultural research reports Human rights commission City government Health planning boards
Social class	Class differences influence the utilization of health services Class composition influences cost of public health services	What percent of the population falls into each social class? What do class differences suggest for health needs and delivery?	State health department Census data Sociological reports

Table 14-3—Continued

Population Variables	Community Health Implications	Community Assessment Questions	Information Sources
Mobility	Mobility of the population affects continuity of care Mobility affects availability of service to highly mobile population	How frequently do members move into and out of the community? How frequently do members move within the community? Are there any specific populations, such as migrant workers, that are highly mobile? How does the pattern of mobility affect the health of the community? Is the community organized to meet the health needs of mobile groups?	State health department Census data Health agencies serving migrant workers Farm labor offices

Table 14-4. Community Profile Inventory: Social System Perspective

Social System Variables	Community Health Implications	Community Assessment Questions	Information Sources
Health system Family system Economic system Educational system Religious system Welfare system Political system Recreation system Legal system Communication system	Each system must fulfill its functions for a healthy community Collaboration among the systems to identify goals and problems affects health of community Undue influence of one system on another may lower the health of the community Agreement on the means to achieve community goals affects community health Communication among organizations in each system affects community health	What are the functions of each major system? What are the major subsystems of each system? What are the major organizations in each subsystem? How well do the various organizations function? Are the subsystems in each major system in conflict? Is there adequate communication among the major systems? Is there agreement on community goals? Are there mechanisms for resolving conflict? Do any parts of the total system dominate the others? What community needs are not being met?	Chamber of Commerce Telephone book City directory Organizational literature Officials in organizations Community self-study Community survey Local library

us consider the six location variables which define, in part, every human community.

BOUNDARY OF COMMUNITY

In order to talk about the community in any sense, you must first discover its boundary. All measurements of wellness and illness within the community depend on knowing the unit under consideration. However, all communities are also related to other communities, and it is important to know about such locations. If you are working in a small community of 5,000 persons, you need to know whether it is part of a huge metropolis or an isolated rural town.

LOCATION OF HEALTH SERVICES

If the members of a town must travel 300 miles to the nearest clinic or dental office, the health of the community will be affected. When assessing a community, you will want to identify the major health institutions and where they are located. In one city, for example, the alcoholism treatment center for skid row alcoholics was located 30 miles outside of the city. This location profoundly affected who volunteered for treatment and how long they remained at the center. The location of services may be restricted from some members who have transportation problems. If a well-baby clinic is located on the edge of a high-crime district, mothers may be discouraged from using it. It is often enlightening to place the major health institutions, both inside and outside the community, on a map that shows their proximity and relation to the community.

GEOGRAPHIC FEATURES

Communities have been constructed in every conceivable physical environment. Mountain communities face problems that are foreign to a desert town. A healthy community takes into consideration the geography of its location, identifies the possible problems and likely resources, and responds in an adaptive fashion.

In Anchorage, Alaska, the community is set in the midst of mountains and almost on top of a geologic fault line. The same is true for San Francisco, where in 1906, a massive earthquake destroyed many buildings and fire swept through the city. Seven hundred persons died. In such places, the health of the community would be partly determined by its preparedness for an earthquake and its ability to cope when such a crisis occurred.

A geographic feature such as a lake offers food supplies for community members. A healthy community uses such a local resource in many ways; for instance, as a source of food, recreation, or water supply. The same resource, however, can also present a public health danger if drownings or contamination of fish occur. Sometimes the contamination comes from far distant communities. In Ontario, Canada, a series of lakes called the Lac la Croix is a valuable resource for the Ojibway Indian communities. They depend on fish from the lakes for their livelihood. However, in recent years, acid rain has begun to affect the lakes and the fish. Coal-burning power plants in the United States and Canada emit large amounts of sulfur dioxide which rise high in the air and are then blown by strong winds over the Lac la Croix chain of lakes. In the atmosphere, the sulfur dioxide reacts with water vapor to form sulfuric acid, which then falls to earth in the rain and snow, eventually finding its way into the lakes. As the acidity of lakes rises, the egg-producing ability of the fish drops. More immediately, the acid in the water changes mercury in the lake sediment into methyl mercury, which is easily absorbed by the fish. A major food supply has thus become contaminated for the Ojibway Indian community.

CLIMATE

The climate also has a direct influence on the health of a community. When Buffalo, New York, is blanketed with deep winter snows, members of this community are sometimes immobilized for days. Deaths from coronary occlusions increase as people attempt to shovel their walks and uncover their cars. The intense summer heat of another location, such as Phoenix, Arizona, can create other health problems. Skin cancer, for example, is highest in states that constitute the Sun Belt. A healthy community will encourage physical activity among its members, but the climate, in turn, affects this activity. Although long cold winters can restrict activity, one community, St. Paul, Minnesota, holds an annual Winter Carnival which includes sporting events. Parades, ice sailing, dog sleds, treasure hunts, and hot air balloon races bring thousands of people out-of-doors at a time when they might otherwise be confined by the weather.

FLORA AND FAUNA

Plant and animal populations in a community are often determined by location. The way a community responds to these populations, whether wild or domestic, can affect the health of the community. In

Covina, California, black widow spiders make up part of the local insect population. The poison from a single bite may cause injury and death. In Seattle, Washington, a bushy, attractive plant, known as deadly nightshade, grows in yards and vacant lots. It has an appealing black berry which appears edible to children. However, it contains the drug belladonna, and people have died from ingesting the berries. The community health nurse will want to know about the major sources of danger from plants and animals in the community. Are there community agencies that provide educational information about these dangers? Does the populace understand their significance? Are emergency services, such as a poison control center, available to community members?

HUMAN-MADE ENVIRONMENT

Every community is located in the midst of an environment created and transformed by human ingenuity. We build houses and other buildings; we dump wastes into streams or vacant lots; we fill the air with gasses; we build dams to control streams. All these human alterations of the environment have important implications for community health.

A community health nurse might improve the health of a community by working for legislation to prevent disposing of waste chemicals into water or landfills. Had such legislation been passed years ago, the disaster at New York's Love Canal, where toxic wastes are still seeping into the homes and yards of victimized citizens, might have been prevented.

One way in which we alter the environment is through agricultural activity. Southern Wisconsin is in the heart of midwest farmland. The rich harvests attract thousands of seasonal workers, farm migrants, every year. Because of their nomadic lifestyle and their rural location, the health of migrants suffers. Community assessment in this area would include a careful examination of the migrant population, the health services available to them, their housing accommodations, and the community's economic resources.

Every community exists in some physical location. This fact has important implications for the community's health and any plans to assess or improve it. Table 14-2 shows the first part of a provisional assessment tool, the Community Profile Inventory. It will help sensitize you to the health implications of geographic location as well as give some direction for assessing any community.

POPULATION

When we consider the community as the client, the second dimension to examine is the population of the total community. As discussed in the previous chapter, one level of practice in community health nursing is working with special population groups. These population groups may be within a community or cut across many communities. For example, health care for the elderly population may be carried out in a city such as Des Moines, Iowa, or in the entire state of Iowa. However, from the perspective of the community itself, the population consists not of a specialized aggregate, but of all the diverse people who live within the boundaries of the community. As Sanders has said, "A community can be viewed as a population, as a collection of people. Health authorities conduct demographic analyses in order to determine the extent of maternity, morbidity, and mortality within a community" [8].

The health of any community is greatly influenced by the population that lives in it. Different features of the population suggest health needs and provide a basis for health planning. A healthy community has leaders who are aware of the population's characteristics, know its different needs, and respond to those needs. Community health nurses can better understand any community by knowing about population size, density, composition, rate of growth or decline, cultural differences, social class, and mobility (Fig. 14-2). Let us consider each of these population variables briefly.

SIZE

The town of Dover, Delaware, with less than 10,000 people, and the city of Los Angeles, California, have radically different health problems. If a single hepatitis case occurred in Dover, health officials would likely learn of it. It would be relatively easy to trace the course, check the few restaurants in town, and interview people about sanitation practices. However, many cases might occur in Los Angeles without the health department's knowledge. Moreover, if these cases were discovered, tracing the source of contamination might involve a long and complicated search. This is only one small way in which population size might affect the health of a community. But it also would influence the presence of slums, heterogeneity of the population, and almost every conceivable area of health need and service. One of the first things community health nurses need to know about a community is its size.

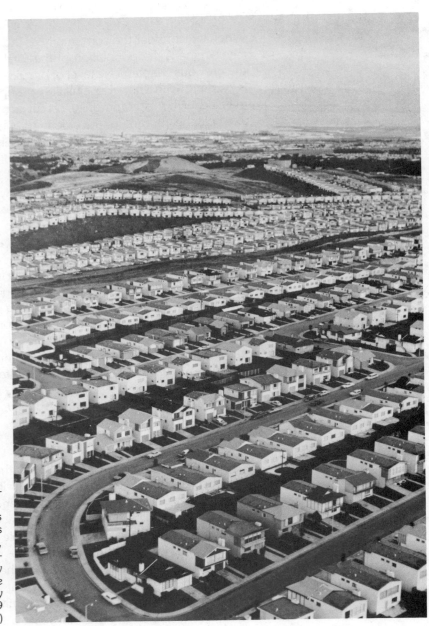

Figure 14-2. A. Many factors affect a community's health. Urban sprawl, shown here in this San Francisco suburb, influences commuting distance to work, pressures to conform to neighborhood standards, and many other variables affecting lifestyle and health. (Photograph by Robert Isaacs for *Time.* © 1969 Time, Inc.)

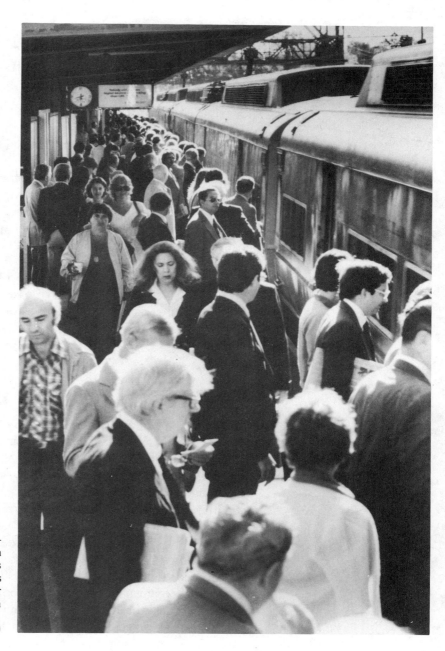

B. A community's resources, including its public transportation system, profoundly affect its health. Here white collar workers crowd together to catch their commuter train. (Photograph by Kevin Byron for *Time*. © 1979 Time, Inc.)

DENSITY

In some communities, thousands of people are crowded into high-rise housing. In others, such as a farm community, people live at great distances from one another. We do not yet know the full impact of living in high density communities, but some research has already shown that crowding affects individual and community health. A study of Ohio farmers, living in low density communities, suggests that the absence of stress from crowding may contribute to their reduced rate of coronary artery disease [5].

A low density community may have other problems. When people are spread out, health delivery may become difficult. There may not be enough resources in the form of taxes to support public health services. Rural communities often suffer from inadequate supply of health care personnel ranging from private physicians to community health nurses. A healthy community will take into consideration the density of its population. It will organize in ways to meet the differing needs created by its density levels; for example, it will recognize differences in density between the inner city and the suburbs, and allocate services accordingly.

COMPOSITION

Communities differ in the types of people who live within their boundaries. A retirement community in Florida whose majority of members are over 65 years of age has one set of problems. A city with a higher number of women in the childbearing years will have another set of problems. A healthy community is one that takes full account of differences in age, sex, educational level, and occupation of its members.

Occupations may be diversified among many industries or concentrated in a single field. In a town where 75 percent of the workers are employed by a textile mill, the community lives under the threat of cotton dust, the cause of brown lung disease. Some textile mill communities ignore this danger, do nothing to inform workers of the dangers they face, and provide little help for older workers who are laid off as a result of contracting this disease. A community nurse working to improve the health of this type of community would need to visit the textile mill, check on safety precautions such as face masks, and work to instigate regular lung examinations for all workers. Community leaders would have to become aware of the problem. Such a nurse might find it necessary to become an advocate for workers and organize them to negotiate with the textile mill managers for improving conditions in the mill. Understanding a community's composition is the first step in determining its level of health.

RATE OF GROWTH OR DECLINE

Community populations change over time. Some grow rapidly, thus putting extreme demands on the delivery of health services. Others, due to economic change, may decline. Any fluctuation in population size can affect the health of the community. As population declines, community leadership may also decline. Even a stable community can have problems; for instance, members may resist needed change because they see little fluctuation in their population.

CULTURAL DIFFERENCES

A community may be composed of a single cultural group. A Pennsylvania farming town may share a common commitment to traditional Pennsylvania Dutch heritage. An Indian reserve in Washington State may reflect a single cultural tradition of Snohomish Indians. In many communities, however, several cultures or subcultures may be present. If a city has a large Hispanic population, a cluster of Native Americans who live in the inner city, and a scattering of Vietnamese refugees, the cultural differences among these members will influence the health of the community. A university town in a southern state had a large influx of students from Iran, Iraq, Greece, Turkey, Saudi Arabia, and other Middle Eastern countries. When Iranian militants in Teheran held American citizens hostage, their action had a direct effect on the university town. A healthy community is aware of such cultural differences and moves quickly to promote understanding between subcultural groups.

SOCIAL CLASS

Some communities appear to be primarily middle-class; others have large numbers of lower-class members. Still other communities may have a sprinkling of each social class. We know that social classes have different health problems, resources for coping with illness, and ways of using health services. A healthy community recognizes these differences and creates a health care delivery system to meet these varied needs.

MOBILITY

American people are a mobile population. We move to go to college, take a new job, or seek new climates upon retirement. This mobility has a direct effect on the health of communities. If the population turnover is extensive, continuity of care may suffer. Leadership for improving the health of the community may change so frequently that concerted action becomes difficult. High turnover may require special attention to health education about local conditions.

Population groups may arrive and depart in seasonal swings; migrant farm workers and college students can both affect a community. The community health nurse will want to identify those populations that are seasonally mobile. They not only present special health needs, but may place an added burden on a community. If a town of 3,000 people has an annual influx of 10,000 students who disappear in the summer, members must prepare to meet this population change. A healthy community neither ignores nor overreacts to this kind of mobility. Rather, it identifies the nature of population change, determines the needs created by such change, and organizes to meet those needs.

As you consider the population dimension of the community, you will take a long step toward uncovering the true character of the community. Each of the variables related to population will suggest clues to the relative health of the community itself. Table 14-3 presents the second part of the Community Profile Inventory. It identifies the seven population variables, suggests some implications for community health, and provides several community assessment questions as well as possible sources of information.

SOCIAL SYSTEM

Every community has a third dimension, a social system. A social system consists of parts, such as the local government, churches, families, and hospitals, that are linked together. The parts interact with and influence each other. Whether you want to assess a community's health, develop new services for the elderly within the community, or promote the health of several families, you need to understand the community as a social system. A community health nurse working in a tiny village in Alaska needs to grasp the social system of that village no less than a nurse working in Washington, D.C. needs to understand the social system of our country's capital.

A social system is an abstraction. For this reason, it can be elusive and difficult to grasp. Let us start with a specific example of a community of 20,000 people, which we will call Centerville. If you visited Centerville, you would not see the social system. It does not exist as a concrete reality, something that you can see, touch, or smell. What you would observe in Centerville is people. They would be walking, talking, playing, paying bills, performing surgery, saying prayers, water skiing, voting, and doing all the other things common in a community. Where, then, is the social system of Centerville? We can see how social scientists conceive of a community's social system by focusing briefly on a single individual.

Consider Marian Branch, mother of four children, director of the Centerville Public Health Nursing Agency. If you followed Marian Branch around for a few days, you would notice that she repeats certain activities. She prepares breakfast for her family each morning; she meets with her staff each day at the agency; she shops for food and clothes. If you expanded your observation to several weeks or months, other patterns of behavior, such as church attendance, participation in a subcommittee of the Centerville City Council, and theater patronage, would appear.

From a social system perspective, these patterns of activities make up the roles that Marian Branch enacts in the course of her daily life. She acts in the capacity of mother, agency director, store customer, church member, and Centerville City Council member. When we take specific actions of a person and group them into patterns, we have identified social roles. Keep in mind, however, that these roles are only abstractions from observable concrete actions.

We can also look for patterns among roles, such as those enacted by Marian and the people whom she encounters. In doing so, we quickly discover that certain roles are closely connected: interaction occurs between mother and daughter, nursing supervisor and staff nurse, customer and sales clerk, and church member and clergyman. These new patterns that emerge among roles form the basis of *organizations*. Some organizations, such as the Branch family, are informal; others, such as the Centerville City Council, are formal. However, all organizations are constructed from roles that are enacted by individual citizens. You can see that by discussing organizations we have moved another rung up the ladder of abstraction.

Patterns of similarity can also be found among organizations. As people move in and out of organizations, playing out their roles, they connect with people from other organizations. When a group of organizations are thus linked, and when they have similar functions, we can begin to refer to systems and subsystems. For example, as a patron at the theater in Centerville, Marian Branch participates in the recreation system of the community. The Centerville Public Health Nursing Agency is linked to the Centerville Health Department, Centerville Hospital, Centerville Nursing Home, and other organizations that make up the health system of this community. The city council is part of the political system; Marian's church is part of the religious system. These systems all interact because people, in their various roles, move in and out of organizations, connecting with other people from still other organizations.

As a rough map of a community's social system, Figure 14-3 shows the ten major systems common to all communities. The people (or population) are represented by the circle at the center. They become part of the social system by virtue of the roles they enact, roles which form organizations and ultimately one or another major community system.

You may ask why it is important to understand Centerville, or any other community, as a social system. Perhaps you consider a social system as merely an abstract idea about a community. It may be abstract, but it reflects an important reality: the various community systems have a profound influence on one another. Because this interaction among parts determines the health of the whole, it is the total system that concerns community health nurses.

Let us consider one aspect of the health of Centerville. The city's department of health reported more than 75 pregnancies among teenage girls, a large number for the size of this community. This situation has placed a marked strain on the families of these girls, as well as caused increased demands for services from the health system. Because the vast majority of these pregnancies are unwanted, they present a problem for the unwed teenage parents, their families, and eventually, the community. What will happen to the babies of these girls? Evidence from research suggests that, in the future, the girls are likely to have larger families, depend more frequently on the welfare system, and have a higher number of health problems than women who were not teenage mothers. How is the community responding to this situation? Their response gives us clues to the overall health of Centerville.

For one thing, the problem has been ignored, a sign of defense rather than adaptation. When it does come to public attention, it divides various groups. Families blame the schools; school officials in turn blame the changing sexual mores represented in motion pictures. Some members of the health system asked Planned Parenthood to set up an office and clinic in Centerville, in an effort to resolve the problem. Almost immediately, however, the religious system entered the picture with groups forming to picket Planned Parenthood facilities because of the association's stand on abortion. Planned Parenthood

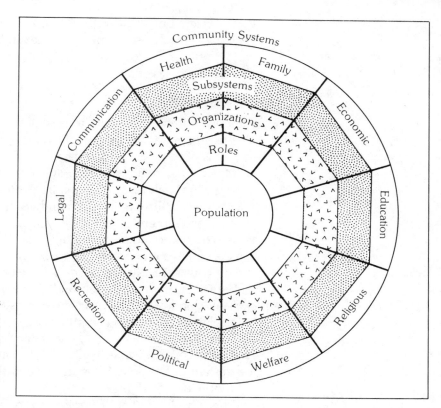

Figure 14-3. The community as a social system. Each of the ten major systems of a community includes a number of subsystems that are made up of organizations. Members of the community occupy roles in these organizations.

set up their office in an old restaurant on the edge of one business district in Centerville. Individuals from the religious and economic system (local businessmen) joined to file suit to prevent Planned Parenthood from occupying the old building. Within months, every major system of this community was involved in the problem, yet it was as far from solution as ever. Indeed, the original problem had almost fallen by the wayside as community members fought over the issues of abortion and the Planned Parenthood headquarters. Vandals set several fires which destroyed part of the building. Pickets daily called attention to this unwanted health agency. Moreover, in the midst of the trouble, more teenagers, some with parents who were deeply involved in the conflict, became pregnant.

Community health nurses work in such community situations. Their goal is to assess the community's level of health, identify needs, set priorities, and then work with community members to raise the level of health. It is a complex yet challenging task. We cannot describe all the ways to assess the community as a social system within the scope of this chapter, but the last part of our Community Profile Inventory (Table 14-4) suggests some of the health implications for each of the major systems. It also offers some suggestions for making an assessment of each system.

THE HEALTH SYSTEM

Although community health nurses must have some understanding of all the systems in a community and how they interact, the health system is of particular importance. Let us compare community assessment, for a moment, with individual health assessment. Then we can examine the health system in greater depth, as an example of how you might conduct a more detailed study of a community.

Initial assessment of individuals begins with a survey of major systems. You do not begin by minutely examining the health of each cell, but concentrate instead on the overall condition of the individual. This survey usually involves a head-to-toe examination during which you look for indications of health and illness in the respiratory, musculoskeletal, glandular, skin, and circulatory systems, among others.

Initial assessment of a community also begins with a survey of major systems. Instead of asking, "Is the traffic policeman doing his job?" or "Is the mayor an effective leader?," you would inquire about the political system as a whole. What are its constituent parts? Are there any signs of health or illness?

When beginning an examination of a single person, you ask whether the major body systems are functioning well or poorly. Pulse rate and blood pressure checks provide information about the level of functioning in the circulatory system. In order to answer questions about a system's level of functioning, you must first know its function, that is, the job it has to do as part of the larger system, the body.

The same holds true for community assessment. You might ask, for example, "How well does the communication system keep members informed about important matters?" This question implies that this system has a basic function, information dissemination. You might also ask, "Does the educational system offer equal education to all children of the community?," which implies that this system's function is to offer learning opportunities to everyone in a particular age group.

Each of the major systems in Figure 14-3 has developed over time in a community to meet the needs of its members. The major function of the health system is to promote the health of the community. Community assessment does not merely ask if, but also how well the system is functioning. What is the level of health promotion as carried out by the health system of a community? In order to answer this question, which can be applied to any system, you need a clear notion about the subsystems, organizations, and roles that make up the system.

Let us say that in examining an individual patient, you have surveyed all the general systems of the body and discovered that the person has an elevated blood pressure. You will now want to move from your initial survey to a more detailed examination of the circulatory system or other parts of the body. Any evidence of inadequate functioning becomes a green light for more careful assessment.

The same rule should be followed in community assessment. The rate of teenage pregnancies in Centerville signals inadequate functioning of some systems; perhaps the family, educational, religious, health, or all these systems need improvement. Thus, you want to take a closer look. What community values influence sexual behavior among adolescents? What sex education programs are available to this population? Does the health system provide information and counseling? Like high blood pressure in a single person, this sign in Centerville may quickly lead to discovery of many other underlying problems. They might require care as simple as regular exercise or as complicated as major surgery, each solution translated into community terms.

What are the components of the health system? Figure 14-4 abstracts one segment from our illustration of the community social system—the health system. It is composed of eight major subsystems, each with one or more organizations. Although the community health nurse must be aware of all the systems in a community, the health system is of central importance. Figure 14-4 shows some representative types of organizations for each of the major subsystems. Keep in mind that each of these organizations also has members with many different roles, and the health of the entire system depends, in part, on how well these roles are carried out.

COMMUNITY DYNAMICS

Our discussion to this point may have suggested that the community is a rigid structure composed of a geographic location, a population, and a social system. Yet every community has a dynamic quality. Think of the diagram in Figure 14-3 as a wheel that turns rather than as a static structure. Two factors in particular affect community dynamics: citizen participation in community health programs, and the power and decision-making structure of the community [4].

In some communities, citizens show little concern about public

Figure 14-4. Components of the health system. (For a detailed discussion of the health system with slightly different categories of subsystems, *see* I. T. Sanders, Public Health in the Community. In H. Freeman, S. Levine, and L. P. Reeder [Eds.], *Handbook of Medical Sociology* [2nd ed.], Englewood Cliffs, N.J.: Prentice-Hall, 1972. P. 411.)

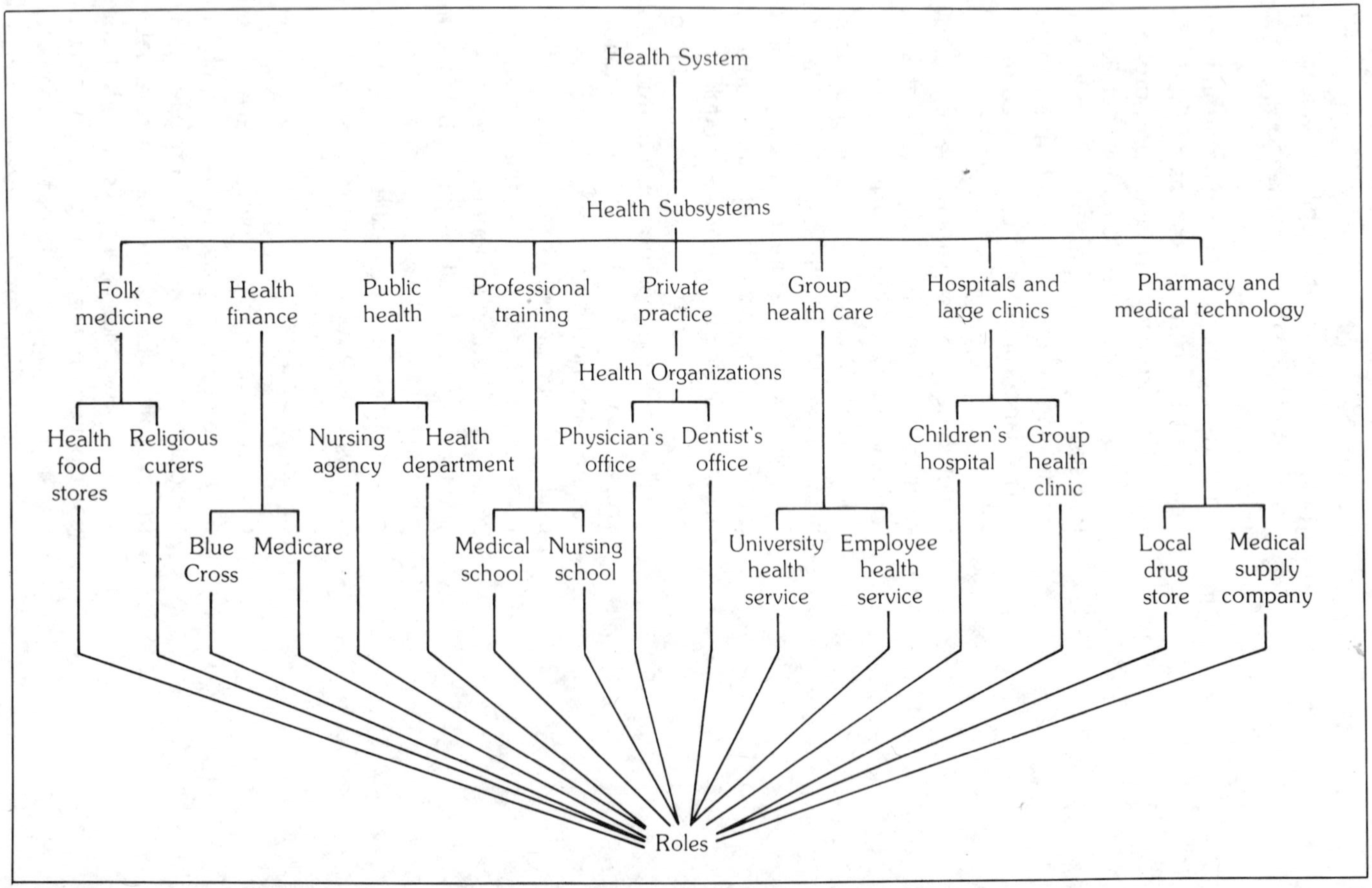

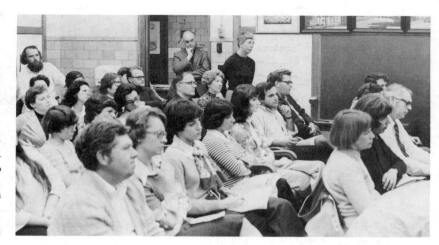

Figure 14-5. A healthy community encourages its citizens to participate in decision making. Here citizens are involved in a town meeting discussion. (Courtesy of the *Mt. Vernon News.*)

health issues. They expect health officials to take entire responsibility: "That's what we pay them to do." When apathy abounds, community health nurses will probably have to work on community education and awareness. In other communities, participation may be widespread but either uninformed or obstructive. Our example of the Planned Parenthood Clinic in Centerville suggests that citizens can block the development of some programs or at least hamper them. It is much more difficult to work in a community where groups have become polarized by issues such as abortion and fluoridation. Assessing the type and extent of citizen participation will be a necessary first step in community work.

The goal of encouraging responsible participation touches on the concept of self-care discussed in earlier chapters. One goal of community nurses when working with families or groups is to encourage people to take responsibility for their own health care. They have the right to make decisions, to have adequate information, and to consult widely about their own health. Our role is to encourage the full development of a self-care attitude. On a community level, self-care occurs when citizens become committed to the goal of a healthy community (Fig. 14-5). Such a commitment includes responsible involvement in assessing, planning, and carrying out programs to meet community needs [3]. Community self-care is our goal.

The second factor, the power and decision-making structure, is a central concern to anyone wishing to bring about change. Our description of the community as a social system may suggest that power and decision making reside primarily in the political system, but that is not

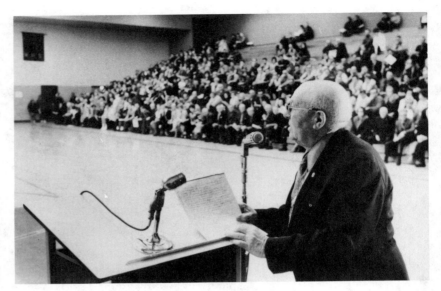

Figure 14-6. Key individuals within every community exert power and influence. (Photograph by Dick Swanson. © 1971 Time, Inc.)

the case. Irwin Sanders has argued against oversimplifying the decision-making process: "In its naivest, simplest terms this [oversimplification] blandly states that (1) every community has an identifiable power clique and (2) that if you get the members on your side, all of your problems will be solved" [8, p. 417].

Decision making in any community is much more complex than this description. Sanders suggests that power is distributed unevenly among members of organizations in various community systems. A *key leader* may have influence in more than one system, but that power will be diffuse (Fig. 14-6). Seldom does a public health official have power in the religious system or a clergyman in the legal system. A *dominant leader* is one who has specific power, but only within a single community system. An *organizational leader* will have power, but only within a single organization, not in the entire system. Sanders also says that key and dominant leaders will often work through other, less powerful leaders, which he calls *functionaries, issue leaders,* and *spokesmen* [4]. We will return to the problem of leadership and the types of leaders in Chapter Fifteen.

Although power and decision making in any community are complex, Sanders does suggest several propositions that we can use as general guidelines for understanding this aspect of a community's dynamics [4]:

1. Because communities differ widely in their power structures, do not assume that what you know about one community will be true of another.

2. The leaders within the health system have different degrees of power and varying spheres of influence; a knowledge of these differences is prerequisite to effective community work.
3. Those leaders whose power is limited to the health system or organizations often have a network of contacts with similar leaders in other systems. Many of the decisions are made informally through this network.
4. Power does not automatically flow through the established bureaucratic channels. Locate the informal patterns of power and decision making.
5. Beware of leaders who speak authoritatively on issues outside their sphere of power. Their power may be more apparent than real.
6. Leaders from the health system may become key leaders with power that extends far beyond the health system.
7. Learn to distinguish between political, economic, and social power; then use the appropriate combination needed to promote community health issues.
8. Do not overestimate the support of key leaders or power cliques; their support may be helpful but still leave much organizational work to be done.
9. Try to encourage participation in the decision-making process at every level, from average citizen to key leader.
10. You can assume that leaders in one part of a community are ignorant of needs and problems in other parts of the system. When you contact such leaders, recognize that you will have to educate them in community health issues.

TYPES OF COMMUNITY ASSESSMENT

When dealing with an individual patient, it is important to know whether you need to record temperature, check all vital signs, or recommend a complete physical examination with thorough laboratory analysis. The same is true for community assessment. In some situations, an extensive community study becomes the first priority. In others, all you need is a study of one system or even one organization. At other times, you may need to familiarize yourself with an entire community without going into any depth; in other words, to perform a cursory examination. The type of assessment will depend on variables such as the needs you think exist, the goals you wish to achieve, and the resources available for carrying out the study. Although it is impossible to make such a decision ahead of time, it will be much easier if you understand the several different types of community assessment.

COMPREHENSIVE ASSESSMENT

This type of study seeks to discover all the relevant community health information. It begins with a review of existing studies and all the data presently available on the community. A survey would compile all the demographic information on the population, such as its size, density, and composition. Key informants would be interviewed in every major system—educational, health, religious, economic, and others. Then more detailed surveys and intensive interviews would yield information on organizations and the various roles in each organization. A comprehensive assessment would not only describe the systems of a community but also how power was distributed throughout the system, how decisions were made, and how change occurred.

Because comprehensive assessment is an expensive, time-consuming process, it is seldom performed. Indeed, in many cases such a thorough research plan might be a waste of resources and repeat, in part, many other studies. A more focused study based on prior knowledge of needs is often a better strategy. Yet knowing how to conduct a comprehensive assessment has an important influence over your approach to a more focused study.

FAMILIARIZATION

The second kind of community assessment is also the most necessary. Familiarization involves studying data already available on a community, and perhaps gathering a limited amount of firsthand data, in order to gain a working knowledge of the community. Such an approach has been used in nursing students' community survey courses [2, 7]. This type of assessment is needed whenever the community health nurse works with families, groups, organizations, or populations. It provides you with a knowledge of the context in which these other aggregates exist.

Consider use of community familiarization when your main concern is a single family. You visit the Angelo family on the edge of Philadelphia's city limits. During your first few visits, you gather information, learning that they are an Italian-American family with four children. The father has been out of work for 6 months; the oldest boy has been in trouble with the juvenile authorities; a younger child is deaf; their house appears run down to you. You assess this family, trying to determine their coping ability, their level of health as a family.

However, even this task is almost impossible without some knowledge of the community. Is theirs an Italian-American neighborhood? What is the extent of unemployment in this city? What are the services for the deaf? Are all the houses in this part of town old and in need of repair? Once you begin working with the family, familiarity with the community becomes even more imperative. You discover that as a result of the Angelos' low income, family conflicts are intense. The family seldom gets out; they make almost no use of the community's recreational system. Before you can help them make use of it, however, you must find out what resources are available. As you familiarize yourself with the community, you discover a group called "Friends of the Deaf," which sponsors a group for parents of deaf children. You can now help Mr. and Mrs. Angelo become part of that group. A quick survey of the religious system in the community reveals two job transition support groups, one of which will welcome Mr. Angelo. In the meantime, you will want to find out about the welfare system and how this family can benefit from its services. Even your own attitude toward the family will change as you study the community. For instance, if you discover that a strike closed down the plant where Mr. Angelo worked for 20 years, you can then view his unemployment from a broader perspective.

However, familiarization will go beyond connecting the family to the community and its resources. Whatever role you play in a community, you will want to be making a continuous study, an ongoing assessment. Whether you become a client advocate, working with the local government, or operate from a nursing agency with the elderly, this kind of assessment is a prerequisite for your work.

PROBLEM-ORIENTED ASSESSMENT

The third kind of assessment begins with a single problem and then assesses the community in terms of that problem. Assume that when you check around for services available for the Angelos' deaf child, you discover that there are none. Confronted with this problem, one family with one deaf child, you could make a problem-oriented community assessment. Your first step would be to seek to discover the incidence of childhood deafness, both in the community and in the state. Second, you might begin interviewing officials in the schools and health institutions to find out what has been done in the past with such problems. You could check the local library to find out what resources are available on the subject of deafness. Do they subscribe to *The Deaf American*? Are there interpreters available for adults who use sign language? How do hospitals and courts approach deafness? Are there any clubs or other organizations for deaf adults? Is there a state school for the deaf and where is it located?

The problem-oriented assessment is commonly used when familiarization is not sufficient and a comprehensive assessment is too expensive. It is the type of assessment that responds to a particular need. The data you collect will be useful in any kind of planning for a community response to the problem.

COMMUNITY SUBSYSTEM ASSESSMENT

In this type of study, the community health nurse focuses on a single dimension of community life. For example, you might decide to survey churches and religious organizations to discover their role in the community. What kinds of needs do the leaders in these organizations believe exist? What services do these organizations offer? To what extent are services coordinated within the religious system and between it and other systems in the community?

The community subsystem assessment can be a useful way for a team to conduct a more thorough community assessment. If five members of a nursing agency divided up the ten systems in the community, and each person did an assessment of two systems, they could then share their findings and create a more comprehensive picture of the community and its needs.

THE HEALTHY COMMUNITY

Throughout this chapter, we have emphasized that our role is to promote the health of the entire community. Included in our discussion were suggestions about the characteristics of a healthy community. However, what is a healthy community? If we are going to assess a community, set goals for community health, plan to improve the health of a community, and work toward our goals, we require some criteria of wellness, health, and competence.

To begin, we can assert that there is no such thing as the perfectly healthy community. All aggregates exist in a relative state of health. New needs emerge every day; the system is threatened or weakened and must respond to maintain homeostasis. Thus, whatever our concept of a healthy community is, it will be a relative idea.

Because of their complexity, criteria for healthy communities must be discussed cautiously. At present, there is not wide agreement on such criteria. We can begin with a classic article, "The Competent Community," by Leonard Cottrell, Jr. [1]. His concept of competence is close to our ideas of health. He argues that a competent community is one whose various systems have four important characteristics:

1. They can collaborate effectively in identifying community needs and problems.
2. They can achieve a working consensus on goals and priorities.

3. They can agree on ways and means to implement the agreed-upon goals.
4. They can collaborate effectively in the required actions.

These general requirements take us closer toward an understanding of a healthy community. However, we must still determine the factors that enable a community's systems to work together in these ways. Cottrell suggests a rather complex list which includes (1) commitment of members, (2) self-awareness and awareness of others among groups, (3) clarity of situational definitions, (4) articulateness of various subgroups, (5) communication, (6) conflict containment and accommodation, (7) participation, (8) management of relations with the larger society, and (9) machinery for effective decision making [1]. Rather than elaborate or attempt to define these characteristics of competence, let us conclude this chapter with a list of our own suggested criteria. Like all such lists, this one must be viewed as a tentative and partial attempt to provide a workable idea rather than as a definitive statement. Use it as a guide as you assess and work in any community, and add to it other characteristics that you think are important.

1. A healthy community is one in which members have a high degree of awareness that "we are a community."
2. A healthy community uses its natural resources while taking steps to conserve them for future generations.
3. A healthy community openly recognizes the existence of subgroups and welcomes their participation in community affairs.
4. A healthy community is prepared to meet crises.
5. A healthy community is a problem-solving community; it identifies, analyzes, and organizes to meet its own needs.
6. A healthy community has open channels of communication that allow information to flow among all subgroups of citizens in all directions.
7. A healthy community seeks to make each of its systems' resources available to all members of the community.
8. A healthy community has legitimate and effective ways to settle disputes that arise within the community.
9. A healthy community encourages maximum citizen participation in decision making.
10. A healthy community promotes a high level of wellness among all its members.

PLANNING FOR THE HEALTH OF A COMMUNITY

Planning for community health is based on assessment of the community. Once we have this essential information, we can determine needs, prioritize them, establish goals and objectives, and develop a plan of

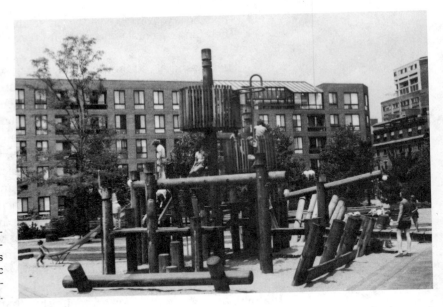

Figure 14-7. Healthy communities provide needed resources for all their citizens. This city park in Boston offers scenic beauty as well as play equipment for active children.

action. The nursing process, detailed in Chapter Five, again becomes an important tool to facilitate our practice, this time with the community as the client. Throughout this chapter, we have discussed elements to consider in planning for community health. We have examined characteristics of a healthy community as a guide to assessing the health of the community we seek to serve. We also need to understand what a healthy community is in order to establish planning objectives; in other words, we need to know what to aim for. A health subsystem with deficient communication patterns, for instance, will require intervention if health care services in the community are to function effectively.

Aggregate level nursing practice requires team work. The job of planning for the health of an entire community or a community subsystem of necessity means that the nurse will be collaborating with other professionals. Working with a health board task force to recommend methods for improved communication between health care agencies is one way the nurse works as a team member in serving the community as the client. All sound public health practice depends on pooling resources, including people, in ways that will best serve the public. Whether health service is aimed at the individual, family, group, organization, population, or community level, the consumer of that service is an equally important member of the team. In planning for a community's health, the community (represented by appropriate individuals and agencies) must be involved. We cannot lose sight of the need for client involvement at all levels and in all stages of community health practice.

SUMMARY

A major mission of community health nursing practice is to promote the health of aggregates of people. A strong value of individualism in the United States distracts nurses from a broad focus. It has led to three pervading myths: (1) community health nursing is only clinical nursing outside the hospital setting, (2) community health nursing employs only the skills of basic nursing when working with community clients, and (3) the primary client in community health nursing is the individual in a family context. Rather, community health nursing is practice with and to the community. It employs basic nursing expertise but adds many important concepts and skills from public health. Moreover, in addition to serving individuals, it is practiced at five aggregate levels—families, groups, organizations, population groups, and communities.

Any community has three important dimensions to consider when assessing its health needs: location, population, and social system. The effect of a community's location may be further analyzed by considering such variables as its boundary, location of health service, geographic features, climate, flora and fauna, and human-made environment. The health of a community is also influenced by its population. Knowledge of features, such as the population size, density, composition, rate of growth or decline, cultural differences, social class, and mobility, helps the community health nurse to better understand the community. The third dimension of a community, its social system, includes ten major systems (including the health system) and many subsystems. Each subsystem is composed of organizations whose members assume various roles. A Community Profile Inventory details the community health implications of each dimension, poses assessment questions for the nurse to ask, and suggests sources of information.

Initial assessment of a community begins with a survey of the major systems to determine how well they are functioning. Evidence of malfunctioning in any part becomes a stimulus for further and more detailed analysis.

Community dynamics, the driving forces that govern a community's functioning, must also be considered when assessing community health. Two factors, in particular, affect community dynamics: citizen participation in community health programs, and the power and decision-making structure. We need to encourage community self-care by promoting community level involvement in, commitment to, and responsibility for, its own health. We also need to recognize the sources of community influence in order to use the system effectively to promote community health.

There are different types of community assessment. A comprehensive assessment surveys the entire community in depth, gathering much original data. A familiarization assessment studies available data, perhaps adding some first-hand data, to gain a general understanding of the community. Problem-oriented assessment focuses on a single problem and studies the community in terms of that problem. Community subsystem assessment examines a single facet of community life.

A healthy community has a number of characteristics which we look for when assessing its health. Among them are a sense of unity, ability to collaborate and communicate effectively, a problem-solving orientation, ability to conserve and utilize resources, and ability to handle crises and conflict.

Planning for community health draws on a thorough assessment and utilizes the nursing process. It involves a team effort by professionals and community personnel.

REFERENCES

1. Cottrell, L. S., Jr. The Competent Community. In B. H. Kaplan, et al. (Eds.), *Further Explorations in Social Psychiatry*. New York: Basic Books, 1976. Pp. 195–209.
2. Flynn, B., Gottschalk, J., Ray, D., and Selmanoff, E. One Master's curriculum in community health nursing. *Nurs. Outlook* 26:633, 1978.
3. Kinlein, L. Nursing and family and community health. *Fam. Community Health* 1(1):57, 1978.
4. Lynd, R. *Knowledge for What? The Place of Social Science in American Culture*. Princeton: Princeton University Press, 1939. P. 60.
5. Nagi, S. Z. Factors related to heart disease among Ohio farmers. *Ohio Agric. Exp. Sta. Res. Bul.* Oct., 1959. P. 842.
6. *Redesigning Nursing Education for Public Health: Report of the Conference.* Bethesda, Md.: U.S. Department of Health, Education, and Welfare (Pub. No. 75–75), 1973.
7. Ruybal, S. E., Bauwens, E., and Fasla, M. Community assessment: An epidemiological approach. *Nurs. Outlook* 23:365, 1975.

8. Sanders, I. T. Public Health in the Community. In H. E. Freeman, S. Levine, and L. G. Reeder (Eds.), *Handbook of Medical Sociology* (2nd ed.). Englewood Cliffs, N.J.: Prentice-Hall, 1972. Pp. 407–434.

SELECTED READINGS

Bertrand, A. *Social Organization: A General Systems and Role Theory Perspective.* Philadelphia: Davis, 1972.

Blum, H. L. *Planning for Health: Development and Application of Social Change Theory.* New York: Behavioral Publications, 1974.

Boyle, J. S. Community Assessment. In A. Reinhardt and M. Quinn (Eds.), *Family-Centered Community Nursing: A Socio-cultural Framework.* St. Louis: Mosby, 1973.

Brill, N. *Teamwork: Working Together in the Human Services.* Philadelphia: Lippincott, 1976.

Burke, E. M. *A Participatory Approach to Urban Planning.* New York: Human Sciences Press, 1979.

Cater, D., and Lee, P. (Eds.). *Politics of Health.* New York: Medcom, 1972.

Cottrell, L. S., Jr. The Competent Community. In B. H. Kaplan, et al. (Eds.), *Further Explorations in Social Psychiatry.* New York: Basic Books, 1976. Pp. 195–209.

Elling, R. H., and Lee, O. J. Formal Connections of Community Leadership to the Health System. In E. G. Jaco (Ed.), *Patients, Physicians, and Illness: A Sourcebook in Behavioral Science and Health* (2nd ed.). New York: Free Press, 1972.

Flynn, B., et al. One Master's curriculum in community health nursing. *Nurs. Outlook* 26:633, 1978.

Frankle, R. T., and Owen, A. Y. *Nutrition in the Community: The Art of Delivering Services.* St. Louis: Mosby, 1978.

Hanchett, E. *Community Health Assessment: A Conceptual Tool Kit.* New York: Wiley, 1979.

Hays, B., and Mockelstrom, N. R. Consumer survey: An approach to teaching consumer participation in community health. *J. Nurs. Educ.* 16:30, Oct. 1977.

Klein, D. C. *Community Dynamics and Mental Health.* New York: Wiley, 1968.

Knight, J. H. Applying nursing process in the community. *Nurs. Outlook* 22:708, 1974.

Kramer, R. M., and Specht, H. (Eds.). *Readings in Community Organization Practice.* Englewood Cliffs, N.J.: Prentice-Hall, 1975.

Logan, R. Assessment of sickness and health in the community—needs and methods. *Med. Care* 2:173, 1964.

McGavran, E. G. Scientific diagnosis and treatment of the community as a patient. *J.A.M.A.* 162:723, 1956.

Milio, N. *The Care of Health in Communities: Access for Outcasts.* New York: Macmillan, 1975.

Moe, E. O. (Ed.). *Fam. Community Health* 1(2):1–108, 1978.

Mullane, M. K. Nursing care and the political arena. *Nurs. Outlook* 23 (11):699, 1975.

National Commission on Community Health Services. *Health is a Community Affair.* Cambridge, Mass.: Harvard University Press, 1967.

Perlman, R., and Gurin, A. *Community Organization and Social Planning.* New York: Wiley, 1972.

Redesigning Nursing Education for Public Health: Report of the Conference. Bethesda, Md.: U.S. Department of Health, Education and Welfare (Pub. No. 75–75), 1973.

Ruybal, S. E. Community health planning. *Fam. Community Health* 1(1):9, 1978.

Ruybal, S. E., Bauwens, E., and Fasla, M. Community assessment: An epidemiological approach. *Nurs. Outlook* 23(6):365, 1975.

Sanders, I. T. The community: Structure and function. *Nurs. Outlook* 11(9):642, 1963.

Sanders, I. T. Public Health in the Community. In H. E. Freeman, S. Levine, and L. G. Reeder (Eds.), *Handbook of Medical Sociology* (2nd ed.). Englewood Cliffs, N.J.: Prentice-Hall, 1972. Pp. 407–434.

Simmons, H. J. Community health planning—With or without nursing. *Nurs. Outlook* 22:260, 1974.

Stokinger, M., and Wallinder, J. A Graduate practicum in health planning. *Nurs. Outlook* 27:202, 1979.

Storck, J. Assessing the community's health in times of change. *Public Health Rep.* 81:821, 1968.

Wax, J. Power theory and institutional change. *Soc. Service Rev.* 45(3):274, 1971.

FOUR

EXPANDING THE NURSE'S INFLUENCE

FIFTEEN

LEADERSHIP AND
PLANNED CHANGE

Leading people to change their beliefs and practices about health lies at the heart of all community health nursing. This aim characterizes work at every level, from individual clients to large organizations and communities. At all levels, to influence change requires knowledge and skill in two closely related areas: leadership and planned change.

How do nurses carry out their roles as both leader and change agent at the community level? With such rapidly expanding opportunities, it is possible to give several examples. One community health nurse becomes a member of the Governor's Commission on the Handicapped. In addition to understanding the entire state as a community and the handicapped as a special population, she urges the commission to formulate new plans for meeting the needs of the handicapped. Another nurse, as a member of a metropolitan health planning board, works to improve health care for a group of Hmong immigrants from Southeast Asia. In a rural community of farms and small towns, another nurse organizes a grass roots committee concerned about a nearby nuclear generating plant. The committee works to develop an emergency evacuation plan in case of radiation leaks from the plant. All three of these nurses are involved in leadership and change at the community level. They are working to change people's beliefs regarding health and health activities, and to involve them in creating organized responses to community problems.

Community health nurses also lead people to change at the organizational level. Let us say that you are a staff nurse in a public health nursing agency, a health delivery organization. Like the other staff members, you feel overburdened by paperwork; you may feel burned out and lack clear goals for your daily tasks. Setting priorities is difficult. Rather than blaming yourself, you recognize that other staff feel the same way; it is an organizational problem. During a staff meeting, you bring up the problem of job stress and suggest that everyone read an article on the subject to discuss at the next staff meeting. The first discussion is so successful that others follow. At your prompting, a regular staff development meeting evolves with rotating leadership. As the months pass, a new sense of direction emerges among the staff; people feel more competent to cope with job stress, and morale improves. Although you worked informally, you acted as a leader to bring about organizational change. The result not only left individuals feeling better able to cope with their jobs, but also improved the health of the organization.

Community health nurses also seek to influence families to achieve new levels of health. One nurse assists a family to improve its communication; another leads a family through the stress caused by incest, helping its members to change and move to a new level of health. You can act in a leadership capacity with groups, perhaps negotiating a contract with a group to quit smoking or to develop a school program on battered children. The list goes on and on, but in every case the pattern of assuming leadership in order to promote change in health practices is the same. Even with individuals you will seek to influence change. You may teach a young mother to care for her handicapped child; you may negotiate a contract regarding regular exercise with a man recovering from a heart attack. Hardly a day goes by for most community health nurses without deep involvement in leadership and change activities at every level of practice.

The roles of leader and change agent both require specialized knowledge and skills to be effective. This chapter examines leadership and the management of change. We will see how they are inextricably linked and how community health nurses incorporate them into practice.

LEADERSHIP

Many nurses do not see themselves as leaders nor do they wish to become leaders; all too often, leadership for these nurses has come to mean they must assume a formal position of being in charge. As leaders, they would have to tell other people what to do. Some nurses feel it means being alone at the top of a group or organization, taking all the risks and being held accountable for the outcomes. Many of these conceptions of leadership, however, are based on false premises.

Leadership is *an interpersonal process in which one person influences the activities of another person or group of persons toward accomplishment of a goal in a specific situation* [7, 12]. In its simplest terms, leadership involves setting the pace, going first, and guiding and directing the way people think and act. It is accomplishing goals with and through people [7]. To lead requires interacting with other people to influence them to achieve the goal. Let us look at three major characteristics of leadership implied in this definition.

LEADERSHIP CHARACTERISTICS

First, leadership is purposeful: it always has a goal. No act of leadership exists without a reason. A mayor wants low-cost housing for the poor; a community nurse wants to see a family change its nutritional habits; a minister wants transportation that is accessible to all the physically handicapped. In each instance, the leader has a purpose and hopes that others will come to share that purpose. A leader will work to achieve goals by making them clear, attainable, specific, and agreeable to the follower constituency.

Second, leadership is interpersonal. It is a social exchange, a transaction between the two parties of leader and follower [11]. These parties share information in a variety of patterns. An authoritarian army general gives direct orders to his military personnel; the president of a garden club makes informal suggestions to club members. In both cases, however, the leader and followers must maintain a relationship that fosters ongoing communication and facilitates the goal-seeking process.

Third, leadership means influencing. In one small community that existed in a larger city, a nurse received reports of several children who had been bitten by rats. A casual survey revealed alleys with piles of garbage and trash which attracted rats. The nurse, as a leader, wanted to influence members of this community to eliminate a public health problem. She could not clean up all the refuse herself, nor would city maintenance crews undertake the responsibility. In order to mobilize the local citizens to achieve this goal, she needed to influence them. She began with the parents of children who had received rat bites, influencing them to call their neighbors together. At that meeting, she spoke about the potential health hazard with a resulting need for eliminating the garbage and trash from alleys; she quietly listened to the discussion and offered suggestions when the group decided to form a committee and hold a clean-up day. As a leader, she offered guidance and direction, thus influencing the ideas and activities of this group of followers.

Leadership, then, in community health means to influence people toward development of an optimally healthy lifestyle and environment. Any purposeful effort to influence behavior is an example of leadership; thus, every community health nurse can act as a leader [7]. Moreover, according to Moloney, all nurses should exercise leadership [12]. She bases her rationale on the fact that nurses must accept responsibility for revitalizing and upgrading professional nursing practice and for improving health services. She declares: "Accountability for professional practice implies that nurses are functioning as leaders in health care. If nurses are to become accountable for practice, they must broaden their view of what responsible leadership entails" [12, p. 3]. Nurses have many opportunities to exercise leadership: in community health, they may lead citizens; in practice, they may lead clients toward optimal health; as nurse managers, they may lead colleagues to improved practice; and, as nurse faculty, they may lead students toward future leadership [12].

LEADERSHIP FUNCTIONS

Leadership functions occur at many levels, each with its own set of activities and sphere of influence. A captain's leadership functions will differ from a corporal's, a governor's from a school board member's, and a corporation president's from an assembly line inspector's. Within community health nursing, the functions of leadership also vary depending upon the nurse's position and work situation. Take, for example, a large community health nursing agency. Listed below are some areas of influence associated with various positions.

Director	Influences organizational policy and decision making
Associate director	Influences management of specific aspects of the organization
Supervisor	Influences structure and process of care delivery
Team leader	Influences day-to-day quality of nursing practice
Staff nurse	Influences client health behavior and environment

In other settings for community health nursing practice, such as rural or occupational environments, there may be only one nurse present to provide leadership that encompasses many, if not all, of these activities. Beyond the agency itself, the leadership role of each nurse extends to influencing those community attitudes, programs, and environmental factors that affect community health. Each nurse must assess the situation and determine the kind and extent of leadership needed.

What are the functions of leadership in community health nursing? Argyris summarizes several functions: "Leaders . . . know how to discover the difficult questions, how to create viable problem-solving networks to invent solutions to these questions, and how to generate and channel human energy and commitment to produce the solutions" [1, p. ix]. More specifically, we can identify five essential functions required for effective leadership at any level: (1) the creative function, (2) the initiating function, (3) the risk-taking function, (4) the integrative function, and (5) the instrumental function. These functions do not occur in any particular order; rather, they operate simultaneously throughout the leadership process.

CREATIVE FUNCTION

Nurse leaders must be able to envision new and better ways to solve problems. This first step in creativity is then followed by developing methods and activities for carrying out the solutions. This function requires ingenuity, innovation, vision, and a future orientation. For instance, a nurse in a rural agency recognized that the home health aid/homemakers could potentially meet more client needs, find their jobs more fulfilling, and better serve the agency through an expanded role. She revised their job descriptions and instituted an expanded role-training program [6]. The creative leadership function is one that includes generation of ideas and development of designs for action.

INITIATING FUNCTION

As a leader, the nurse introduces change and sets its process in motion. This function includes convincing clients or followers of the need for change, starting the problem-solving process, and launching the activities needed to carry out the plan. Like all the other leadership functions, it requires decision-making skills. For example, after seeing an increased number of pregnancies, a nurse who works in a high school convinces the girls to start a prenatal counseling group and originates a series of sex education seminars. The initiating function begins the process toward goal accomplishment; it is the stimulus or "push" that starts clients or followers on their course of action.

RISK-TAKING FUNCTION

Every leader is faced with uncertainty, and to proceed under uncertain conditions is to take risks. What nurse, working with a family or group in the community, has not encountered a number of unpredictable variables during the process of planning with clients for health goals? Will this diet control the disease? Will client self-disclosure in this group therapy lead to group acceptance and understanding or to open ridicule and deteriorated self-image? Will the new drug counseling clinic significantly reduce the problem, or will county funds have been spent needlessly, thus jeopardizing future funding requests? Leaders cannot guarantee outcomes. The leadership process requires careful planning based on all available data and the creation of scenarios in order to predict all possible obstacles and outcomes. It even requires preparation of alternative courses of action, should earlier plans fail. Nevertheless, some variables cannot be predicted beyond a certain point, and leaders must be willing to take chances. They have to "go out on a limb," to expose themselves to possible failure and embarrassment. Taking chances also means they will expose clients or followers to potential negative outcomes. No leader throughout history has operated without taking risks. Effective leaders, however, take calculated risks; they weigh the pros and cons and potential consequences of each action before proceeding. Their concern is to minimize harmful exposure to followers.

INTEGRATIVE FUNCTION

This aspect of the leadership role focuses on strengthening collective ties and uniting clients or followers through a strong sense of purpose. The leader reminds the followers of their goals, encourages pride in their group identity, stablizes intragroup relations, and mediates interpersonal conflict. Community health nurses working with families and groups frequently find members at odds or cross-purposes with one another. Individuals in any group setting tend to have their own hidden agendas and separate needs. One of the nurse leader's jobs is to keep the client group on target by clarifying and reinforcing the goals they have mutually identified. The integrative function requires good interpersonal skills for establishing positive relationships with, as well as between, followers. This function supports the aim of promoting member commitment and cooperation.

INSTRUMENTAL FUNCTION

Leaders must also keep followers moving in the right direction, the purpose of the instrumental or facilitative function. As Schaefer puts it, a leader is "capable of moving others in the direction the leader is moving" [13, p. 16]. For nurse leaders, this function involves good

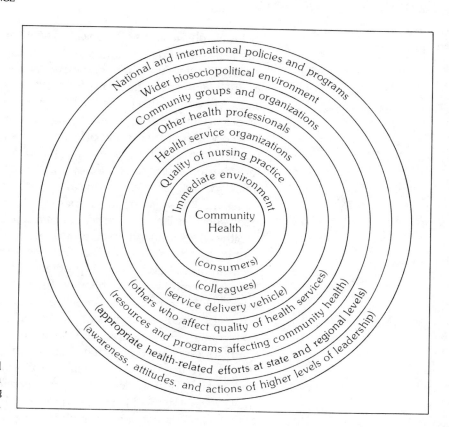

National and international policies and programs
Wider biosociopolitical environment
Community groups and organizations
Other health professionals
Health service organizations
Quality of nursing practice
Immediate environment

Community
Health

(consumers)
(colleagues)
(service delivery vehicle)
(others who affect quality of health services)
(resources and programs affecting community health)
(appropriate health-related efforts at state and regional levels)
(awareness, attitudes, and actions of higher levels of leadership)

Figure 15-1. Areas of potential leadership influence within community health nursing practice.

communication. We must keep in constant touch with clients or followers, make certain that goals and activities are understood and agreed upon, and encourage both negative and positive feedback. Leaders further stimulate followers to progress toward achievement of goals by reinforcing desired behaviors and by setting the pace themselves. The latter is particularly important for gaining followers' respect and sustained commitment. To set the pace means to demonstrate your competence, practice what you preach, and show your followers that you believe in them and in what you are asking them to accomplish.

AREAS OF INFLUENCE

Community health nurses exercise the functions of leadership in ever-widening spheres of influence, as is shown in Figure 15-1. The central aim of this leadership role is to influence community health. A first area of focus is to improve the immediate environment, which includes physical, psychological, social, and spiritual factors, by influencing consumer health-related behavior. Community health nurses exercise leadership when they influence the quality of nursing practice of their coworkers through, for instance, peer consultation and review. They may also influence the service delivery vehicle, the agency or organization through which care is offered, by accepting a higher-level position or by serving on committees and taking an active part in quality control. Other professionals involved in the health delivery system are an additional target of community health nurses' leadership influence. Ongoing communication with colleagues from other disciplines may serve to stimulate these professionals' awareness of health needs and facilitate development of appropriate services. Community health nurses may influence groups and organizations that affect community health, such as clubs, churches, or the legislature, by keeping them informed about health problems and suggesting ways they can improve community health levels. Extending their leadership influence even wider, community health nurses may focus on the wider biosociopolitical environment of the city, county, state, or regional community. For example, the nurse may support anti-smoking programs or campaign for proper disposal of nuclear waste. Finally, community health nursing leadership may extend to influencing national and international policies and programs that affect health, such as those of the World Health Organization. Participating in citizens' lobbies, serving on national committees, or contacting senators and representatives of the United States Congress are some of the many possible actions one could take. The number of spheres in which the nurse exercises a leadership role varies, depending on health needs, the work situation, the nurse's abilities, and time.

LEADERSHIP STYLES

Some nurses effectively influence people's behavior. Others do not. What causes the difference? What accounts for effective leadership? Some researchers, assuming that certain individuals acquire or are born with leadership qualities, have sought to identify the personality traits of leaders. These efforts have been unsuccessful in establishing any one group of traits that would predict leadership effectiveness [12].

More recent research has focused on the behavior of leaders during interaction with followers. This approach views leader behavior, rather than leader personality, as the chief determinant of leadership effectiveness. From this research, several taxonomies of leadership styles have evolved. We will consider one that identifies three styles: (1) autocratic leadership, (2) participative leadership, and (3) laissez-faire leadership [6, 12, 16].

AUTOCRATIC STYLE

The autocratic style is authoritarian. Leaders who adopt this style use their power (usually the power of their position) to influence their followers. The autocratic leader gives orders and expects others to obey without question. Suggestions from followers are not, as a rule, invited or accepted. The leader is dominant; the followers have little power or freedom of choice. In times of extreme crisis, an autocratic style may enhance survival. Sometimes a nurse finds that members of a group will expect to be led in an autocratic style; they may see the nurse as the only qualified expert.

PARTICIPATIVE STYLE

The participative style, a supportive approach, is sometimes called the democratic style. This form of leadership has become increasingly popular in recent years as leaders have sought to involve followers in the decision-making process. This style tends to promote followers' self-esteem and to increase motivation and productivity (Fig. 15-2). Leaders utilizing this style sometimes find it difficult to maintain control and prevent followers from taking charge while remaining democratic. Some participative leaders permit their followers more freedom and power than others; generally, however, this leadership style allows followers considerable freedom to make choices.

LAISSEZ-FAIRE STYLE

The laissez-faire style means giving the followers free rein to do whatever they wish. The leader maintains a "hands off" policy that gives complete freedom of choice to the group members, who set their own goals, carry out their own activities, and are essentially independent of the leader. This style may be effective in a group whose members have both the motivation and competence to achieve the goals. Although someone is formally the leader, this style uses little or no direct influence, and some people would argue against its classification as a style of leadership.

TASK- AND RELATIONSHIP-ORIENTED STYLES

We discussed earlier that leadership is accomplishing goals with and through people. Consequently, leaders must be concerned with tasks

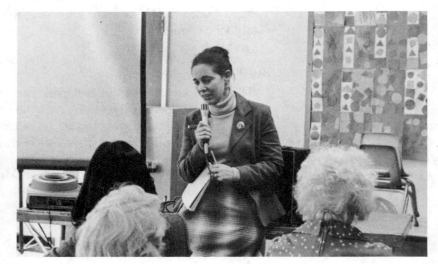

Figure 15-2. As a leader, the nurse seeks to influence clients toward a healthier state. Here the nurse involves a class of senior citizens in a discussion about their health. She uses a participative leadership style. (Courtesy of Beth Israel Hospital, Boston. Photograph by Michael Lutch.)

(in order to achieve goals) and with relationships (to show concern for people) [7]. These two dimensions, tasks and relationships, become opposite points of emphasis on a continuum of leader behavior, as is illustrated in Figure 15-3. Research has shown that autocratic leaders tend to be concerned about goals and are task-oriented, whereas participative leaders are concerned about people and stress relationships. These two emphases have led to a new taxonomy of leadership styles as either task-oriented or relationship-oriented [7].

Leader behavior research has demonstrated that leadership style has a significant influence on leadership effectiveness. However, since many variables, such as leader personality, follower needs and resources, or the situation, influence effectiveness, no one style can be advocated as best.

SITUATIONAL LEADERSHIP

The situational approach to study of leadership behavior has yielded the most promising results to date. Based on a recognition that leadership is a relationship between leader, followers, and the situation, it is unrealistic to assume a single, ideal type of leader behavior. A participative style of leadership used in one organization is not always successful in another, similar organization. An integrated style that shows high concern for both tasks and relationships might be appropriate in one setting but not in another. Researchers pursuing the situational approach have concluded that the situation dictates the style of leadership one should use. Because every situation is unique,

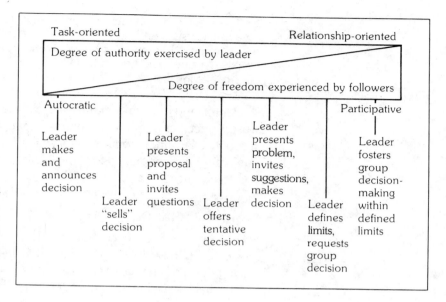

Figure 15-3. Leadership behavior continuum. (Adapted from P. Hersey and K. Blanchard, *Management of Organizational Behavior: Utilizing Human Resources* [3rd ed.]. Englewood Cliffs, N.J.: Prentice-Hall, 1977. P. 92.)

leadership becomes a dynamic process of adapting one's style to the demands of the situation. Hersey and Blanchard refer to this process as "adaptive leader behavior" [7, p. 101]. Its implications for community health nursing can be stated thus: The more nurses adapt their style of leader behavior to meet the particular situation and the needs of clients or followers, the more effective they will be in reaching health-related goals.

The most effective leadership style, then, is an adaptive one. Nurses will need to determine the most appropriate style by assessing the unique qualities of each situation, followers' needs and degree of independence, and their own personalities and abilities.

CONDITIONS FOR EFFECTIVE LEADERSHIP

The ultimate test of nurse leadership is in the outcomes. Are goals met? What did the leader accomplish? To reach a successful outcome involves certain factors; adherence to these factors will contribute to positive results, while violation of one or more of them will create negative results. They form the conditions necessary for leadership to be effective [11]:

1. Followers must understand the suggestion, advice, or directive, in order to make compliance possible.
2. Followers must be able to carry out the suggestion; they must have, or be supplied with, the needed resources or abilities.

3. The required action must be consistent with the followers' personal values and interests.
4. The required action must be consistent with the followers' collective purposes, values, and norms; that is, followers must be in tune with group or organizational goals.

Central and most important to effective leadership is a relationship of trust, respect, and mutual exchange between leader and followers. It is through this transactional relationship that community health nurses can satisfy the conditions for effective leadership and accomplish positive outcomes.

NATURE OF CHANGE

"To lead means to effect change" [12, p. 87]. When we suggest that postcoronary clients adopt a new, healthier pattern of living, we are asking them to change. Teaching diabetic children how to give themselves insulin is introducing a change. Revising home health aid/ homemakers' responsibilities, again, requires that those individuals change. Since our responsibility in leadership is to accomplish goals and thus promote change, we cannot lead without introducing change. Therefore it becomes imperative for community health nurses to understand the nature of change, how people respond to it, and how to manage it.

What is change? For some analysts, change means that things are out of balance; they refer to it as an upset in a system's equilibrium [2]. For instance, when the mother of a family becomes ill, that family's normal functioning is thrown off balance. Adjustments are required; new patterns of behavior become necessary. Others view change as the process of adopting an innovation [15]. Something different, such as a new diet, is introduced; change occurs when the innovation is accepted, tried, and integrated into daily living. Lippitt defines change as "any planned or unplanned alteration of the status quo in an organism, situation, or process" [9, p. 37], thus reminding us that change may occur either by design or by default. Still others view change in terms of its effect on behavior. They say change is both the altering of a situation and, depending upon how people define the new situation, the way behavior is altered to fit it [17]. We can see that change requires adjustment in thinking and behavior and that people's responses to change vary according to their perceptions of it. Change threatens the security that people feel when following established and familiar patterns. It generally requires the adoption of new roles. Change is disruptive.

KINDS OF CHANGE

The way people respond to change depends, in part, on the kind of change it is. We can describe the change process as occurring along a continuum between two opposites, evolutionary change and revolutionary change [5].

EVOLUTIONARY CHANGE

Evolutionary change tends to be gradual and requires adjustment on an incremental basis. It modifies rather than replaces a current way of operating. Becoming parents, stopping smoking by gradually cutting back on the number of cigarettes smoked each day, and losing weight by eliminating desserts and sweets are examples of evolutionary change. Since it is gradual, this kind of change does not require radical shifts in goals or values; in fact, it may enhance current goals or values. Less threatening and more readily adopted than revolutionary change, evolutionary change is sometimes considered reform; it resembles variations on a musical theme.

REVOLUTIONARY CHANGE

Revolutionary change, in contrast, is more rapid, drastic, and threatening. It may completely upset the balance of the system. It involves different goals and perhaps radically new patterns. This kind of change resembles a whole new musical theme. A sudden job change, stopping smoking overnight, losing a limb in an accident, or suddenly removing a child from abusive parents are examples of revolutionary change. In each instance, the people affected have little or no advance warning and time to prepare. High levels of psychic energy and rapid behavior change are required in adapting to revolutionary change; as a result, incapacitation, resistance, or denial of the new situation frequently occurs.

The impact of a proposed change on a system will clearly depend on the degree of its evolutionary or revolutionary qualities, a factor to be considered in planning for change. Some situations lend themselves better to one kind of change than the other. A community in need of improved facilities for the handicapped, such as ramps and wider doors, can introduce this change on an evolutionary, incremental basis; whereas a community involved in an unsafe, intolerable, or life-threatening situation, such as a serious epidemic, may require revolutionary change.

STAGES OF CHANGE

The process of change occurs in three stages described by Lewin as unfreezing, moving, and refreezing [10].

UNFREEZING

Unfreezing, the first stage, occurs when a need for change develops. People are motivated to change either intrinsically or by some external force. During this stage the need for change creates disequilibrium in the system. A system in disequilibrium is more vulnerable to change. People have a sense of dissatisfaction; they feel a void which they would like to fill. Like an amputee eager to use a prosthesis or a community concerned about safe intersections, they are ready for change. Thus, the unfreezing stage involves initiating the change.

Unfreezing may occur spontaneously. A family requests help in solving a problem with alcoholism; a group seeks help in adjusting to retirement. However, the nurse/change agent may need to initiate the unfreezing stage by attempting to motivate clients to see the need for change.

MOVING

Moving, the second stage of the change process, occurs when people examine, accept, and actually try out the innovation. For instance, this is the period when participants in a prenatal class are learning the exercises or when the elderly in a senior citizens center are discussing and trying out ways to make their apartments safe from falls. During the moving stage, people experience a series of attitude transformations, ranging from early questioning of the innovation's worth to full acceptance and commitment to accomplishing the change. The change agent's role during this stage is to help clients see the value of the change, encourage them to try it out, and assist them in adopting it for use.

REFREEZING

Refreezing, the third and final stage in the change process, occurs when the change is established as an accepted and permanent part of the system. The rest of the system has adapted to it. Since it is no longer viewed as disruptive, threatening, or even new, people no longer feel resistant to it. As the change is integrated, the system becomes refrozen and stabilized. We know that refreezing has occurred when weight loss clients, for instance, are regularly following their diets and losing weight, or when the senior citizens have installed grab bars in their bathrooms and removed the scatter rugs, or when the community has erected stop signs and established cross-walks at dangerous intersections.

Refreezing involves integrating or internalizing the change into the system and then maintaining it. Simply because a change has been accepted and tried does not guarantee that it will last. Often there is a tendency for old patterns and habits to return; consequently, the change agent must take special measures to assure maintenance of the new behavior. We will discuss ways to stabilize a change in the next section.

PLANNED CHANGE

Planned change can be defined as *a purposeful, designed effort to effect improvement in a system with the assistance of a change agent.* Several characteristics in this definition distinguish planned change from unplanned change. First, the change is purposeful and intentional; there are specific reasons or goals prompting the change. These goals give the change effort a unifying focus and a specific target. Unplanned change occurs haphazardly, and its outcomes are unpredictable. Second, the change is by design, not by default. Thorough, systematic planning provides structure for the change process, a map to follow toward a planned destination. Third, planned change in community health aims at improvement. That is, it seeks to better the present situation, to promote a higher level of efficiency, satisfaction, or productivity. Just as not all movement is forward, not all change is positive or growth-producing. Planned change, however, aims to facilitate growth. Finally, the change is accomplished by means of an influencing agent. The change agent serves as a catalyst in developing and carrying out the design; it is a leadership role.

PLANNED CHANGE PROCESS

Before initiating planned change, community health nurses need to consider the dynamics of change in the context of system functioning. Any system seeks to achieve and maintain a relative state of equilibrium. It is in the nature of a system to seek this stability in order to maximize its ability to function. Yet the internal and external forces acting upon every system create new needs which, in turn, demand change in order to restore the system to a new level of functioning and equilibrium. For example, toxic fumes emanating from a derailed freight train forced community residents in a southern town to flee. The introduction of this external force upset the community's equilibrium and ability to function. Every effort was made to remove the source of danger and restore the community to normal functioning. The creation of a new need (to eliminate the toxic fumes) led to a change effort (the cleanup process) in order to restore system balance (normal community living). Community health nurses, as leader/change agents, are responsible for seeing that the needs of clients are met through some kind of change and that a new equilibrium is achieved as soon as possible. You can meet those needs, effect change successfully, and restore your clients to a stable state by conducting planned change.

Planned change involves a systematic sequence of activities. We shall consider eight basic steps to follow in the successful management of change [14]. They are: (1) recognize the symptoms, (2) diagnose the need, (3) analyze alternative solutions, (4) select a change, (5) plan the change, (6) implement the change, (7) evaluate the change, and (8) stabilize the change. Figure 15-4 shows how forces acting on a system create a need for change. When we recognize that need, we have begun the change process. This model also illustrates what happens when the nurse fails to respond to the need for change. The need remains and, in fact, may increase. The client system (those involved and affected by the change) and the change agent must work together throughout the entire planned change process. Their respective roles will vary depending upon the situation, but no planned change will be truly effective without recognition and utilization of this helping relationship. The model depicts the client system as variable and vacillating (wavy arrow) because the client system is generally composed of a number of people. It may be an entire community; thus it will experience many fluctuations in its involvement with the change process. The change agent (straight arrow), as a good leader and manager, analyzes the situation thoroughly, plans carefully, and sets a steady course for effecting the change.

STEP 1. RECOGNIZE THE SYMPTOMS

The first step in managing change is to realize that there is a need for change by listing all the need's indicators. In this step, one should gather and examine the presenting evidence, not diagnose or jump ahead to treatment. For instance, let us say that several clients request help with parenting. Before we can diagnose or plan, we must determine all the indicators of a need. We cannot assume that these clients

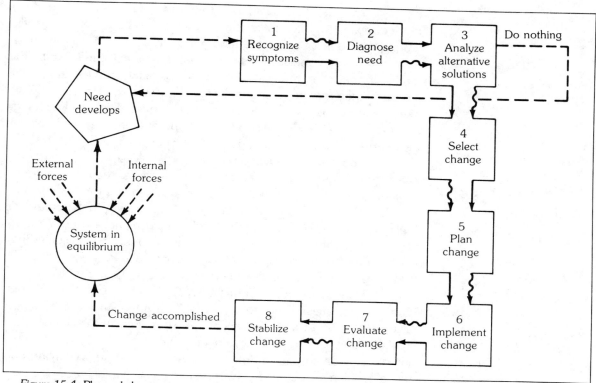

Figure 15-4. Planned change model. The change agent (solid line) and the client system (wavy line) must work together to effect change.

feel inadequate in the parent role, nor can we assume that they lack information about parenting or are having difficulty with their children. One, all, or perhaps none of these assumptions may be true. Therefore, we first look for symptoms and discover that some of the parents have trouble talking to their teenagers, others wonder if their children's behavior is normal, a few question how strictly they should set limits, and still others are not certain about how to handle punishment. These symptoms are pieces of evidence that we will analyze in the next step. Before moving on, however, we need to ask ourselves as change agents what our motives are for pursuing this change. Inappropriate motives, such as wanting to be needed, can cloud judgment and interfere with effective management of change.

STEP 2. DIAGNOSE THE NEED

Diagnosis means to analyze the symptoms and reach a conclusion about what, if anything, needs changing. First, describe the situation as it is now (the real) and compare it to the way it should be (the ideal). For example, you may notice a great deal of loud arguing and conflict among members of a client family. Although your ideal may be quiet harmony, noisy conflict may be normal, functional behavior for this family. In that case, there is no discrepancy between the real and the ideal and therefore no need for change. If, however, there is a discrepancy between the real and the ideal, then a need exists and a change effort is justified [7]. From speaking with the parents, we recognize that their behavior and concerns indicate a possible lack of information about, and confidence in, the parenting role. A gap clearly exists between their present and ideal situations; therefore, there is a need.

Next, determine the exact nature and cause of the need. Gathering data by means such as questioning clients, checking the literature, or seeking consultation is important for making a more accurate diagnosis. We question the parents in more detail about the difficulties they are having with their children. How do they feel about being parents? What are the most difficult aspects of parenting for them? Have they read any books or used any other resources to help them in their parenting activities? Who do they talk to, if anyone, about parenting problems? When they have a problem handling the raising of their children, how do they usually solve it? We also check the literature ourselves to determine the most effective approaches to solving parenting problems. We consult with an expert on family life to get ideas about what this group of parents might need, given the symptoms we have seen. We need to come to a conclusion about what specific changes are needed for these parents. Unless the diagnosis is made accurately, the entire change effort may be addressing its attention to the wrong problem. Also, when possible, the client system should help diagnose. We ask the parents to help us determine what, exactly, it is that they need.

Finally, we must narrow the findings down to a single diagnostic statement that also includes the cause. The parents, we discover after data collection, are insecure in their parenting roles. They believe the insecurity is caused partially by lack of knowledge about how to carry out parental responsibilities. Primarily, however, they are convinced that the cause is lack of a supportive reference group. Most of them live some distance from relatives or no longer maintain close ties with relatives. Our diagnosis for these parents is insecurity in the parenting role. We define the cause to be lack of support as well as some lack of knowledge.

STEP 3. ANALYZE ALTERNATIVE SOLUTIONS

Once we know the diagnosis and its cause, we are ready to identify solutions or various alternative directions to follow. Like the physician who has studied the patient's symptoms and diagnosed the patient as having a duodenal ulcer, the next decision must involve what general treatment direction to follow. Should it be surgery, diet, medication therapy, or a lifestyle change approach? At this point the physician does not decide on a specific treatment regimen. That step comes later. Brainstorming is helpful at this point, and the client system should be involved as much as possible in the process. Make a list of all the reasonable broad alternatives, and then analyze them thoroughly to determine the advantages, disadvantages, possible consequences, and risks involved in each. For the parents, we could consider general alternatives such as family counseling, a support group, or education in family life. Each of these alternatives has some advantages and disadvantages toward meeting the parents' need for confidence in their roles.

Next, we analyze each alternative. For example, the counseling solution could provide insight and awareness into family behavior. It would give family members opportunities to express feelings and gain understanding of how other members feel. However, it would not provide a frame of reference that they could use to compare their own parenting behaviors with other acceptable ones. Nor would it provide adult peer support for the parents. The consequences of this alternative would most likely be to promote parents' self-understanding and better family communication. Risks would include the possibility that children, especially teenagers, might not be willing to participate and that parents might not gain self-confidence in their roles. We study each alternative to determine its usefulness and feasibility. We also go to the literature again and to other resources, such as consultants, to learn all we can about the best ways to meet the parents' need for change.

STEP 4. SELECT THE CHANGE

Having carefully analyzed all the alternatives, we now select the best solution. The parents agree with us that the best solution seems to be a parenting support group. We re-examine the risks involved in the change choice; sometimes a possible course of action may be too costly in time, money, or potential for failure. Also, there may be ways to reduce the risks.

It is important to know what the change is aiming to accomplish; we need a clearly stated goal. For the parenting group, our mutually agreed-upon goal is to provide a supportive, reinforcing climate while increasing members' parenting skills.

STEP 5. PLAN THE CHANGE

This step is at the heart of planned change because it is now that the change agent prepares the design, the blueprint that guides the change action. In steps 1 through 4, data are gathered, a diagnosis made, resources assessed, and a goal established, all preparatory actions for planning the change. The plan tells the change agent and client system how to meet that goal. Preferably they develop the plan together.

We talk with the parents about ways to meet their goal, considering such possibilities as weekly discussion groups on selected topics, monthly meetings with an informed speaker, or reading books and articles on parenting with regular sessions to discuss their application. After analysis and discussion, we decide to meet one evening a month, rotating the location between members' homes. Group sessions will include a variety of approaches: a speaker will be invited every 3 months; a book or article discussion will be held quarterly; and the remaining meetings will be spent on topics of the group's choice. All sessions will provide opportunities for parents to discuss their concerns or problems. We design this plan around a set of objectives.

The most important activity in planning is to have clear, specific objectives. They should be measurable and preferably stated as outcomes. For example, the objective, "by the end of the second session, each parent in the group will have participated in the discussion at least once," is measurable and describes an outcome. Make a list of activities to help you accomplish each objective and develop a time plan. It is also important to assess the potential costs in terms of time, money, number of people and materials needed and to determine the resources available. Design the evaluation plan and start a list of ways to stabilize (refreeze) the change.

During planning, it is useful to perform a force field analysis, a technique developed by Kurt Lewin for examining all the positive and negative forces in a change situation [8].

In any situation, there are both driving and restraining forces which influence change. Driving forces push for change. Examples might be clients' desire to be healthier, more productive, or have a safe environment. These are influencing forces in favor of change. Restraining forces, such as apathy, fear of something new, or hostility, work against change, decreasing its possibility. When the strength of the driving

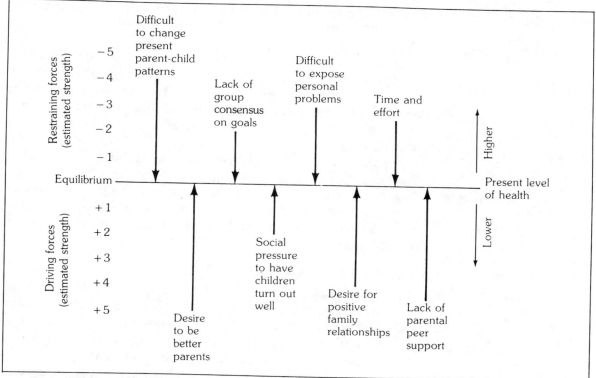

Figure 15-5. Analysis of restraining and driving forces. (Adapted from P. Hersey and K. Blanchard, *Management of Organizational Behavior: Utilizing Human Resources* [3rd ed.]. Englewood Cliffs, N.J.: Prentice-Hall, 1977. P. 122.)

forces is equal to the strength of the restraining forces, equilibrium exists. To introduce a change and move the client system to a higher level, that balance must be altered. To do so, the change agent either increases the driving forces, decreases the restraining forces, or both. Force field analysis is a technique which the change agent utilizes to study both sets of forces and to develop strategies to influence them in favor of the change (see Fig. 15-5).

The procedure for conducting a force field analysis follows a few simple steps. As change agent, you may conduct it alone; preferably, you will consult with your clients or a change-planning resource group, such as your nursing team or both. The steps for force field analysis are:

1. Brainstorm a list of all driving and restraining forces. (For the parenting group, one driving force is their desire to be better parents; a restraining force might be lack of group agreement on discussion topics.)
2. Estimate the strength of each force.
3. Plot them on a chart such as the one shown in Figure 15-5.
4. Note the most important forces; then research and analyze them.

5. List and document possible responses or action steps that might strengthen each important driving force or weaken each important restraining force.

Finally, as a consideration in planning the change and in analyzing the driving and restraining forces, study the social network and interaction of the system involved in the change. The change agent needs to be aware of formal and informal leaders, cliques within larger groups, influential persons, the grapevine, and all the other possible social network influences on the change process. For instance, one nurse attempting to change the infant-feeding practices of a young mother failed to consider the strong influence of the grandmother living next door. Another nurse was making no headway with a group of teenage drug addicts until she discovered that their real leader was one of the boys who always sat in the back, not the "captain" appointed by the center director.

STEP 6. IMPLEMENT THE CHANGE

The implementation step involves enacting the change plan. Because their objectives and activities have been clearly defined, change agent and client system know exactly what needs to be done and now proceed to do it. The parenting group and their nurse/change agent, for instance, can start the discussion sessions since they know what they want to accomplish and how to go about it. The change plan tells them where they will meet, how often, what they will discuss, and who will be involved. As they move through implementation, they will also know when their objectives have been met and will have a ready-made plan for evaluation and stabilization of the change, once it has been completed.

At the start of implementation, it is important to make certain that all persons concerned are prepared for the change. When working with a family, for example, the nurse may do most of the planning with one or two key members. Do the other family members, who will also be affected by the proposed change, know what to expect? Do they understand the meaning of the change and what will be required of them in adapting to it? An unprepared client system, especially in a large group or organization, may often spell disaster; no matter how well it is planned, people who are unprepared for a change effort may resist it strongly and render it useless.

In some instances, such as introduction of a mass immunization program or a new clinic procedure, it is helpful to do a pilot study. The study is done to try out the change on a small scale, iron out the problems, and revise the change before implementing it into the whole system. One advantage of a pilot study is that it demonstrates to the client system how the change will work on a scale that is small enough not to require any major adaptation or pose any serious threats to present security. It gives people time to adjust their thinking and to discover that the change may not be so bad after all. It is another way of introducing evolutionary change.

STEP 7. EVALUATE THE CHANGE

The success of this step also depends on how well the change is planned. Well-written objectives with specific criteria for their measurement will make the evaluation step much simpler. However, evaluation does not end with saying whether or not the objectives were met. Each objective requires analysis in terms of: (1) was it met, (2) what evidence (documentation) shows that it was met, and (3) were the best means used to accomplish it, or would some other method have been better? The objective mentioned earlier for the parenting group could be evaluated by saying, yes, it was met. The fact that every person had entered into the discussion by the end of the second session, a point noted by the nurse/leader, would be evidence that the objective was met. However, the method used to encourage participation might have been to call on individuals who were not contributing, thus in a sense coercing them into participation. A better method would have been to suggest that some individuals seem more involved than others and that the more active ones might like to solicit ideas from those who had not had an opportunity to speak. Finally, based on the evaluation, the change agent makes needed modifications in the change before stabilization.

STEP 8. STABILIZE THE CHANGE

The final step in the planned change process requires taking measures to reinforce and maintain the change. A well-developed change plan includes a design for stabilization. The change agent actively encourages continued use of the innovation by establishing two-way communication; thus any future resistance can be overcome and the client's full commitment to the change can be maintained. Stabilization occurs through soliciting reactions from the client system. Do they perceive any potential problems? Do they have doubts? Reinforcing the desired behavior and following up on the change as long as necessary will help assure its permanence. Alcoholics Anonymous, for example, stabilizes the change to nondrinking by providing a regular support group that reinforces the nondrinking pattern. They reward compliance with praise and replace drinking with other satisfying experiences, such as social acceptance, to keep the alcoholic from returning to the old behavior. We stabilize our parenting group's changed behavior by calling attention to their increased confidence in their parenting roles and by pointing out the greater number of successes they are having in coping with their children. The group itself decides to give a Parent of the Month plaque to the member who demonstrates the most growth in his or her parenting skills. They also agree to nominate one member as Parent of the Year in the community newspaper contest. When stabilization occurs, the system achieves a new equilibrium (see Fig. 15-5), and the change agent-client system relationship, at least for this particular change effort, can be terminated.

We have viewed the planned change process primarily in the context of introducing change to smaller aggregates. Community health nurses also utilize these eight steps when managing change at the organization, population group, and community levels. For example, a nurse may suspect that there is a widespread lack of confidence among young parents. This hypothesis could be tested through an epidemiologic survey to determine parenting needs among the entire population group of young parents. If symptoms are present (step 1), the nurse, in collaboration with health department personnel or other appropriate professionals, could analyze the symptoms and reach a diagnosis (step 2), perhaps that a large percentage of young parents in this community are lacking in confidence and knowledge of parenting skills. Several approaches to meet this need could be considered, such as instituting a parenting center in the community with satellite clinics, organizing churches or clubs, or both, to sponsor parenting support groups, or working through the community college system to hold workshops and classes on parenting skills (step 3). The most feasible and useful alternative could be selected (step 4) and a parenting program for the community planned (step 5) and implemented (step 6). The nurse, with the other professionals involved, would then evaluate the outcomes (step 7), and make any necessary adjustments in the parenting program before finally stabilizing it (step 8), making certain that this change, undertaken to meet a population group need, remained an established and effectively functioning service.

PLANNED CHANGE STRATEGIES

The literature describes three general change strategies [2, 4, 17]. In any given situation, the change agent may use one or a combination of these strategies to effect a change. They are: (1) empirical-rational, (2) normative-reeducative, and (3) power-coercive.

EMPIRICAL-RATIONAL

This set of strategies assumes that men and women are rational. When presented with empirical data, people will adopt a new practice because it appears to be in their own best interest. To use this approach, which is common in community health, one simply offers or makes new information available to clients. For instance, most family-planning programs use empirical-rational strategies [4]. Clients are given basic information on reproductive anatomy and physiology, and they are told about the benefits of contraception with an explanation of a variety of birth control methods. Health workers hope that once clients have this information, they will adopt some form of birth control. Some clients respond well to this approach, while others do not. The difference lies in client ability and interest in self-help. The nurse/change agent uses empirical-rational strategies with clients who can assume a relatively high degree of responsibility for their own health. In some respects, this set of strategies parallels the participative leadership style, described in Figure 15-2, which fosters maximum client autonomy.

NORMATIVE-REEDUCATIVE

A second set of change strategies goes beyond merely informing to actively influencing the client system. This approach assumes that attitudes and practices are determined by cultural norms, thus knowledge is necessary but not enough to change behavior [3]. Nurse/change agents who use this set of strategies seek to modify the normative orientations of clients through reeducation. They directly influence clients' values, attitudes, skills, and relationships as well as present new information. This approach attempts to strengthen client self-understanding, self-control, and commitment to new patterns through direct persuasion or manipulation. For example, a health-teaching program that aims to increase safety practices in an industrial setting will, if employing normative-reeducative strategies, not only provide safety information such as posters and warning signs but will also use persuasive tactics such as individual rewards for safe practices, division recognition for minimum number of accidents, or discipline for noncompliance. We use normative-reeducative strategies with clients who have a measure of self-care skill but, at the same time, need external assistance to effect lasting behavior change. This type of client is found in teaching, counseling, and therapy situations.

POWER-COERCIVE

The third set of change strategies uses power to effect change. Change agents may derive power from the *law* (such as health regulations or administrative policies), from *position* (such as political, social, or managerial positions), from a *group* (such as a social, work, or professional group), or from *personal power* (such as personal magnetism, competence, or respect of followers). They use this power to coerce change; the result is more or less forced compliance by the client system. Some situations, particularly those that are life-threatening, may require power-coercive strategies. In community health practice, power-coercive strategies may be used with people who cannot help themselves or in situations which threaten the public's health. If officials find a restaurant in violation of health codes, for example, they will most likely require forced compliance or close down the restaurant. Occasionally clients cannot exercise responsibility, perhaps because they are experiencing temporary physical or psychological incapacitation caused, for example, by severe illness or family abuse. In such cases, the nurse may need to use power along with an authoritarian leadership style to effect changes that are in the clients' best interests. While power-coercive strategies are appropriate in some situations, they should be used with caution since they rob clients of opportunities to grow in autonomy and capacity for self-care.

Planned change strategies may be combined; for instance, a normative-reeducative approach might have a power backup. We see this combination in programs that, for example, educate and persuade groups of people to be immunized against an impending epidemic or to keep their garbage contained to avoid insect and rodent infestation. Behind this normative-reeducative strategy is an implied power threat of official disapproval, or worse, for noncompliance.

The effectiveness of a change strategy, then, varies with each situation and particularly with the degree of client capacity for self-care. As in the approach to leadership styles discussed earlier in the chapter, the nurse/change agent adapts strategies to fit each change situation.

PRINCIPLES FOR MANAGING CHANGE

Community health nurses introduce change every day that they practice. Every effort to solve a problem, prevent another from occurring, meet a potential community need, or promote optimal client health requires changes. To make these changes truly successful so that desired outcomes are reached, they must be managed well. We shall examine six principles which provide some guidelines for effective management of change.

INVOLVE PERSONS AFFECTED BY THE PROPOSED CHANGE

Persons affected by a proposed change should participate as much as possible in every step of the planned change process. This involvement is important for several reasons. Collaboration with those who have a vested interest in the change can produce a wealth of ideas and insights that can greatly improve the change plan. Furthermore, such participation can help remove obstacles and reduce resistance. Participation ensures a greater likelihood of the change's acceptance and maintenance. One nurse, for instance, when planning for a grandmother's care, involved all the family members, including the grandmother; as a result, she automatically secured their support and cooperation, gained many helpful suggestions which she herself had not considered, and discovered that the grandmother was happier and more responsive to care because the change plan was specifically tailored to her needs (Fig. 15-6).

BE PREPARED FOR RESISTANCE TO CHANGE

Because all systems instinctively preserve the status quo, the change agent can expect people to resist change. The homeostatic mechanism operating in any system seeks to maintain equilibrium; change poses a threat to that stability and security. Furthermore, all systems experience inertia, that is, they resist beginning movement. People do not undertake a change until they are convinced of its worth. Resistance may also come from conflict over goals and methods or from misunderstanding about what the change will mean and require. Involving clients in the planned change process, discussed in the last section, is one way to overcome resistance. Another way is establishing and maintaining open lines of communication in order to make ideas clearly understood and to resolve disagreements quickly. Prepare people thoroughly for the change, provide support and patience during the changing process, and encourage response and expression of feelings.

PROPER TIMING IS IMPORTANT IN PLANNING FOR CHANGE

The Bible says, "for everything there is a time and a season." Sometimes a change, even a well-designed and much needed one, must be postponed because the present is not the right time to effect it. The

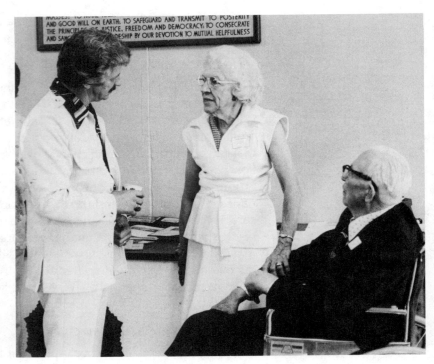

Figure 15-6. Planned change involves introducing new practices that may be difficult to accept or learn. Clients who participate in the planning are more likely to carry out and accept the change. (From C. Schuster and S. Ashburn, *The Process of Human Development: A Holistic Approach.* Boston: Little, Brown, 1980.)

client system may now be experiencing too many other changes to handle the stress of another change. Other projects or activities in which the client system is currently engaged may compete for energy and other resources, depleting those needed to make the proposed change successful. For example, some young mothers, eager to start a book club that focused on discussion of child raising, had to postpone the project because Christmas was approaching. Shopping, entertaining, and vacations made it impossible to give the kind of time and energy needed to make the book club effective.

Proper timing is as important to a planned change as proper seed planting is to a good harvest. The change idea must be appropriate, the change recipient prepared, the climate right, and the resources available before the change can be fostered to grow into full maturity and usefulness.

VIEW CHANGE IN TERMS OF POTENTIAL IMPACT ON SYSTEMS OR SUBSYSTEMS

Every system has many subsystems that are intricately related to, and interdependent upon, one another. A change in one part of a system affects its other parts, and a change in one system may affect other systems. A county community nursing agency made a change in its use of home health aids. Because many home-bound clients needed more care than the agency staff could provide, the agency contracted with a private home-care service for extra home health aids. These aids worked in the homes of agency clients, supplementing the care given by agency staff. The private company preferred to supervise its own aids, whereas the county agency had a policy of community health nurse supervision of aids. The county agency was legally responsible and professionally accountable for the quality of care given to clients. The private company wanted to retain control of its workers. The matter was resolved by contracting with another private service. The change, however, had affected the roles of nurse and aids within the system as well as the relationships between the two systems.

This principle reminds the nurse that change does not take place in a vacuum. When parents learn new practices associated with their parental roles, their relationships with each other, with their children, and possibly with their own parents may easily be affected. One must anticipate and prepare for the impact of the proposed change on the clients involved, other persons, departments, organizations, or even geographic areas.

BE FLEXIBLE

Unexpected events can occur in every situation. This fifth principle emphasizes two points; first, you need to be able to adapt to unexpected events and make the most of them. Perseverance and flexibility are the marks of a good change manager. One community health nurse had tried unsuccessfully to contact a young mother who was reportedly abusing her two-year-old son. After several phone calls and visits to an empty house, she finally found the mother at home but accompanied by a neighbor who insisted on staying for the entire visit. At first the nurse was angry that the neighbor was interfering with her goal of getting to know the mother. Then she realized that this situation offered an opportunity to learn more about the mother through an acquaintance's eyes and possibly to influence another client as well. She included them both in the discussion, explained what she had to offer in terms of health teaching and support, and eventually won their mutual respect and confidence.

The second point to remember about flexibility is that a good change planner anticipates possible blocks or problems by preparing strategies and alternate plans. During step 3 of the planned change process, it is helpful to rank order the alternative solutions considered.

Then, if the first choice does not work out for some reason, a second alternative is ready to be put into action. Flexibility involves a willingness to consider a variety of options and suggestions from many sources.

KNOW YOURSELF

Self-understanding is essential for an effective change agent. As a leader and change agent, how do you define your role, and how do others see it? What are your values and motives in relation to each change that you ask clients to make? What is your personality like and how will it affect the change process? What is your typical leadership style, the one that you most often revert to when not consciously adapting it to the situation? The answers to these questions about yourself will give you much insight into personal behaviors which you may wish to alter, and must be considered when planning for change in community health.

SUMMARY

Community health nurses, at every level of practice, are leaders and change agents. They influence individuals and families to adopt healthier behaviors. They lead groups of people to change their health practices. Formally or informally, they act as leaders to bring about organizational change. At the community level, they are involved in changing people's health beliefs and practices and in promoting organized responses to community health problems.

Leadership is an interpersonal process in which one person influences the activities of another person or group of persons toward accomplishment of a goal in a specific situation. It has three major characteristics. First, it is purposeful; it always has a goal. Second, it is interpersonal; it always involves a social transaction. Third, it means influencing; it always affects other people by altering their beliefs and practices in some manner. Community health nursing leadership aims to influence people toward optimal health as well as upgrade professional nursing practice.

Effective leadership incorporates five essential functions. Exercising the *creative function,* the leader generates ideas and develops innovative plans for action. With the *initiating function,* the leader introduces changes and sets their processes in motion. Good leaders take calculated risks, evidence of the *risk-taking function.* They use the *integrative function* to strengthen the ties among their followers and unite them through a strong sense of purpose. Finally, with the *instrumental function,* effective leaders facilitate the movement of followers in the right direction. Community health nurses utilize these leadership functions in the context of ever-widening spheres of potential influence. They influence consumers, other nurses, health service organizations, other professionals, resources and programs affecting health, and state, regional, national, and even international programs and organizations.

Leadership styles have been studied for many years. The original view that some individuals are born with leadership qualities has been refuted. More recent research supports the fact that leader behavior, rather than leader personality, determines effectiveness. From this research we have drawn three styles of leadership. *Autocratic* leadership is authoritative; orders are given that people are expected to follow. *Participative* leadership is democratic and involves followers in the decision-making process. This style tends to promote the self-esteem and to increase the productivity of followers. *Laissez-faire* leadership, the third style, gives followers complete freedom of choice; they are essentially independent of the leader. Some would argue that this style is not a form of leadership at all.

Leadership encompasses two important dimensions: a concern for accomplishing goals and a concern for relationships with people. The different leadership styles emphasize these dimensions to varying degrees. An autocratic style tends to be task-oriented, while a democratic style tends to be relationship-oriented. Situational leadership integrates both task and relationships by emphasizing one or the other depending upon the situation. This more recent leadership approach has evolved as the most effective to date because it tailors the style of leadership one should use to each situation.

Change is an outcome of leadership. Our job in community health nursing is to effect change by preventing illness and promoting health. Change, however, is disruptive. Evolutionary change is gradual and requires adjustment on an incremental basis. We introduce this kind of change in many situations. Revolutionary change tends to occur suddenly and is more drastic. It may be necessary to introduce revolutionary change under certain conditions, such as an emergency.

Change occurs in three major stages. First, there is *unfreezing.* It is during this stage that the need for change develops. People become receptive. *Moving,* the second stage, occurs when people accept and try out the innovation. The third stage, *refreezing,* involves maintaining the change as an accepted, established part of the system.

Planned change is a purposeful, designed effort to effect improvement in a system with the assistance of a change agent. It involves a process of eight steps which nurses can follow to manage change:

1. Recognize the symptoms that indicate a need for change.
2. Diagnose the need by analyzing the symptoms and reaching a conclusion about what needs changing.
3. Analyze alternative solutions by first identifying a variety of possible general directions to pursue and then analyzing each of these in relation to their advantages, disadvantages, and possible outcomes and risks.
4. Select the change alternative that is most feasible and most likely to meet the identified need. Decide on the goal for this change project.
5. Plan the change by developing specific objectives and a set of activities to meet the stated goal. Force field analysis is a useful tool to facilitate change planning.
6. Implement the change by enacting the change plan, making certain that the client system is properly prepared.
7. Evaluate the change, measuring its outcomes and making needed adjustments.
8. Stabilize the change, instituting measures to reinforce and maintain (refreeze) the change.

During planned change, we can use one or a combination of three major strategies. *Empirical-rational* strategies provide basic information and assume that people are rational and will act on this new knowledge because to do so serves their own best interest. *Normative-reeducative* strategies not only give information but also directly influence people to change. *Power-coercive* strategies use power to force change.

Six principles provide community health nurses with guidelines for managing change:

1. Involve the persons affected by the proposed change.
2. Be prepared for resistance to change.
3. Proper timing is important in planning for change.
4. View any change in terms of its potential impact on systems or subsystems.
5. Be flexible.
6. Know yourself.

REFERENCES

1. Argyris, C. *Increasing Leadership Effectiveness.* New York: Wiley, 1976.
2. Bennis, W. G., Benne, K. D., and Chin, R. (Eds.). *The Planning of Change* (3rd ed.). New York: Holt, Rinehart & Winston, 1977.
3. Chin, R., and Benne, D. General Strategies for Effecting Changes in Human Systems. In W. Bennis, K. Benne, R. Chin, and K. Corey (Eds.).

The Planning of Change (3rd ed.). New York: Holt, Rinehart & Winston, 1976. P. 31.

4. Fischman, S.   Change strategies and their application to family planning programs. *Am. J. Nurs.* 73:1771, 1973.

5. Gerlach, L., and Hine, V.   *Lifeway Leap: The Dynamics of Change in America.* Minneapolis: University of Minnesota Press, 1973.

6. Hennes, K., Sr.   Expansion of the Aide's Role in Home Care. Unpublished project, University of Minnesota, 1979.

7. Hersey, P., and Blanchard, K.   *Management of Organizational Behavior: Utilizing Human Resources* (3rd ed.). Englewood Cliffs, N.J.: Prentice-Hall, 1977.

8. Lewin, K.   Frontiers in group dynamics: Concept, method, and reality in social science; social equilibria and social change. *Hum. Relations* 1:5, 1947.

9. Lippitt, G. L.   *Visualizing Change: Model Building and the Change Process.* La Jolla, Calif.: University Associates, 1973. P. 37.

10. Lippitt, R., Watson, J., and Westley, B.   *The Dynamics of Planned Change.* New York: Harcourt, Brace & World, 1958. P. 130.

11. Merton, R. K.   The social nature of leadership. *Am. J. Nurs.* 69:99, 1969.

12. Moloney, M.   *Leadership in Nursing: Theory, Strategies, Action.* St. Louis: Mosby, 1979.

13. Schaefer, M. J.   Managing complexity. *J. Nurs. Adm.* 5:16, 1975.

14. Spradley, B.   Managing change creatively. *J. Nurs. Adm.* 10: May, 1980.

15. Spradley, J., and McCurdy, D.   *Anthropology: The Cultural Perspective.* New York: Wiley, 1975. P. 565.

16. Uris, A.   *Techniques of Leadership.* New York: McGraw-Hill, 1964.

17. Zaltman, G., and Duncan, R.   *Strategies for Planned Change.* New York: Wiley, 1977.

SELECTED READINGS

Aeschleman, D.   A strategy for change. *Nurse Pract.* 1(1):121, 1976.

Argyris, C.   *Increasing Leadership Effectiveness.* New York: Wiley, 1976.

Argyris, C., and Schon, D. A.   *Theory in Practice: Increasing Professional Effectiveness.* San Francisco: Jossey-Bass, 1974.

Ashley, J.   Power, freedom and professional practice in nursing. *Superv. Nurse* 6(1):12, 1975.

Ashley, J.   This I believe about power in nursing. *Nurs. Outlook* 10(10):637, 1973.

Aspree, E. S.   The process of change. *Superv. Nurse* 6:5, 1975.

Bennis, G., et al. (Eds.).   *The Planning of Change* (3rd ed.). New York: Holt, Rinehart & Winston, 1977.

Bohm, S. M. ⎸Toward 2002: A community perspective. *N. Z. Nurs. J.* 71:24, 1978.

Brooten, D., Hayman, L., and Naylor, M.   Leadership for change: A guide for the frustrated nurse. *Am. J. Nurs.* 78:1526, 1978.

Brooten, D., Hayman, L., and Naylor, M.   *Leadership for Change: A Guide for the Frustrated Nurse.* Philadelphia: Lippincott, 1978.

Chin, R., and Benne, D.   General Strategies for Effecting Changes in Human Systems. In W. Bennis, et al. (Eds.), *The Planning of Change* (3rd ed.). New York: Holt, Rinehart & Winston, 1976.

Conway, M. E.   Clinical research: Instrument for change. *J. Nurs. Adm.* 8(12):27, 1978.

Deal, J.   The timing of change. *Superv. Nurse* 8(9):73, 1977.

Diers, D.   A different kind of energy: Nurse-power. *Nurs. Outlook* 26(1):51, 1978.

Douglass, L. M., and Bevis, E. O.   *Nursing Leadership in Action—Principles and Application to Staff Situations.* St. Louis: Mosby, 1974. (See Chapters 6 and 7 on changing and leadership behavior.)

Dyer, W. G.   Planning Change in the Family. In A. Reinhardt and M. Quinn (Eds.), *Family-Centered Community Nursing: A Socio-Cultural Framework.* St. Louis: Mosby, 1973.

Fischman, S.   Change strategies and their application to family planning programs. *Am. J. Nurs.* 73:1771, 1973.

Fordyce, J. K., and Weil, R.   *Managing with People.* Reading, Mass.: Addison-Wesley, 1971.

Gerlach, L., and Hine, V.   *Lifeway Leap: The Dynamics of Change in America.* Minneapolis: University of Minnesota Press, 1973.

Green, L. W.   Change process models in health education. *Public Health Reviews* 5(1):5, 1976.

Grissum, M.   How you can become a risk taker and a role breaker. *Nursing '76* 6(11):89, 1976.

Havelock, R. G., and Havelock, M. C.   *Training for Change Agents: A Guide to the Design of Training Programs in Education and Other Fields.* Ann Arbor, Mich.: University of Michigan, Institute for Social Research, 1973.

Hersey, P., and Blanchard, K.   *Management of Organizational Behavior: Utilizing Human Resources* (3rd ed.). Englewood Cliffs, N.J.: Prentice-Hall, 1977.

Kalisch, B.   The promise of power. *Nurs. Outlook* 26:42, 1978.

Leary, P. A.   The change agent. *J. Rehabil.* 1:30, 1972.

Lewis, J.   Conflict management. *Nurs. Digest* 5:78, 1979.

Lippitt, G. L.   *Visualizing Change: Model Building and the Change Process.* La Jolla, Calif.: University Associates, 1973.

Lippitt, R., Watson, J., and Westley, B.   *The Dynamics of Planned Change.* New York: Harcourt, Brace & World, 1958.

Longest, B.   Managing Change: The Management Imperative. In B. Longest, *Management Practices for the Health Professional.* Reston, Va.: Reston Publishing, 1976. Pp. 223–238.

Mirvis, P. H., and Berg, D. N.   *Failures in Organization Development and Change: Cases and Essays for Learning.* New York: Wiley, 1977.

Moloney, M.   *Leadership in Nursing: Theory, Strategies, Action.* St. Louis: Mosby, 1979.

Rodgers, J.   Theoretical considerations involved in the process of change. *Nurs. Forum* 12(2):161, 1973.

Rothman, J.   *Planning and Organizing for Social Change: Action Principles from Social Science Research.* New York: Columbia University Press, 1974.

Rubin, I., Plovnich, M., and Fry, R.   Initiating planned change in health care systems. *J. Appl. Behav. Sci.* 10:107, 1974.

Sanders, I. T.   Professional Roles in Planned Change. In R. M. Kramer and H. Specht (Eds.), *Readings in Community Organization Practice* (2nd ed.). Englewood Cliffs, N.J.: Prentice-Hall, 1975.

Schaefer, M. J.   Managing complexity. *J. Nurs. Adm.* 5:16, 1975.

Schaller, L. E.   *The Change Agent: The Strategy of Innovative Leadership.* Nashville: Abingdon, 1972.

Sims, L. S.   The community nutritionist as change agent. *Fam. Community Health* 1(4):83, 1979.

Spradley, B.   Managing change creatively. *J. Nurs. Adm.* 10(5):32, 1980.

Stevens, B. J.   Effecting change. *J. Nurs. Adm.* 5(2):23, 1975.

Uris, A.   *Techniques of Leadership.* New York: McGraw-Hill, 1964.

Veninga, R.   The management of conflict. *Nurs. Digest* 5:72, 1977.

Watzlawick, P., Weaklund, J., and Fisch, R.   *Change: Principles of Problem Formation and Problem Resolution.* New York: Norton, 1974.

Wheelis, A.   *How People Change.* New York: Harper & Row, 1973.

Zaltman, G., and Duncan, R.   *Strategies for Planned Change.* New York: Wiley, 1977.

Zaltman, G., Duncan, R., and Holbek, J.   *Innovations and Organizations.* New York: Wiley, 1973.

Zimmerman, B. M.   Changes of the second order. *Nurs. Outlook* 27(3):199, 1979.

INDEX

INDEX

437

TO THE STUDENT

One of the most important aspects of publishing a book is learning how the book is received by its readers. In the past, we have relied on instructors for comments about the quality of a text as well as perceptions of how their students feel about the book. The following questionnaire is an attempt to get the student's viewpoint directly. We'd like to know if you liked or disliked **Community Health Nursing: Concepts and Practice,** and why; if you found it interesting or dull; what you learned or what you felt the book passed over too lightly.

We hope to use your comments as the basis for making improvements in subsequent editions, and we will appreciate all you have to say about **Community Health Nursing.**

SCHOOL

COURSE TITLE

INSTRUCTOR

1. What is your general impression of this text? _____

_____

_____

2. What are the book's major strengths? _____

_____

3. What are its major weaknesses? _____

_____

4. Please give us your reaction to the following elements of **Community Health Nursing:**

	poor	fair	good	very good	excellent
a. Writing style					
b. Explanations of terms and concepts					
c. Appearance (cover, layout, use of illustrations)					
d. Selected readings					

5. Please comment on the illustrations:

a. Were the drawings clear and easy to understand? _____

_____

Did they add to your understanding of the concepts? _____

_____

How might they be improved? _____

_____

b. Did the photographs contribute to your understanding of community health nursing? _____

In what ways? _____

_____

6. Did you find valuable the author's use of case studies and examples to illustrate key ideas and concepts? Were there enough of these? Too many?_____

_____

_____

7. One of the author's primary goals was to explain fully the concept of the aggregate. Did you gain a clear understanding of this concept? _____

_____

Do you feel you are now able to apply it in practice? _____

_____

8. Do you think your instructor should continue to assign this text? Why or why not? _____

9. Please add any further comments or suggestions on how we might improve the book. _____

_____

_____

10. (Optional)

_____   _____
Name   Address

_____
Date

May we quote you in promotion for this book? Yes____ No____

Please mail to:

Nursing Editor
Medical Division
Little, Brown and Company
34 Beacon Street
Boston, MA 02106